THE ALOPECIAS

Previous Books by Pierre Bouhanna

Soigner et préserver ses cheveux : Les nouveaux traitements du cheveu, Editions ALPEN, Paris, 2006.

Les alopécies: de la clinique au traitement, Collection Guide Pratique de Dermatologie, Editions MED'COM, Paris, 2004.

Capelli e calvizie: I nuovi trattamenti, Springer Italia, Rome, 2001.

Garder et retrouver ses cheveux: Les nouveaux traitements, Editions Springer, Paris, 2000.

Pathologie du cheveu et du cuir chevelu, Editions Masson, Paris, 1999.

Cabello y Calvicie, Las novedades médicas y quirurgicas para un problema que afecta a hombres y mujeres, Garsi, Madrid, 1998.

Cabello e Calvicie, As novidades médicas cirurgicas na mulher e no homem, Andréi, Sao Paulo, 1997.

Hair Replacement Surgery: Textbook and Atlas, Springer-Verlag, Berlin, Heidelberg, 1996.

Cheveux et Calvitie, Les nouveautés médicales et chirurgicales chez la femme et chez l'homme, Editions SIMEP, Masson, Paris, 1994.

Chirurgie de la Calvitie, Editions Springer Verlag, Paris, 1994.

THE ALOPECIAS

DIAGNOSIS AND TREATMENTS

EDITED BY

PIERRE BOUHANNA, MD, FISHRS

Private Practice in Hair Restoration Surgery
Director, University Diploma, Hair Pathology and Scalp Surgery (Paris VI)
Consultant, Hôpital Saint-Louis de Paris (Centre Sabouraud)
Paris, France

ERIC BOUHANNA, MD

Private Practice in Plastic Surgery and Hair Restoration Surgery
Paris, France

CRC Press
Taylor & Francis Group
Boca Raton London New York

CRC Press is an imprint of the
Taylor & Francis Group, an **informa** business

MIX
Paper from responsible sources
FSC® C014174

CRC Press
Taylor & Francis Group
6000 Broken Sound Parkway NW, Suite 300
Boca Raton, FL 33487-2742

Printed on acid-free paper
Version Date: 20150831

International Standard Book Number-13: 978-1-4822-1275-4 (Hardback)

Visit the Taylor & Francis Web site at
http://www.taylorandfrancis.com

and the CRC Press Web site at
http://www.crcpress.com

Contents

Preface

The appearance of hair plays an important role in a person's overall physical appearance and self-perception. Physicians frequently encounter patients complaining about hair alterations and alopecia of various types, while the etiology of these conditions often remains unclear. In fact, disorders of hair growth are among the most common problems confronted in the practice of dermatology.

In this book, we review basic hair biology, the clinical features and pathophysiology of the major disorders of hair growth including alopecia, and the medical and surgical therapies available. We are fortunate to have internationally recognized experts contributing to this volume, and to them we express our appreciation. Special concentration has been placed on ethnicity and hair diseases, and specific medical–surgical treatments have been emphasized. Most men and women with pattern baldness will seek a remedy, and virtually all would have a full head of hair if all they had to do was snap their fingers to obtain it. As a result, we have dedicated a large portion of our practice to the restoration of hair for this group of patients.

This book is organized into 19 chapters that can be schematically divided into four major categories. The first category deals with biology and hair investigations. The second category is dedicated to clinical pathology; it describes various hair diseases including all major pathological conditions of the scalp affecting hair growth. The third category emphasizes the role of aesthetic and reconstructive hair transplantation or scalp surgery. The fourth category is devoted to hair cosmetology and hair cell treatments.

With this book, dermatologists, students, internists, hair transplant surgeons, endocrinologists, pediatricians, obstetricians–gynecologists, those in the pharmaceutical and cosmetic industries, laboratory workers, and any physicians who see hair loss in their regular practice are given the opportunity to understand the basic pathophysiology, clinical presentation, and various effective treatment options for patients with hair growth disorders. It is hoped that the general mission of this textbook to make the diagnosis and treatment of hair disorders concise, clear, and eminently practical, has been accomplished.

Pierre Bouhanna, MD, FISHRS
Director of the University Diploma of Paris for Scalp Pathology and Surgery

Contributors

Aurora Alessandrini
Department of Experimental Diagnostic and Specialty Medicine
University of Bologna
Bologna, Italy

Gilbert Amgar
Private Practice
Paris, France

Alfonso Barrera
West Houston Plastic Surgery Clinic
Houston, Texas

Ulrike Blume-Peytavi
Department of Dermatology and Allergy
Clinical Research Center for Hair and Skin Science
Charité–Universitätsmedizin Berlin
Berlin, Germany

Eric Bouhanna
Private Practice in Plastic Surgery and Hair Restoration Surgery
Paris, France

Pierre Bouhanna
University Diploma of Hair and Scalp Surgery
University Paris VI
and
Hair Bouhanna Center, Private Practice
and
Hospital Saint-Louis de Paris (Centre Sabouraud)
Paris, France

Claude Bouillon
Paris, France

Sophie Casadio
Private Practice
Marseille, France

Jerry E. Cooley
The Hair Center
Charlotte, North Carolina

Juan Ferrando
Department of Dermatology Hospital Clínic
Universitat de Barcelona
Barcelona, Spain

Joseph Greco
Greco Medical Group
Sarasota, Florida

Varvara Kanti
Department of Dermatology and Allergy
Clinical Research Center for Hair and Skin Science
Charité–Universitätsmedizin Berlin
Berlin, Germany

Gerardo A. Moreno-Arias
Department of Dermatology Hospital Clínic
Universitat de Barcelona
Barcelona, Spain

L. Alheli Niebla
Mexican Institute of Tijuana
Tijuana, Mexico

Damkerng Pathomvanich
Center for Cosmetic and Hair Surgery
Bangkok, Thailand

Bianca Maria Piraccini
Department of Experimental, Diagnostic, and Specialty Medicine
University of Bologna
Bologna, Italy

Fabio Rinaldi
Private Practice in Dermatology
Milan, Italy

Lidia Rudnicka
Department of Dermatology
Medical University of Warsaw
Warsaw, Poland

Ralph M. Trüeb
Department of Dermato-trichology
Center for Dermatology and Hair Diseases
Zurich-Wallisellen, Switzerland

Michèle Verschoore
L'Oréal Research & Innovation
Asnières sur Seine, France

Salvador Villablanca
Department of Dermatology Hospital Clinic
University of Barcelona
Barcelona, Spain

Annika Vogt
Department of Dermatology and Allergy
Clinical Research Center for Hair and Skin Science
Charité–Universitätsmedizin Berlin
Berlin, Germany

1 Biology of the hair follicle

Ulrike Blume-Peytavi, Varvara Kanti, and Annika Vogt

INTRODUCTION

The spectrum of physiological functions of hair ranges from protection, e.g., from ultraviolet (UV) radiation, insulation against cold, and mechanical protection, to sensory and tactile as well as decorative and gender defining functions. Hair growth plays an important role in social and sexual communication, and hair loss may have a detrimental impact on quality of life, with significant impairment of life perceived by the affected patients. Understanding the biology of the hair follicle, its growth activity, including hair cycle regulation, is key for hair loss counseling and management.

Despite the development of new treatments, hair cycle regulation and its dysregulation leading to alopecia are not yet fully understood and controllable. A greater understanding of hair biology and pathogenetic mechanisms of hair disorders could lead to new therapeutic approaches for the management of hair disorders. The majority of clinically relevant hair diseases are caused by disturbances of hair cycle regulation, differentiation and keratinization, pigmentation, and immunology of the hair follicle. Generally, the complex mechanisms of hair follicle biology are only rudimentarily understood; our current knowledge is predominantly based on structural and morphological investigations as well as on functional characterization of single cell populations. The identification of mediators and elucidation of the complex cell–cell interactions in hair cycle regulation could open up new diagnostic and therapeutic possibilities. The aim of this chapter is to present current aspects of hair follicle biology and pathophysiology and carve out their clinical relevance.

HAIR FOLLICLE DEVELOPMENT

The hair follicle is composed of epidermal and dermal components; the latter includes the dermal papilla and the dermal fibrous sheath that are derived from an aggregate of mesenchymal cells that forms directly beneath the epithelial hair germ at the onset of follicular development. The epidermal hair germ grows downward and forms the hair peg as a result of complex epidermal–dermal interactions, which involve many pathways known from embryonic development, e.g., Hedgehog (Hh) and Wingless (Wnt) signaling. The full development of the hair follicle further requires a complex sequence of autocrine, paracrine, and endocrine signals both within and between the epidermis and the dermis. The development and differentiation of hair follicles during embryogenesis are classically divided into eight stages, characterized by distinct morphologies (Figure 1.1).

ANATOMY OF THE PILOSEBACEOUS UNIT AND HAIR FOLLICLE TYPES

More than 20 different cell populations are involved in the structure of the pilosebaceous unit, which includes the hair follicle, together with the sebaceous gland and the arrector pili muscle as well as the adjacent vascular supply of the hair follicle (Figure 1.2).

Hair follicles compose a permanent upper segment of follicular infundibulum and isthmus and a

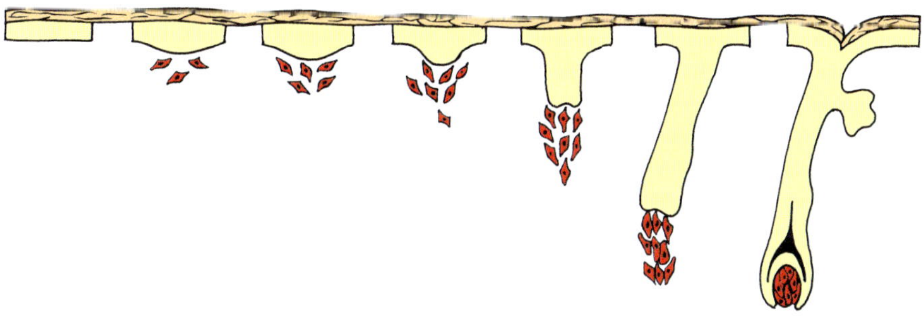

Figure 1.1 **Morphogenesis of the human hair follicle. Hair follicle formation is the result of complex sequential signaling events between the dermal mesenchyme and the overlying epithelium. Morphologically, induction, organogenesis, and cytodifferentiation phases can be determined. (With kind permission from Springer Science+Business Media: *Hair Growth and Disorders*, Biology of the hair follicle, 2008, 1–22, Berlin: Springer, Vogt A, McElwee KJ, and Blume-Peytavi U.)**

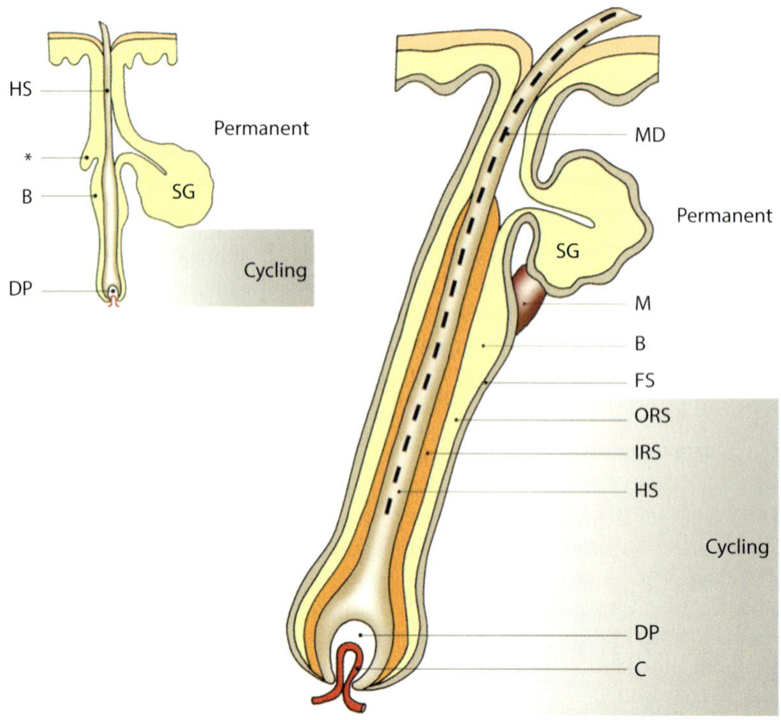

Figure 1.2 Anatomy of the pilosebaceous unit. All hair follicles follow a common architecture. Together with the sebaceous gland (SG) and the arrector pili muscle (M), the hair follicle is part of the so-called "pilosebaceous" unit. The fibrous sheath (FS) and the epithelial outer and inner root sheaths (ORS, IRS) form concentric layers, which ensheathe the hair shaft (HS). Hair growth results from the proliferative activity of matrix keratinocytes in the bulb, which sit on the dermal papilla (DP). The dermal papilla is a condensate of specialized mesenchymal cells with important inductive properties. It also provides nutrition via a capillary loop (C), which is especially prominent in terminal hair follicles. The permanent, superficial component has to be differentiated from the transient cycling component of the hair follicle, which includes the bulb. The morphological dividing line between these two components lies below the bulge (B) region and the insertion of the arrector pili muscle (M). Size and shape of the hair follicles, however, vary with the body location and potential functions. In anagen phase, for example, vellus hair follicles from the retroauricular region (left) are approximately six times shorter than scalp hair terminal follicles (right). Each hair follicle has characteristic features. Vellus hair shafts, in contrast to terminal hair shafts, are usually devoid of a medulla (MD). Skirt-like epithelial structures (*), however, can only be found in vellus hair follicles. (With kind permission from Springer Science+Business Media: *Hair Growth and Disorders*, Biology of the hair follicle, 2008, 1–22, Berlin: Springer, Vogt A, McElwee KJ, and Blume-Peytavi U.)

nonpermanent, variable lower segment of the hair follicle and bulb, which undergoes continuous renewal during the hair cycle. The morphological dividing line between these two components lies just below the bulge region and insertion of the arrector pili muscle.

The infundibulum extends from the skin surface to the point of the sebaceous gland duct opening to the hair canal. The superficial section of the hair follicle infundibulum, the acro-infundibulum, is lined by intact epidermis including a well-developed stratum corneum and a stratum granulosum. Continuous loss of epidermal differentiation occurs toward the isthmus of the lower infundibulum, the infrainfundibulum.

The isthmus extends from the arrector pili insertion (bulge area) down to the entry of the sebaceous duct. The bulge region represents a specialized compartment of the outer root sheath, which forms a niche for epithelial and neuroectodermal stem cells as well as various immature cell populations including immature Langerhans cells, mast cells, and melanocyte precursors.

The hair bulb is defined by the position of the dermal papilla and contains specialized mesenchymal cells with important inductive properties and a capillary loop to provide nutrition. The papilla is surrounded by undifferentiated, actively proliferating hair matrix cells, which give rise to the hair shaft and the inner root sheath. The fibrous sheath and the epithelial outer and inner root sheaths form concentric layers, which ensheathe the hair shaft. The outer root sheath extends from the matrix cells in the hair bulb up to the entry level of the sebaceous duct. Outer root sheath cells contain clear vacuolated cytoplasm filled with large amounts of glycogen. Below the isthmus, the outer root sheath is not keratinized. However, at the level of the isthmus, where the inner root sheath disintegrates, the outer root sheath keratinizes without forming granules. Outer root sheath cells express a large diversity of mediators, hormones, and receptors. The inner root sheath consists of three layers, the Henle, Huxley, and cuticle, all of which keratinize and provide the form to the hair shaft. The mesenchymal sheath is separated from the epithelial root sheaths by a vitreous or basal membrane. This whole complex is surrounded by a dense vascular network. Free nerve endings form a cuff and provide the basis for intensive piloneural interactions.

The hair fiber is formed of keratin proteins, which are organized as a two-phase intracellular composite consisting of the keratin fibers embedded in a sulfur-rich matrix. The visible hair shaft of terminal hair follicles consists of three layers: cortex, cuticle, and medulla. The hair fiber cortex contains melanosomes, which determine the color of the hair fiber. Homogenous oval eumelanin granules and lamellar pheomelanin granules, in variable composition and density, form the wide spectrum of dark to fair hair. The outermost layer of the hair fiber, the cuticle, consists of multiple layers of corneocytes. It is thin and translucent allowing light to penetrate to the cortex pigments.

The total number of hair follicles in an individual is determined at the time of birth to be between 2 and 5 million, 100,000–150,000 of which are located on the scalp. The number of scalp hair follicles varies depending on the individual's skin, hair color, and ethnicity (Table 1.1). All hair follicles form during embryonic development, and no additional follicles are formed after birth in humans. Consequently, hair follicle density changes in different body regions with age (Tables 1.2 and 1.3). Furthermore, the hair type varies depending on age, sex, and localization of the hair follicle (Table 1.4). Structurally and

Table 1.1 Typical Numbers of Scalp Hair Follicles

Type	Number
Blonde-haired Caucasian	130,000
Dark-brown/black-haired Caucasian	110,000
Red-haired Caucasian	90,000
African (African American)	90,000
Asian (Far East)	90,000

Source: With kind permission from Springer Science+Business Media: *Hair Growth and Disorders*, Biology of the hair follicle, 2008, 1–22, Berlin: Springer, Vogt A, McElwee KJ, and Blume-Peytavi U.

Table 1.2 Hair Follicle Density with Age (Absence of Alopecias)

Location	Mean Density of Hair Follicles in Skin
Full-term fetal scalp	1135/cm^2
Adult scalp	615/cm^2
Full-term fetal forehead	1060/cm^2
Adult forehead	765/cm^2
Full-term fetal thigh	480/cm^2
Adult thigh	55/cm^2

Source: With kind permission from Springer Science+Business Media: *Hair Growth and Disorders*, Biology of the hair follicle, 2008, 1–22, Berlin: Springer, Vogt A, McElwee KJ, and Blume-Peytavi U.

Table 1.3 Estimated Number of Hair Follicles in the Skin by Body Region

Location	Number of Follicles
Head	1,000,000
Trunk	425,000
Arms	220,000
Legs	370,000
Approximate total	2,000,000

Source: With kind permission from Springer Science+Business Media: *Hair Growth and Disorders*, Biology of the hair follicle, 2008, 1–22, Berlin: Springer, Vogt A, McElwee KJ, and Blume-Peytavi U.

Table 1.4 Different Types of Terminal Hair in Humans

Type	Length—Typical Range	Description
Scalp hair	100–1000 mm	Medullated with tapered tip in uncut hair
Eyebrows and eyelashes	5–10 mm	Medullated and curved with punctuate tip
Beard and moustache	50–300 mm	Complex medullary processes, more irregular in structure, blunt tip
Body hair	5–60 mm	Irregularly medullated, fine tip
Pubic hair	10–60 mm	Coarse, kinked, irregular, and asymmetrical cross section
Axillary hair	10–50 mm	Coarse, less kinked than pubic hair, blunt tip, often abraded due to friction

Source: With kind permission from Springer Science+Business Media: *Hair Growth and Disorders*, Biology of the hair follicle, 2008, 1–22, Berlin: Springer, Vogt A, McElwee KJ, and Blume-Peytavi U.

functionally, a distinction is made between lanugo, vellus, and terminal hair, which are differentiated by means of hair shaft diameter, hair length, pigmentation, and characteristics of the multiple concentric cell layers forming the hair shaft (the fibrous sheath and the epithelial inner and outer root sheaths) (Table 1.5). All hair follicle types present the same compartments of the pilosebaceous unit but differ in size and relation of the pilus and the sebaceous contributing parts. Lanugo hair, the first body hairs formed in the embryo, are fine, soft, silky in texture, poorly pigmented, and have no central medulla. Vellus hairs have a diameter of up to 30 μm and are nonmedullated, fine, and poorly pigmented, and normally do not grow longer than 2 cm. Vellus hair follicles are small and reach down only in the upper third of the dermis. The mostly pigmented, terminal hair follicles reach into the lower dermis and often into the subcutaneous fat and produce hair with a diameter of typically 50–100 μm; average hair fiber diameters are smaller in blonde-haired than in dark-haired individuals and larger overall in African and Asian populations (Table 1.6). Furthermore, depending on ethnic origin, elliptical to round hair shafts can be found.

Eyelashes constitute a specialized hair type: they have the largest diameter of all body hair, they have a relatively short active growth phase, and their strong pigmentation is normally preserved into old age.

Table 1.5 Typical Hair Characteristics

Type	Diameter	Length
Lanugo hair	<30 μm	>2 cm
Vellus hair	<30 μm	<2 cm
Intermediate hair	30–60 μm	>2 cm
Terminal hair	>50 μm	>2 cm

Source: With kind permission from Springer Science+Business Media: *Hair Growth and Disorders*, Biology of the hair follicle, 2008, 1–22, Berlin: Springer, Vogt A, McElwee KJ, and Blume-Peytavi U.

Table 1.6 Terminal Hair Diameter

Type	Diameter—Typical Range
Blonde-haired Caucasian	40–80 μm
Dark-brown/black-haired Caucasian	50–90 μm
Red-haired Caucasian	50–90 μm
African (African American)	60–100 μm
Asian (Far East)	80–120 μm

Source: With kind permission from Springer Science+Business Media: *Hair Growth and Disorders*, Biology of the hair follicle, 2008, 1–22, Berlin: Springer, Vogt A, McElwee KJ, and Blume-Peytavi U.

HAIR GROWTH CYCLE

The hair cycle (Figure 1.3) includes a complex remodeling and regeneration of the complete inferior nonpermanent portion of the hair follicle. In humans, hair cycle regulation is not synchronized; each individual hair follicle cycles continuously during its life span through stages of growth (anagen), regression (catagen), and rest (telogen). Recently, an additional phase was recognized, during which the hair shaft is actively shed from the telogen follicle (exogen). The following interval of the hair cycle, in which the hair follicle remains empty after the telogen hair has been extruded and before a new anagen hair emerges, has been named *kenogen*.

Anagen

During the anagen phase, the hair is actively growing and materials are deposited in the hair shaft by cells found in the follicle. Metabolically active and dividing cells above and around the dermal papilla of the follicle, arising from the matrix keratinocytes grow upward during this phase to form the hair shaft. The anagen phase includes hair growth and proliferation of all hair follicle cells in all epithelial compartments, with the highest activity and sensitivity to noxes and toxic events observed in matrix cells.

Catagen

The anagen phase is followed by a short regression phase, the catagen, characterized by a cessation of protein and pigment production, involution of the hair follicle, and fundamental restructuring of the extracellular matrix. Massive apoptosis (programmed cell death) in the infrabulbar transient portion of the hair follicle leads to regression of the hair follicle and formation of a fibrous streamer. Catagen is the first component of the first hair cycle after morphogenesis.

Telogen

In telogen, the hair follicle has completely regressed, leading to total interruption between the permanent and the nonpermanent compartments of the hair follicle, to about half of its previous size and does not extend beyond the upper dermis. The hair root sheaths have retracted to form the club hair. The rounded up dermal papilla is located distantly, having migrated downward in the dermis waiting for the next signal in early anagen to migrate via the down-growing lower portion of the permanent hair follicle compartment. Epithelial cells of the lower telogen follicle do not show significant DNA or RNA synthesis, and the volume of the dermal papilla extracellular matrix is much reduced. The telogen club hair can be retained for months in this epithelial sac until the exogen starts.

Exogen

Recent research suggests that shedding of the hair fiber is a highly controlled, active process (exogen phase)

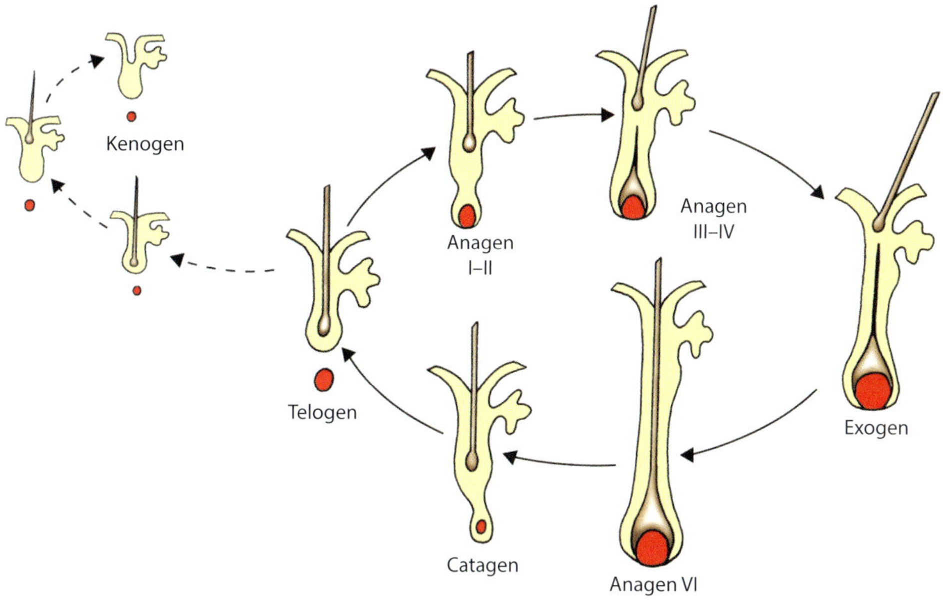

Figure 1.3 **Hair cycle. During one hair cycle a complete remodeling of the nonpermanent portion of the hair follicle occurs, which is controlled by finely tuned changes in the local signaling milieu. Traditionally, three phases of hair growth are recognized: growth phase (anagen I–III), regression phase (catagen), and resting phase (telogen). Recent research suggests that the shedding of the hair fiber is an active process, which has led to the introduction of the term *exogen* to describe this event. As another novel phenomenon in hair cycling, empty hair follicles after shedding of the hair fiber were reported. This interval of the hair cycle in which the hair follicle remains empty after the telogen hair has been extruded and before a new anagen hair emerges has been named *kenogen*. (With kind permission from Springer Science+Business Media: *Hair Growth and Disorders*, Biology of the hair follicle, 2008, 1–22, Berlin: Springer, Vogt A, McElwee KJ, and Blume-Peytavi U.)**

that differs from the quiescence normally found during the telogen phase. In fact, more detailed studies on this process suggest that the former concept, based on the assumption that the newly formed hair fiber pushes the resting shaft outward to effect shedding, is unlikely. It was shown that while anagen and telogen hairs are firmly anchored to the follicle, exogen hairs are passively retained within the follicles. The different morphology of the exogen and telogen hair root suggests that the exogen process involves a proteolytic event that occurs between the moving cells of the telogen shaft base.

Kenogen

Empty hair follicles after shedding of the hair fiber have been found using phototrichograms, and the term *kenogen* has been suggested to describe this interval of the hair cycle in which the hair follicle remains empty after the telogen hair has been extruded and before a new anagen hair emerges. Kenogen can be reproducibly observed in healthy skin; however, frequency and duration have been reported to be greater in men and women with androgenetic alopecia, and only a portion of the hair follicle undergoes this phase. It is yet unclear which signals decide for the occurrence of kenogen.

Duration of the hair cycle

Durations of the different phases depend on the type and localization of the hair follicle (Tables 1.7 and 1.8). Normally, 80%–85% of the scalp hair is in anagen, with the rest either in catagen (2%) or telogen phase (10%–15%). The anagen phase of scalp hair follicles typically persists for 2–6 years and is a major determinant of maximal hair length. But anagen may persist for just a few weeks in terminal hair follicles on the extremities. The anagen phase of hair follicles of the eyebrows is only 70 days, while eyelashes grow for 100–150 days. The duration of telogen in hair follicles is also an important consideration in understanding the consequences of changes in the hair growth cycle. Body hair follicles are characterized by an increased telogen frequency and duration as compared to scalp hair follicles. Under physiological conditions, each hair follicle continues to cycle throughout life, but with reduced anagen phase duration while undergoing the aging process.

HAIR GROWTH REGULATION

Cyclical growth is a characteristic of the hair follicle. Even though all scalp hair follicles are in the same hair cycle phase during the fetal period, the hair cycles of the

Table 1.7 Hair Cycle Duration Depending on Body Location

Location	Hair Growth State	Typical Time Duration
Scalp	Anagen	2–6 years
	Catagen	2–3 weeks
	Telogen	3 months
Beard	Anagen	4–14 weeks
	Telogen	10–18 weeks
Arms	Anagen	6–12 weeks
	Telogen	7–13 weeks
Legs	Anagen	19–26 weeks
	Telogen	13–34 weeks

Source: With kind permission from Springer Science+Business Media: *Hair Growth and Disorders*, Biology of the hair follicle, 2008, 1–22, Berlin: Springer, Vogt A, McElwee KJ, and Blume-Peytavi U.

Table 1.8 Rate of Terminal Hair Growth in Adults

Location	Typical Hair Growth per Day
Chin	0.38 mm
Scalp	0.35 mm
Axillary	0.30 mm
Thigh	0.20 mm
Eyebrows	0.16 mm

Source: With kind permission from Springer Science+Business Media: *Hair Growth and Disorders*, Biology of the hair follicle, 2008, 1–22, Berlin: Springer, Vogt A, McElwee KJ, and Blume-Peytavi U.

individual hair follicles run asynchronously in humans, as opposed to in other mammalian species. The regulation of hair growth has been extensively revised in current literature. We aim to summarize key knowledge of the involvement of the major signaling pathways in hair cycling. Essential for the coordinated regulation of the hair cycle are epithelial–mesenchymal interactions between hair follicle stem cells and dermal papilla cells. The inner root sheath has essential pattern formation functions. The outer root sheath perceives regulatory functions through close contact with antigen-presenting cells and melanocytes.

Reciprocal interactions between epithelial and mesenchymal cell populations are well known from the organogenesis; accordingly, components of signal transduction pathways concerned with pattern formation are expressed in the adult hair follicle. The ligand "sonic hedgehog" (Shh) is expressed in the distal part of the epithelial section of the hair follicle, and the expression of associated target genes, such as transcription factor Gli, could be found in adult hair follicles. The coordination of the different signaling pathways is essential for the proper course of the hair cycle. The transient expression of Shh can induce the anagen phase, but the permanent activation of this signal transduction pathway is an important factor in the pathogenesis of basal-cell carcinoma. A wide spectrum of growth factors, including EGF, FGF, HGF, IGF, and TGFβ, as well as various cytokines, play a role in hair cycle regulation, while overlapping interactions between the different signal transduction pathways are mostly the case, e.g., convergence between EGFR and Wnt/β-catenin signaling pathways: EGF regulates transcription of E-cadherin through Src kinase activation, thus enabling the regulation of Wnt-mediated signals through β-catenin.

The dermal papilla is the central place of regulation, supplying the adjacent germinative epithelial cells and the matrix keratinocytes via the strongly pronounced vessel system. The mesenchymal cells of the dermal papilla express vascular endothelial growth factor (VEGF) and are probably involved in the cyclical restructuring of the vascular system and the extracellular matrix. Dermal papilla cells show in vitro basal expression of nitrogen monoxide (NO). This could be stimulated by 5α-dihydrotestosterone, thereby highlighting the importance of hormonal stimuli for hair cycle regulation.

Hormonal influence

The same hair follicle is able to produce lanugo hair in the fetal period, vellus hair in infancy, and terminal hair in adulthood. Abnormal increases in the serum levels of androgens, such as in the case of hirsutism in adrenal hyperfunction, or of estrogens, progesterone, and prolactin, lead to a prolongation of the anagen stadium. The different receptors and hormone-metabolizing enzymes determine the complex and partially contradictory reaction pattern of the hair follicle depending on age, localization, and gender. For example, there is a graded response of regional hairs to androgens: temporal and occipital scalp hairs as well as eyebrows and eyelashes are insensitive to androgens. Inguinal and axillary follicles are stimulated to grow under low androgen levels, while the androgen-dependent facial hairs in men are stimulated to grow only under high levels of androgen. The inherent specific sensitivity to hormonal stimuli is retained after hair transplantation, a principle called *donor dominance*. Therefore, androgen independent/insensitive hair follicles from the occipital scalp can be successfully transplanted to sites of androgen-sensitive hairs, affected by male pattern baldness (frontal, parietal, coronal areas) and retain their occipital growth behavior. Human hair follicles express a wide variety of steroid metabolizing enzymes, such as aromatase, 5α-reductase, steroid sulfatase, 5,3β-hydroxysteroid dehydrogenase, and 17β-hydroxysteroid dehydrogenase. The activity of these enzymes can locally influence the perifollicular hormone level, depending on the particular isoform as well as availability of the substrate. Hence, usually local imbalances in this equilibrium without changes in the hormone serum levels can lead to clinically relevant hair growth disorders like androgenetic alopecia.

Hair pigmentation

Pigmentation is also hair cycle dependent and underlies endocrine, paracrine, and autocrine regulatory mechanisms. Although melanocytes can be found in different compartments of the anagen hair follicle, melanogenetically active cells are primarily located in the hair bulb. Hair follicle melanogenesis is tightly coupled to the hair growth cycle as a result of closely coordinated epithelial, mesenchymal, and neuroectodermal interactions. Toward the end of each hair cycle, melanocytes reduce melanin production and retract their dendrites, thus leading to a transient "canities"—an unpigmented proximal end of telogen hair fibers. During aging, melanocyte activity decreases, as does the number of dopa-positive melanocytes, resulting in gray and white hair. Furthermore, follicular melanocytes are able to replace interfollicular melanocytes. In pigmentation disorders, such as vitiligo, follicular melanocytes are actively involved in the repigmentation of the interfollicular epidermis. Proopiomelanocortin (POMC) α-, β-, and γ-MSH, and corticotropin (ACTH) are important pigmentation regulators, and polymorphisms of the melanocortin 1 receptor are associated with hair color characteristics. Apart from this receptor, the coexpression of corticotropin-releasing hormone (CRH) and mRNA from α-MSH and even ACTH could be found in the human hair follicle. These findings support results from experimental studies in animals, indicating that the hair follicle is not only a target organ for melanocortins, but also a synthesis site for CRH and POMC peptide. This could be considered as an expression of a potential follicular control system, involved not only in pigmentation regulation but also in hair growth, the perifollicular immune system, and local mediation of the stress response. The dense perifollicular adrenergic and sensory nerve network, as well as the presence of perifollicular Merkel cells and neurotrophin-sensitive mast cells all being with the highest density around the bulge region, also highlights the importance of piloneural interactions in hair follicle cycling and control.

Immune system

The hair follicle represents a physiological break in the skin barrier. Accordingly, antigen-presenting cells can be found at particularly high densities around the upper portion of the hair follicle, which is thus acting as a site for intensive interactions between the immune system and microbial invaders or allergens. The hair follicle constitutes a reservoir of dendritic cells, from which follicular Langerhans cells can contribute to the repopulation of areas of skin that are exposed to UVB. In contrast to the high density of antigen-presenting cells in the upper portion of the hair follicle, very low numbers of intraepithelial T cells, Langerhans cells, and major-histocompatibility-complex-I-(MHC-I-)molecules are found in the anagen hair bulb. Ultrastructural investigations indicate a potential role of Langerhans cells in pigment sequestration in the early catagen stage. An overexpression of MCH-I as well as melanogenesis-associated autoantigen presentation with activation of CD 8^+ cells was found in hair follicles of patients with alopecia areata. Therefore, dysfunctions with collapse of the peribulbar immune privilege have been suggested as a possible factor in the pathogenesis of alopecia areata.

Follicular stem cells

The hair follicle is able to regenerate a variety of cell populations during each new hair cycle. This enormous plasticity is accomplished by the presence of multipotent adult stem cells, which reside in rather undifferentiated, quiescent states and form precursors, transient amplifying cells, which provide further proliferation and differentiation into the different cell types. Furthermore, the reepithelialization of epidermal defects often emanates from the hair follicle. The exact localization of the responsible stem cells has not yet been clarified. Experimental data revealed that the slowest cycling cells within the skin reside in the bulge region. The outer root sheath has also been discussed as the location of the stem cell reservoir. The possible role of mesenchymal stem cells is becoming the focus of scientific interest. In experimental studies in animals with high follicle density, cycle-related/dependent differences were found in wound healing. Mesenchymal hair follicle cells also seem to positively influence the quality of wound healing, so that the fibrous sheath has been suggested to be a possible site for progenitor cells. The mesenchymal cells of the dermal papilla exhibit a high inductive potency and are capable of inducing folliculogenesis after transplantation through interaction with epithelial cells of the host tissue. Moreover, mesenchymal cells of the dermal papilla and the fibrous sheath actively produced hematopoietic cells in vivo and in vitro, whereas follicle epithelial cells did not.

Follicular penetration

With a density of more than 400 vellus hairs per square centimeter on the forehead and more than 93 per square centimeter on the back, hair follicles account for a significant share of the skin surface area. The epithelium of the acro-infundibulum is keratinized and relatively impermeable, like the epithelium of the interfollicular epidermis, whereas the corneocytes in the underlying portions of the follicle are rather fragile and small and only form an incomplete barrier. Experimentally, it could be shown that implantation of dissected hair follicles into reconstructed skin significantly increases the penetration of substances like hydrocortisone. Furthermore, a correlation has been observed between penetration of topically applied substances and sebum production as well as growth activity of the hair follicle. This observation provided the rationale for the development of particular drug formulations and carrier systems to specifically target hair follicles. Therefore, these findings on penetration in and through the hair follicle depending on localization, gender, and growing activity are of high practical relevance and provide implications for the dermatological external therapy and for the development of transcutaneous application systems.

CLINICAL RELEVANCE

The development of new strategies to control the hair follicle cycle is currently in the spotlight of hair research, and a wide range of novel molecules and delivery systems are currently being developed. The investigative challenges in alopecia treatment involve understanding and controlling signal transduction events and their regulatory genes in order to induce and/or prolong anagen and to shorten telogen. A profound knowledge of hair follicle biology could facilitate the targeted control/selective influence of the local regulation systems and the development of novel hair loss therapeutic approaches based on molecular evidence rather than pure empirical evidence.

BIBLIOGRAPHY

1. Baker RE, Murray PJ. Understanding hair follicle cycling: A systems approach. *Curr Opin Genet Dev.* 2012;22:607–612.
2. Blume-Peytavi U, Vogt A. Human hair follicle: Reservoir function and selective targeting. *Br J Dermatol.* 2011;165(suppl 2):13–17.
3. Breitkopf T, Leung G, Yu M, Wang E, McElwee KJ. The basic science of hair biology: What are the causal mechanisms for the disordered hair follicle? *Dermatol Clin.* 2013;31:1–19.
4. Conrad F, Ohnemus U, Bodo E, Bettermann A, Paus R. Estrogens and human scalp hair growth—Still more questions than answers. *J Invest Dermatol.* 2004; 122:840–842.
5. Courtois M, Loussouarn G, Hourseau S, Grollier JF. Periodicity in the growth and shedding of hair. *Br J Dermatol.* 1996;134:47–54.
6. Das BM. A study of cross sections of head hair from some caucasoid and mongoloid populations of Assam, India. *Z Morphol Anthropol.* 1974;65:324–328.
7. Das-Chaudhuri AB, Chopra VP. Variation in hair histological variables: Medulla and diameter. *Hum Hered.* 1984;34:217–221.
8. Driskell RR, Clavel C, Rendl M, Watt FM. Hair follicle dermal papilla cells at a glance. *J Cell Sci.* 2011; 124:1179–1182.
9. Duverger O, Morasso MI. To grow or not to grow: Hair morphogenesis and human genetic hair disorders. *Semin Cell Dev Biol.* 2013;25–26:22–33.
10. Elliott K, Stephenson TJ, Messenger AG. Differences in hair follicle dermal papilla volume are due to extracellular matrix volume and cell number: Implications for the control of hair follicle size and androgen responses. *J Invest Dermatol.* 1999;113:873–877.
11. Fuchs E. Scratching the surface of skin development. *Nature.* 2007;445:834–842.
12. Fuchs E, Horsley V. More than one way to skin. *Genes Dev.* 2008;22:976–985.
13. Ito T. Hair follicle is a target of stress hormone and autoimmune reactions. *J Dermatol Sci.* 2010;60:67–73.
14. Jahoda CA, Christiano AM. Niche crosstalk: Intercellular signals at the hair follicle. *Cell.* 2011;146: 678–681.
15. Kligman AM. The human hair cycle. *J Invest Dermatol.* 1959;33:307–316.
16. Kligman AM. Pathologic dynamics of human hair loss. I. Telogen effuvium. *Arch Dermatol.* 1961;83:175–198.
17. Krause K, Foitzik K. Biology of the hair follicle: The basics. *Semin Cutan Med Surg.* 2006;25:2–10.
18. Lademann J, Otberg N, Richter H et al. Investigation of follicular penetration of topically applied substances. *Skin Pharmacol Appl Skin Physiol.* 2001; 14(suppl 1):17–22.
19. Lako M, Armstrong L, Cairns PM, Harris S, Hole N, Jahoda CA. Hair follicle dermal cells repopulate the mouse haematopoietic system. *J Cell Sci.* 2002; 115:3967–3974.
20. Langbein L, Schweizer J. Keratins of the human hair follicle. *Int Rev Cytol.* 2005;243:1–78.
21. Li A. The biology of melanocyte and melanocyte stem cell. *Acta Biochim Biophys Sin (Shanghai).* 2014;46:255–260.
22. Loussouarn G, El Rawadi C, Genain G. Diversity of hair growth profiles. *Int J Dermatol.* 2005;44(Suppl 1):6–9.
23. Maderson PF. Born in a follicle—A historical perspective. *Differentiation.* 2004;72:466–473.
24. Mecklenburg L, Tobin DJ, Muller-Rover S et al. Active hair growth (anagen) is associated with angiogenesis. *J Invest Dermatol.* 2000;114:909–916.
25. Messenger AG. The control of hair growth: An overview. *J Invest Dermatol.* 1993;101:4S–9S.
26. Mikkola ML. Genetic basis of skin appendage development. *Semin Cell Dev Biol.* 2007;18:225–236.
27. Mirmirani P. Hormonal changes in menopause: Do they contribute to a "midlife hair crisis" in women? *Br J Dermatol.* 2011;165(Suppl 3):7–11.
28. Nishimura EK. Melanocyte stem cells: A melanocyte reservoir in hair follicles for hair and skin pigmentation. *Pigment Cell Melanoma Res.* 2011;24:401–410.
29. Ohyama M, William J. Cunliffe scientific awards. Advances in the study of stem-cell-enriched hair follicle bulge cells: A review featuring characterization and isolation of human bulge cells. *Dermatology.* 2007;214:342–351.

30. Otberg N, Richter H, Schaefer H, Blume-Peytavi U, Sterry W, Lademann J. Variations of hair follicle size and distribution in different body sites. *J Invest Dermatol.* 2004;122:14–19.
31. Pasolli HA. The hair follicle bulge: A niche for adult stem cells. *Microsc Microanal.* 2011;17:513–519.
32. Patzelt A, Lademann J. Drug delivery to hair follicles. *Expert Opin Drug Deliv.* 2013;10:787–797.
33. Paus R, Arck P, Tiede S. (Neuro-)endocrinology of epithelial hair follicle stem cells. *Mol Cell Endocrinol.* 2008;288:38–51.
34. Paus R, Foitzik K. In search of the "hair cycle clock": A guided tour. *Differentiation.* 2004;72:489–511.
35. Paus R, Peters EM, Eichmuller S, Botchkarev VA. Neural mechanisms of hair growth control. *J Investig Dermatol Symp Proc.* 1997;2:61–8.
36. Pecoraro V, Astore I, Barman JM. Cycle of the scalp hair of the new-born child. *J Invest Dermatol.* 1964;43:145–147.
37. Peters EM, Arck PC, Paus R. Hair growth inhibition by psychoemotional stress: A mouse model for neural mechanisms in hair growth control. *Exp Dermatol.* 2006;15:1–13.
38. Plonka PM, Passeron T, Brenner M et al. What are melanocytes really doing all day long…? *Exp Dermatol.* 2009;18:799–819.
39. Rancan F, Blume-Peytavi U, Vogt A. Utilization of biodegradable polymeric materials as delivery agents in dermatology. *Clin Cosmet Investig Dermatol.* 2014; 7:23–34.
40. Randall VA, Botchkareva NV. The biology of hair growth. In: Ahluwalia G, ed. *Cosmetics Applications of Laser & Light-Based Systems.* Boston: Elsevier Science; 2009:3–35.
41. Randall VA, Hibberts NA, Thornton MJ et al. The hair follicle: A paradoxical androgen target organ. *Horm Res.* 2000;54:243–250.
42. Randall VA, Hibberts NA, Thornton MJ et al. Do androgens influence hair growth by altering the paracrine factors secreted by dermal papilla cells? *Eur J Dermatol.* 2001;11:315–320.
43. Rippa AL, Vorotelyak EA, Vasiliev AV, Terskikh VV. The role of integrins in the development and homeostasis of the epidermis and skin appendages. *Acta Naturae.* 2013;5:22–33.
44. Rogers GE. Hair follicle differentiation and regulation. *Int J Dev Biol.* 2004;48:163–170.
45. Rook A. Hair II: Racial and other genetic variations in hair form. *Br J Dermatol.* 1975;92:599–600.
46. Schlake T. Determination of hair structure and shape. *Semin Cell Dev Biol.* 2007;18:267–273.
47. Schneider MR, Schmidt-Ullrich R, Paus R. The hair follicle as a dynamic miniorgan. *Curr Biol.* 2009; 19:R132–R142.
48. Schwartz JR, Shah R, Krigbaum H, Sacha J, Vogt A, Blume-Peytavi U. New insights on dandruff/seborrhoeic dermatitis: The role of the scalp follicular infundibulum in effective treatment strategies. *Br J Dermatol.* 2011;165(Suppl 2):18–23.
49. Schweizer J, Langbein L, Rogers MA, Winter H. Hair follicle-specific keratins and their diseases. *Exp Cell Res.* 2007;313:2010–2020.
50. Sehgal VN, Srivastava G, Aggarwal AK, Midha R. Hair biology and its comprehensive sequence in female pattern baldness: Diagnosis and treatment modalities: Part I. *Skinmed.* 2013;11:39–45; quiz 45.
51. Shimomura Y, Christiano AM. Biology and genetics of hair. *Annu Rev Genomics Hum Genet.* 2010;11: 109–132.
52. Slominski A, Wortsman J, Plonka PM, Schallreuter KU, Paus R, Tobin DJ. Hair follicle pigmentation. *J Invest Dermatol.* 2005;124:13–21.
53. Stenn K. Exogen is an active, separately controlled phase of the hair growth cycle. *J Am Acad Dermatol.* 2005;52:374–375.
54. Stenn KS, Paus R. Controls of hair follicle cycling. *Physiol Rev.* 2001;81:449–494.
55. Tadeu AM, Horsley V. Epithelial stem cells in adult skin. *Curr Top Dev Biol.* 2014;107:109–131.
56. Tobin D. Gerontobiology of the hair follicle. In: Trüeb RM, Tobin DJ, eds. *Aging Hair.* Berlin: Springer; 2010: 1–8.
57. Tobin DJ, Paus R. Graying: Gerontobiology of the hair follicle pigmentary unit. *Exp Gerontol.* 2001;36: 29–54.
58. Vogt A, Blume-Peytavi U. [biology of the human hair follicle. New knowledge and the clinical significance]. *Hautarzt.* 2003;54:692–698.
59. Vogt A, Blume-Peytavi U. Selective hair therapy: Bringing science to the fiction. *Exp Dermatol.* 2014; 23:83–86.
60. Vogt A, Hadam S, Heiderhoff M et al. Morphometry of human terminal and vellus hair follicles. *Exp Dermatol.* 2007;16:946–950.
61. Vogt A, Mandt N, Lademann J, Schaefer H, Blume-Peytavi U. Follicular targeting—A promising tool in selective dermatotherapy. *J Investig Dermatol Symp Proc.* 2005;10:252–255.
62. Vogt A, McElwee KJ, Blume-Peytavi U. Biology of the hair follicle. In: Blume-Peytavi U, Tosti A, Trüeb RM, eds. *Hair Growth and Disorders.* Berlin: Springer; 2008:1–22.
63. Westgate GE, Botchkareva NV, Tobin DJ. The biology of hair diversity. *Int J Cosmet Sci.* 2013;35: 329–336.
64. Yang CC, Cotsarelis G. Review of hair follicle dermal cells. *J Dermatol Sci.* 2010;57:2–11.

2 Hair and scalp investigations

Pierre Bouhanna

INTRODUCTION

For the diagnosis of hair loss or alopecia, it is important to record a complete clinical history to guide the clinical examination. There are additional investigations to quantify the hair loss and confirm its pathological character, to clarify its etiology, to assess the extent of the possible associated alopecia, and finally to objectively measure the effectiveness of specific treatments (Table 2.1).

HISTORY

Diagnosis of alopecia usually proceeds from a good history-taking that analyzes the personal history, the family history, and the history of the disease.[1–3]

Personal history

Many kinds of alopecia are due to underlying or concomitant diseases. Those kinds differ from both scarring alopecia, which results in concomitant follicular and irreversible skin damage, and other nonscarring types of alopecia, which cause reversible alteration of the follicle and skin without final alteration. Nonscarring alopecia (androgenetic alopecia, alopecia areata, trichotillomania, etc.) is an increasingly common reason for consulting a physician (Figure 2.1). In the case of abrupt hair loss (effluvium), we must take careful note of the patient's medications, such as cytostatics, anticoagulants, lithium, antithyroid, vitamin A, etc. Various alopecias are encountered due to endocrinopathies (hypo- and hyperthyroidism, androgen syndrome, Cushing syndrome, etc.), iron deficiency, etc. (see Chapters 5 through 8).

Family history

Family history should be taken systematically, particularly in male and female androgenetic alopecia. The importance of a family history is greater in the diagnosis of certain abnormalities such as congenital or hereditary hypotrichoses (e.g., Marie Unna syndrome), genodermatosis such as anagen loose hair syndrome, or pilar dysplasia (monilethrix, woolly hair, etc.) (see Chapter 4).

Table 2.1 Management of a Hair Loss

History

- Personal history:
  - Initial aspect
  - Concomitant symptoms
  - Evolution
  - Concomitant diseases
- Medications such as:
  - Cytostatics, anticoagulants, lithium, antithyroid, etc.
- Family history about hair and alopecia disease

Methods of clinical exploration

- Pull-test
- Global photography
- Trichoscopy
- Trichogram
- Digital phototrichogram
- Multifactorial classification parameters

⇓

Diagnosis of the hairloss

↓

Schema of treatment

↓

Precise follow-up

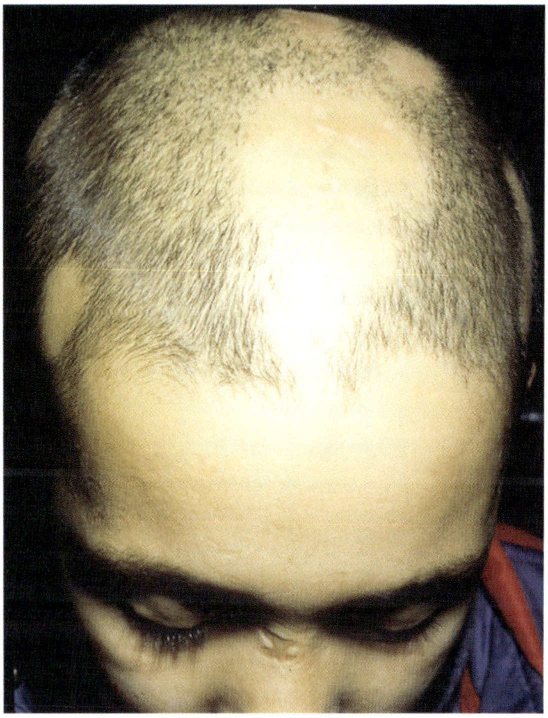

Figure 2.1 Patches of alopecia areata.

History of the disease

The clinician will need to check on the aspects the problem displayed initially, the associated clinical signs, and the disease's evolution (Table 2.2).

Initial aspects include the following: hair loss can be acute and diffuse (effluvium in anagen and telogen), acute and focal (in traumatic alopecia, Figure 2.1), chronic and diffuse (androgenetic alopecia), or chronic and focal (pseudopelade, alopecia areata, trichotillomania). It is important to note the age at onset of the first signs: early (pilar dysplasia, congenital hypotrichoses), postpubertal (androgenetic alopecia), or late (acquired diseases) (see Chapter 5).

Associated signs include:

- Seborrhea, acne, hirsutism, and alopecia (SAHA) syndrome for androgenetic alopecia and alopecia.
- Localized inflammation for decalvans folliculitis or ringworm.
- Alterations in the nails, bones, eyes, or teeth for follicular hyperkeratosis (monilethrix, keratosis pilaris decalvans) or elsewhere in different types of ectodermal hair dysplasias.

Table 2.2 Hair Loss Description

Early form	Diffuse and acute	Telogen or anagen effluviums Alopecia areata
	Diffuse and chronic	Androgenetic alopecia
	Focal and acute	Alopecia areata Traumatic alopecia
	Focal and chronic	Pseudopeladic alopecia of Brocq Trichotillomania
Associated symptoms	Seborrhea	Androgenetic alopecia Female constutional hyperandrogenism (SAHA)
	Inflammation	Folliculitis decalvans Tuft folliculitis Tinea capitis Lichen planopilaris Lupus erythematosus
	Follicular hyperkeratosis	Follicular keratosis decalvans Monilethrix
	Ectodermic alterations	Ectodermic dysplasia
Evolution	Progressive	Androgenetic alopecia
	Successive eruptions	Alopecia areata
	Irreversible	Cicatricial alopecia
	Autoinvolutive	Anagen or telogen effluviums Patchy alopecia areata

- Progression that is slow for androgenetic alopecia, advances in pushes for alopecia, is irreversible for scarring alopecia, or is idiosyncratic for telogen effluvium and alopecia areata.[2]

CLINICAL EXPLORATION

Clinical examination of the hair and scalp provides valuable information about alopecia, indicating the morphological appearance of the hair and scalp as well as the form and extent of alopecia.[1–4]

Morphology of the hair

The morphology of the hair is very important to recognize, as it can provide information not only on the type of alopecia in question but also on the mode of progression. Thus, the presence of hair with normal appearance and texture does not have the same meaning as dry and dull hair (pilar dysplasia, hypotrichoses, malnutrition, deficiency diseases). It is very important to observe if there are hairs of smaller thickness or that are shorter and thinner (intermediate hairs) on the frontoparietal recession or the tonsure. These intermediate hairs correspond to miniaturized hair, becoming thinner and thinner through successive hair cycles under androgenetic alopecia (Figure 2.2). In alopecia areata, "exclamation mark" hairs are found, under the microscope, at the edge of the bald patches (Figure 2.3).

Distribution of alopecia

Alopecia can be diffuse (hypotrichoses, androgenetic alopecia, effluvium) or in patches (alopecia areata, pseudopelade, trichotillomania).

Skin appearance

Examination of the skin surface of the scalp allows a physician, in most cases, to recognize scarring alopecia (irregular bald patches where there remain hairs of normal appearance, with skin changes involving erythema, fibrosis, and atrophy) or nonscarring alopecia (round and

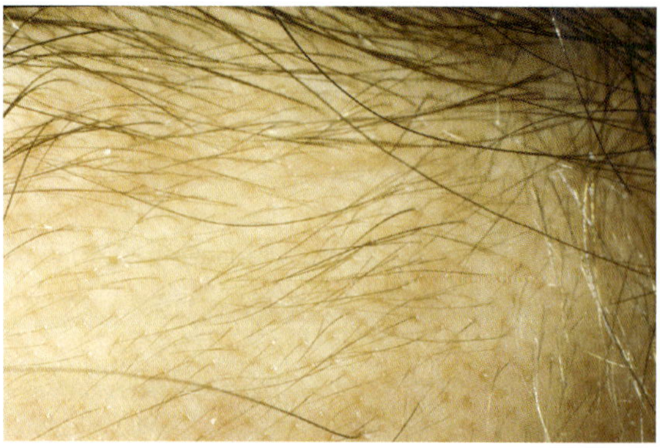

Figure 2.2 **Miniaturized hairs (vellus and intermediate) on the frontal hairline pathognomonic of the androgenetic alopecia.**

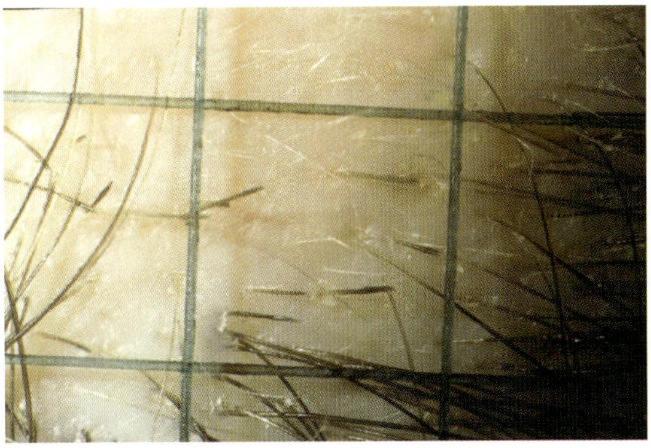

Figure 2.3 **Characteristic dystrophic anagen aspect of "exclamation mark hair," pathognomonic of alopecia areata visible on trichoscopy.**

regular patches with a normal-looking skin surface where all the hair has disappeared).

Types of alopecia

Abnormal hair loss can be acute or chronic, diffuse or localized.[2–4]

Four types of alopecia can be identified schematically (see Chapter 5):

1. Alopecia at the frontotemporal recession or of the crown is characteristic of androgenetic alopecia.
2. Diffuse alopecia is of uniform distribution over the entire scalp and includes effluvium in anagen and telogen phases, and female androgenetic alopecia (especially if it is a lower form with localization to the temporooccipital region). It is not unusual for two types of alopecia to coexist in this group.
3. Alopecia in a band along the edge of the scalp is especially visible in ophiasis alopecia areata, traction alopecia, and frontal fibrosing alopecia.
4. Alopecia in patches is characterized by one or more patches of different shapes and sizes. Several clinical features are present; the most significant are alopecia areata, ringworm, follicular mucinosis, trichotillomania, and pseudopelade.

INVESTIGATIONS

More specific types of investigation to carry out can be divided into two categories: additional clinical tests and laboratory tests aimed at individual cases.

Laboratory tests when hair loss has been observed

A specific blood test is required to detect hematological and biochemical changes.[1–3] It is possible to identify a lack or deficiency of metabolic components of the hair follicle or even whether there is a disease responsible for the androgenetic alopecia or hyperandrogenism.

In women, it is important to carry out first-line investigations for any hair loss, such as a complete blood count (CBC), erythrocyte sedimentation rate (ESR), and serum ferritin and/or iron saturation (total iron-binding capacity, TIBC).

We will suspect a hormonal imbalance if there is facial hirsutism or excess hair (with or without dysmenorrhea or amenorrhea). There should therefore be a prescribed dose blood tests of male hormones such as testosterone (T), dehydroepiandrosterone sulfate (DHEA-S), the Δ4-androstenedione or female hormones such as prolactin (PRL), follicle-stimulating hormone (FSH), and prolactin dehydrogenase (LDH).

It is also advisable to look into a possible thyroid origin, checking FT4 and thyroid-stimulating hormone (TSH).

In men, however, it is not necessary to perform first-line blood tests in male pattern androgenetic alopecia, except in cases of diffuse alopecia of the female type; however, check CBC, ESR, and TIBC in patients with a history or suspicion of anemia.

Clinical tests in routine practice

Critical examinations performed when confronted by any hair loss are the pull-test, standardized global photography, a trichogram, a dermatoscopy or trichoscopy, a digital phototrichogram,[5] and the possible measurement and recording of all parameters in the multifactorial classification[6] in the case of male or female androgenetic alopecia (see Chapter 5).

The pull-test

The pull-test allows for confirmation of hair loss (Table 2.3).[1] It consists of a gentle traction between the thumb and forefinger on a lock of 50–60 hairs on a scalp that had not been washed for 48 hours at three different locations on the scalp. The result is normal if less than six hairs are removed. If the number of hairs that are removed on traction is greater than six hairs per sampling point, we can consider that the patient has abnormal hair loss, as in effluvium in the anagen or telogen phase or alopecia areata (Figure 2.4). The value of this exam is relative to the individual patient and the same examiner.

The standardized global photography

Standardized global photography consists of global photographs of the vertex,[4] frontal, and temporal regions performed in a standardized manner (Figure 2.5). The patient places his or her chin on a stereotactic positioning device. The camera is mounted on a metal rod and fixed at a known distance to allow taking photographs of the vertex, frontal, and temporal regions. This system, developed by Canfield Scientific (Fairfield, New Jersey), allows for an accurate monitoring of alopecia areas and hairy areas.

For better control of the treatment's efficacity on androgenetic alopecia, we suggest that the global photographs

Table 2.3 Hair-Pull Test for Various Hair Diseases

Disease	Hair-Pull Test
Normal	0–5 hairs can be pulled; a test with ≥6 hairs is positive
Alopecia areata	Positive ≥6 hairs on light microscopy show dystrophic anagen and telogen stage
Androgenetic alopecia	Mostly normal; in active AGA, positive on the top of the scalp, negative in occipital area
Acute anagen or telogen effluvium	Positive in active phases with increased numbers of anagen or anagen dysphastic hairs or normal telogen hairs
Chronic telogen effluvium (CTE)	Positive only in active phase of CTE always with 6–8 telogen roots when examined with light microscopy
Trichotillomania	Negative with no pluckable hairs
Loose anagen syndrome	Highly positive; up to 100% when hairs are examined under the microscope; anagen hair root mostly lacking the hair sheath (anagen dysplastic)

Source: With kind permission from Springer Science+Business Media: *Hair Growth and Disorders: With 85 Tables*, 2008, Berlin Heidelberg: Springer, Blume-Peytavi U.

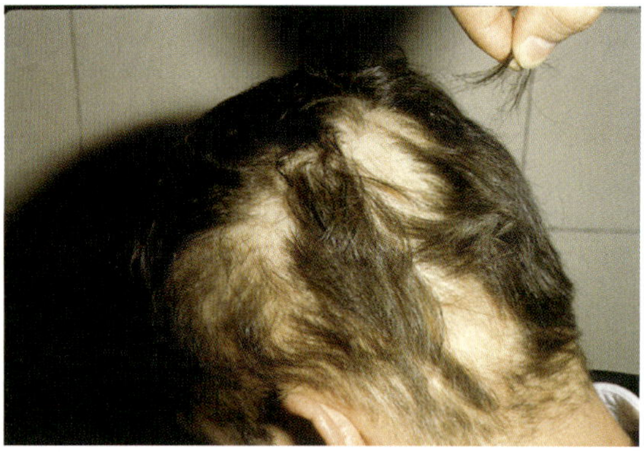

Figure 2.4 **Positive plucking test (+++) performed on a patient with very extensive alopecia areata progressing to total alopecia.**

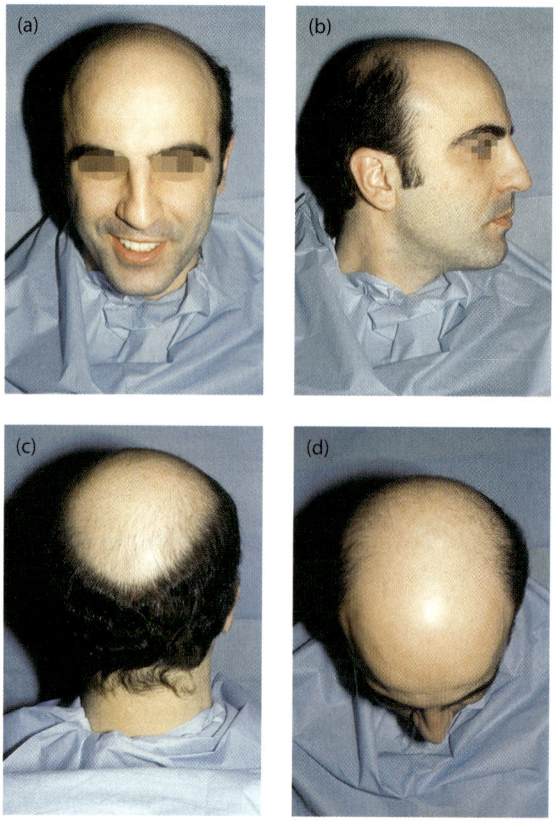

Figure 2.5 **Global photographs: (a) front view, (b) side view, (c) back view, and (d) vertex view of a patient with androgenetic alopecia.**

be taken with wet hair combed forward to eliminate the artifactual effect (Figure 2.6).

The trichogram

This type of investigation allows us to determine the hair formula—that is, the distribution of hair as a percentage,[5,7] in each hair phase.

In adulthood, the number of hairs on a normal scalp varies from 100,000 to 150,000. They grow on average from 0.35 to 0.44 mm/day, and growth is cyclical.

The hair cycle consists of three phases (Figure 2.7): a growth or anagen phase, a transition or catagen phase, and a falling or telogen phase. Each telogen hair, once fallen, is replaced by a new anagen hair, and the balance of anagen/telogen hair remains constant.

Schematically, the anagen phase lasts an average of 3 years (2–4 years in males and 4–6 years for women), the catagen phase 3 weeks, and the telogen phase 3 months.

This explains that at every moment of the hair cycle, 80%–85% of hair is in the anagen phase, 1%–2% in the catagen phase, and 15%–20% in the telogen phase.

The percentage of anagen hair is more important in women (85%–90%) with 10%–15% of hair in the telogen phase. Normal drop is on average 25–60 hairs a day.

Sampling is effected with the aid of a curved Kocher clamp with jaws coated with rubber. A row of about fifty hairs is pulled sharply in the direction of their emergence from the skin in three different areas: occipital, frontotemporal and temporoparietal (Figure 2.8). It is important to take the sample on hair that has not been washed for three days, as washing or brushing removes telogen hair and thus leads to an overestimation of the anagen/telogen ratio. Plucking hair in the direction of the emergence

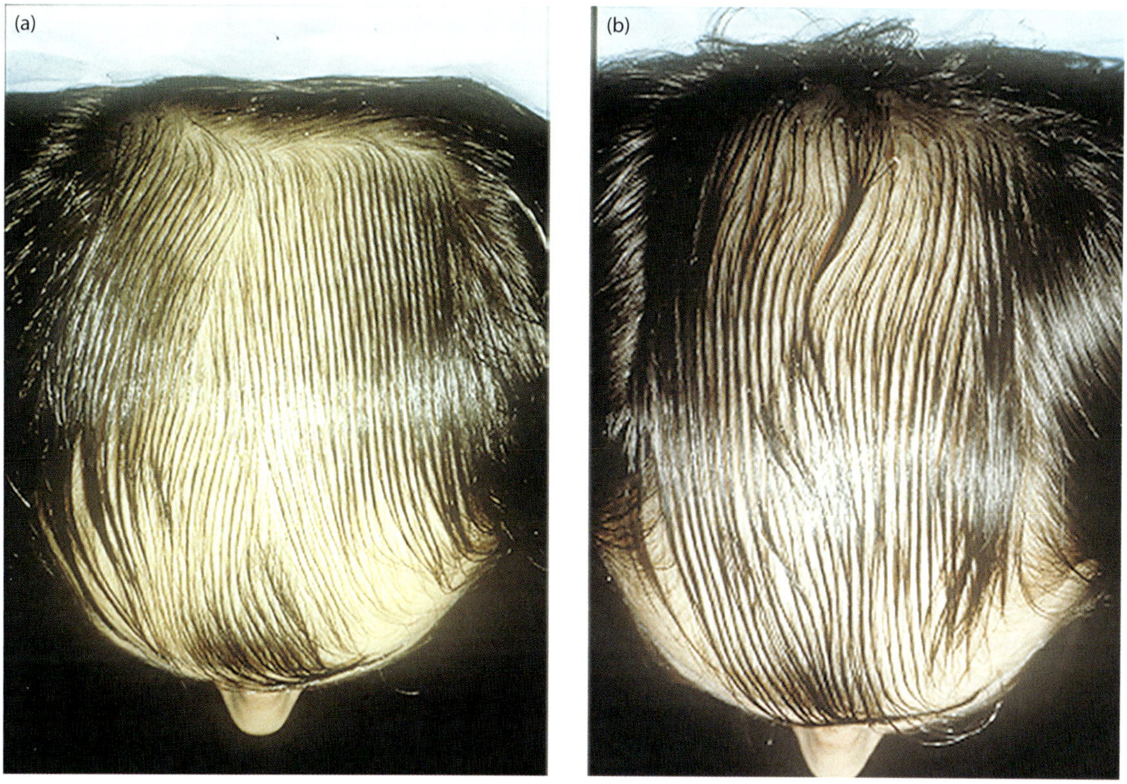

Figure 2.6 **(a) Global photography of an androgenetic alopecia (with hair wet and combed forward to eliminate artifactual effects), (b) the same patient with clinically visible regrowth after 6 months of treatment with 2% minoxidil treatment.**

of hair shafts can minimize the number of broken hairs. These hairs are cut about 1 or 2 cm from the root and placed between a slide and a cover slip (Figure 2.9). The reading is made on a microfiche reader or a microscope at low magnification; the image, magnified 20–40 times, allows detailed analysis of the root and part of the hair shaft (Figures 2.10 and 2.11).

Microscopic aspects

- *Normal microscopic aspects.* Three types of hair roots are visible:
  - *Anagen hair* has a large pigmented bulb (Figure 2.12).[3,5] In the early anagen phase, the bulb is at its largest with a pyramid shape; it then becomes quadrangular and narrower, and pigmentation remains strong. When the epithelial ducts are present, they are visible and clear; when these are absent, the anagen hairs are "naked."
  - *Telogen hair* has a rounded bulb, which is very obvious and easily identifiable by the appearance as a "golf club" or "cotton swab" (Figure 2.13). In early telogen phase, epithelial ducts form a transparent bag that covers the bulb. Later, when the telogen phase is concluding, ducts are not visible (or scarcely visible) with a marked depigmentation.
  - *Catagen hair* is in an intermediate phase. It is purely a transitional period of short duration during which the bulb is narrower and has already begun to lose pigmentation. Epithelial ducts are narrower, more irregular, and cover a smaller part of the bulb (Figure 2.14).
- *Modified microscopic aspects.*
  - *Dysplastic (distorted) anagen hair.* Plucking can distort the anagen hair, giving it the appearance of the "handle of a walking stick." The bulb is discolored, and ducts are often absent. These hairs do not have any bad significance.
  - *Broken hair.* This is most often caused by plucking rather than by a break caused by traction on dystrophic anagen hair. A percentage greater than 10% indicates a faulty technique.
- *Abnormal microscopic aspects.*
  - *Dystrophic anagen hair.* These are thin, nongrowing anagen hair, most often secondarily to

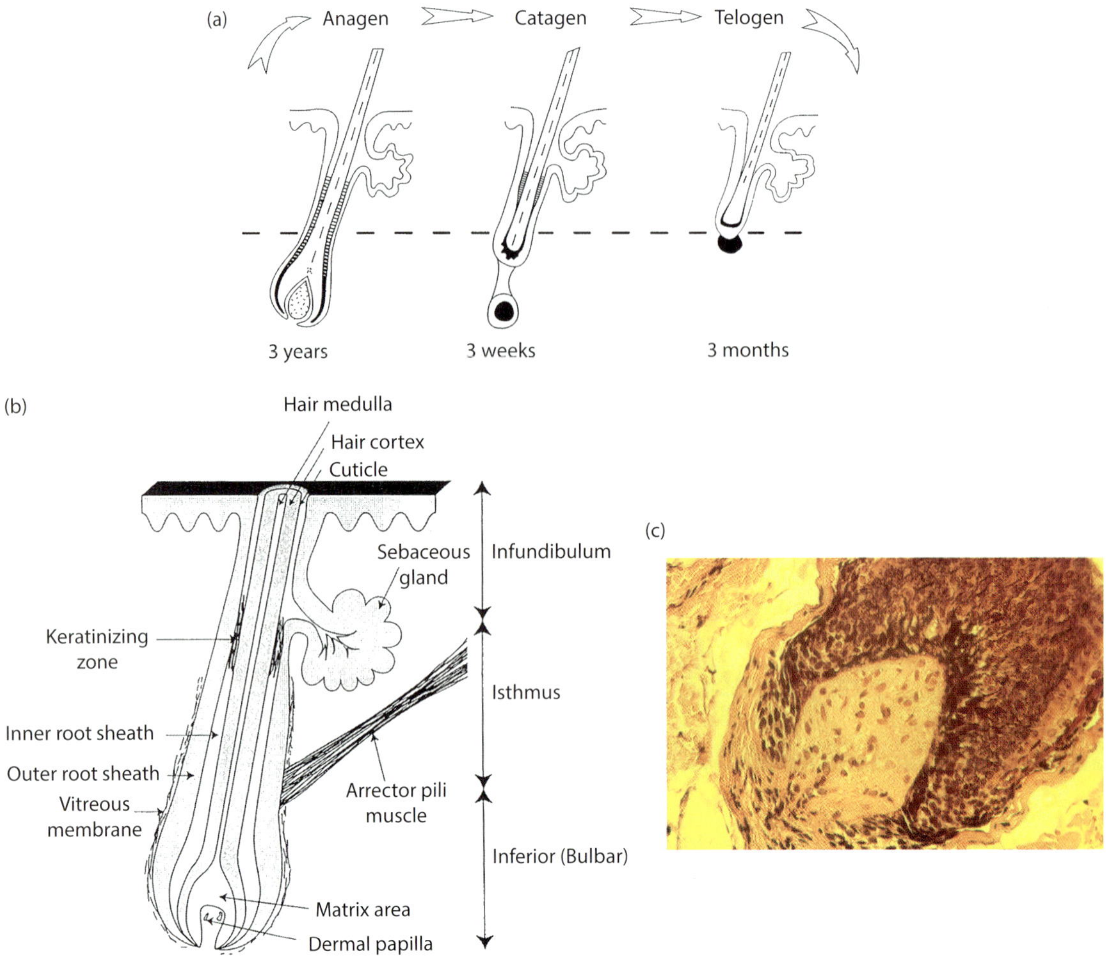

Figure 2.7 **Hair cycle (a) and schematic aspect of the hair follicle (b). (c) Histological view of the lower segment of the hair follicle, with the matrix.**

an assault. This anagen hair has a tapered end, is without a matrix, is without a sheath, and is often discolored. The keratinization is defective. This appearance is rare on a normal hair (Figure 2.15).

- *"Exclamation mark hair" in alopecia.* This is an anagen hair that is approximately 3 cm from the base, fringed fracture above a terminal bulge (Figure 2.15). It is almost visible in evolutive alopecia areata (Figures 2.3 and 2.4).

Whatever their form, dystrophic hair without sheaths and with little pigmentation does not represent more than 5% of normal hair.

Results of a normal trichogram

The anagen phase lasts 3 years, the catagen stage 3 weeks, and the telogen stage 3 months.

The normal hair formula for young adults is 80%–85% of hair in anagen, 1%–2% in catagen, and 14%–20% in telogen.

There are normally 20% of dysplastic anagen hairs called "naked anagen hair" (without ducts) and less than 2% of dystrophic anagen hair. In children, the number of anagen hairs is at least 90%. The number of telogen hairs is also very high in the newborn and the infant.

Physiological changes on the trichogram

The number of telogen hairs is higher on the frontoparietal regions, and the percentage of telogen hairs is highest for patients between 50 and 60 years.

Note that the formula for hair cycles varies with the seasons: in summer, the anagen stage is longer; falling telogen hair is up in March to April and September to October; while telogen hair falls out least during the months of January and July.

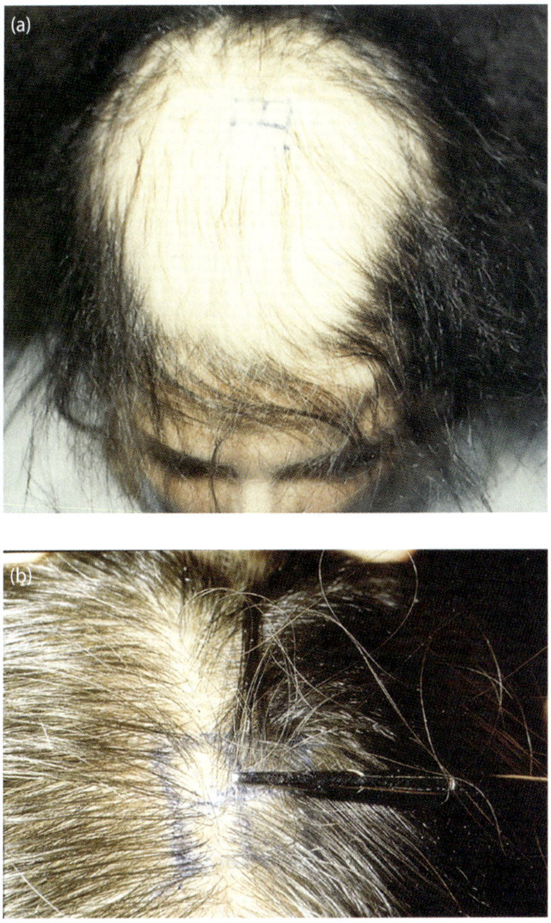

Figure 2.8 Area of hair to be sampled for a trichogram: (a) choice for sampling in a patient with type III female androgenetic alopecia, (b) the tuft of hair is separated out in an area bounded by tattooing at four points and divided into four quarters.

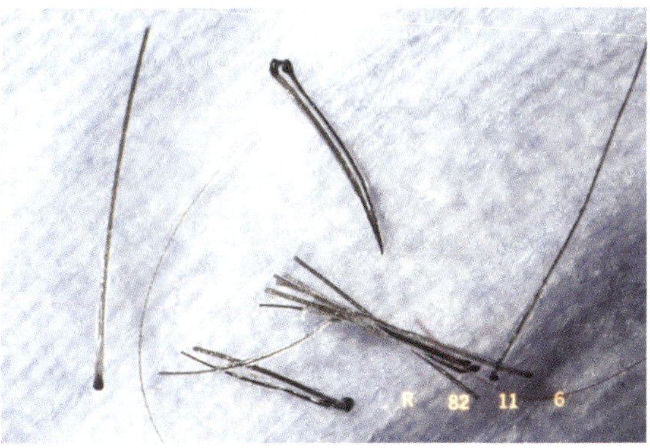

Figure 2.9 Tuft of hair taken before alignment between the slide and cover slip.

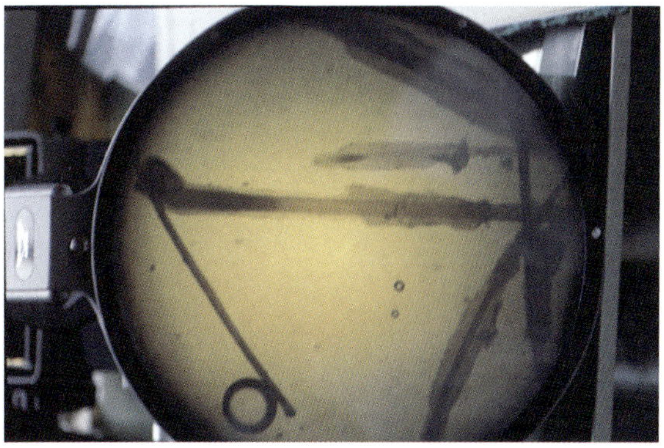

Figure 2.10 Microprojector view for a trichogram.

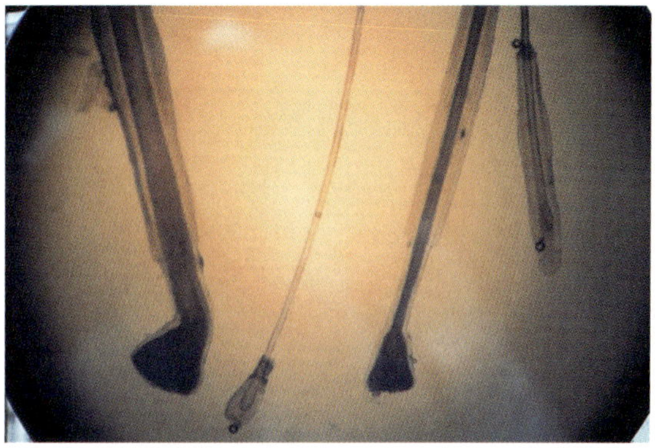

Figure 2.11 View of the three hair evolution stages (anagen, catagen, and telogen).

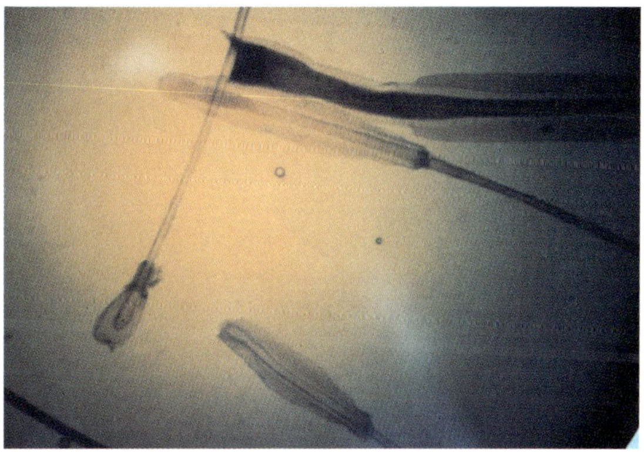

Figure 2.12 Microscopic aspect of the three types of hair under magnification (×25): two anagen hairs, one catagen hair, and one telogen hair.

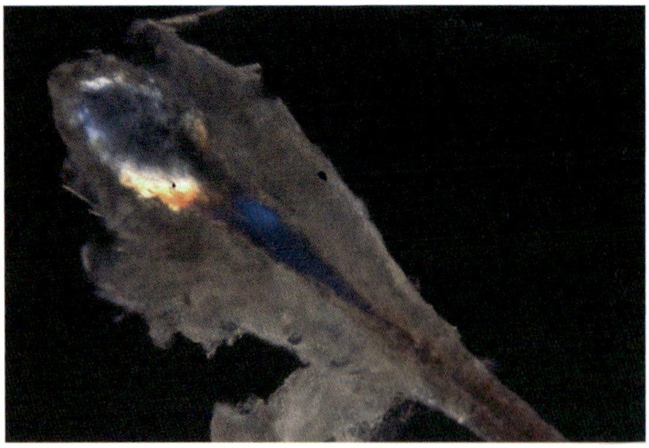

Figure 2.13 **Microscopic view of a telogen hair (in polarizing light).**

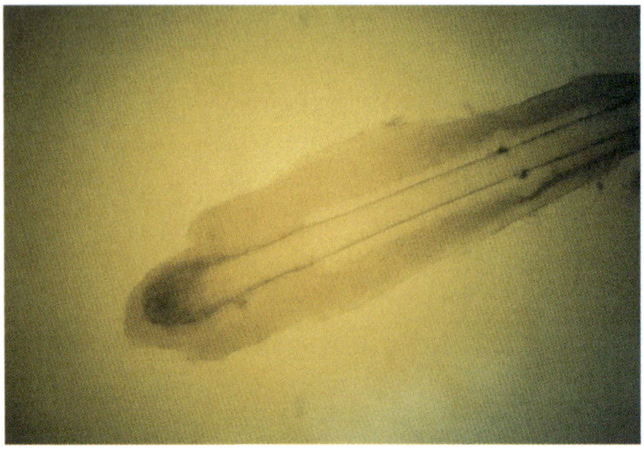

Figure 2.14 **Microscopic view of a catagen hair.**

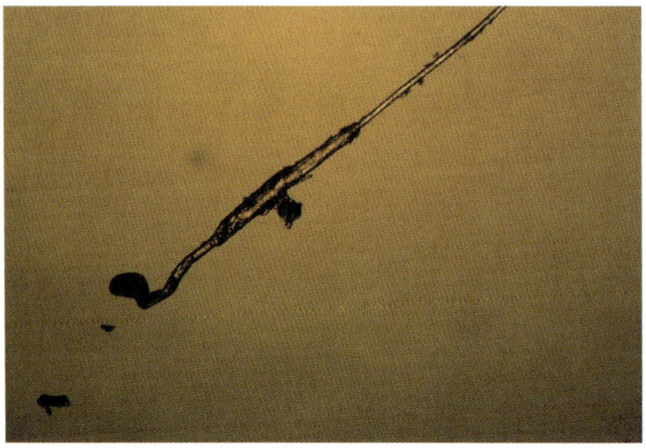

Figure 2.15 **Dystrophic anagen hair visible in alopecia areata.**

Pathological changes on the trichogram

One can observe three types of abnormal hair cycle percentages:

- The telogen type in which the percentage of telogen is increased (>20%–25%); this is telogen effluvium.
- The dystrophic type in which the number of dystrophic anagen hairs is increased at the expense of normal anagen; this is anagen effluvium (e.g., in highly developed alopecia).
- The most common mixed dystrophic telogen type, in which there is an increase in both dystrophic anagen and dystrophic telogen (e.g., in androgenetic alopecia).

The trichogram is used to assess the diameters of the hair shafts and to highlight a decrease in the size of hair follicles, which shows the miniaturization characteristic of the androgenetic alopecia.

The goal of the trichogram

The trichogram has a role that is both diagnostic and prognostic. It is indicated in five situations:

1. In the case of any hair loss for physiological reasons, a normal trichogram can reassure anxious patients.
2. In case of any diffuse hair loss without alopecia, it can decide between telogen effluvium, androgenetic alopecia, and diffuse alopecia.
   a. Telogen effluvium (pregnancy, iron deficiency, acute infection, hemorrhage, accident, general anesthesia, weight loss, emotional distress, etc.) is characterized by the abrupt and synchronized passage of many follicles into the telogen phase, resulting in hair loss 2–3 months later. The trichogram shows at that time a large number of telogen hairs (>20% or 25%) in all regions of the scalp examined.
   b. Anagen effluvium (toxic or drug-induced, chemotherapy alopecia) is due to an abrupt halt in the growth of hair in the anagen phase without passage into the the telogen phase. The loss of hair occurs 4–6 weeks later. Thus, we find in the trichogram a high number of dystrophic anagen hairs. In alopecia areata, there may be a dystrophic form of hair cycle percentages, or a mixed dystrophic telogen type.
   c. In androgenetic alopecia, the formula for hair cycle percentages is normal on the occipital area, while the number of telogen hairs and therefore the anagen/telogen ratio decreases gradually as one moves toward the front area. In addition, the hairs have diameters of different sizes, with the presence of miniaturized hair. The trichogram has a prognostic value in androgenetic

alopecia: a very reduced anagen/telogen ratio and the presence of a large number of dystrophic anagen hairs have a poor prognosis.
3. In the case of localized alopecia, the trichogram can help distinguish trichotillomania. In both cases, one can see dystrophic hair and broken hair; however, in trichotillomania, there are no telogen hairs because they were all torn, and the trichogram is normal when performed on nonaffected areas. In some cases, only histology will decide.
4. In children with suspected hair dysplasia, the trichogram can contribute to the diagnosis, but examination in polarized light directed to a lock of hair that has been cut and not torn will specify the type of hair dysplasia (see Chapter 4). However, trichogram does confirm the hair dysplasia diagnosis of loose anagen hair syndrome in which a majority of anagen hair devoid of epithelial sheaths is observed.
5. The trichogram is used to assess the effectiveness of various treatments, particularly during androgenetic alopecia. By repeating it after 6 months or 1 year of treatment, where treatment is effective it will show a decreased percentage of dystrophic anagen and telogen, with an increase or normalization of the anagen/telogen ratio.

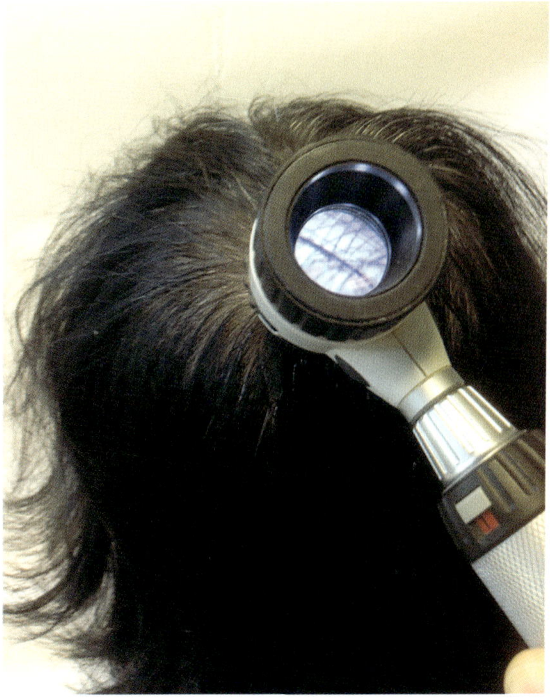

Figure 2.16 **Trichoscopy with the dermatoscope.**

The trichogram may be subject to certain criticisms: the technique of sampling and examination of different bulbs can vary from one examiner to another, and it does not allow study of the density of hair coverage, which is a fundamental criterion for the assessment of the severity of alopecia. However, the trichogram deserves a place in clinical practice to confirm and quantify hair loss.

Trichoscopy (scalp dermatoscopy)

The usefulness of trichoscopy (scalp dermoscopy) has been reported for hair loss diseases (see Chapter 3).[6,8–10] Here, characteristic trichoscopic features of common hair loss diseases are described using a DermLite II pro or Epilight eight (Figure 2.16).

Using the dermatoscope in clinical practice

The dermatoscope can provide:

- An objective check of the efficiency of a treatment to prevent hair loss (in androgenetic alopecia).
- Monitoring of the effectiveness of treatment (in progressive scarring alopecia).
- Confirmation to undertake reconstructive surgery when there has been stability for over 6 months (in stabilized scarring alopecia).

Interpretating dermatoscopy in clinical practice

A small change in the number of hairs, of about 5%, is not significant and can reflect natural changes such as a seasonal variation or the natural loss of telogen hair. In addition, a loss of more than 5% of hair may indicate either a natural worsening or a lack of efficacy in the treatment:

1. *Alopecia areata:* Characteristic trichoscopic features of alopecia areata are black dots, tapering hairs (exclamation mark hairs) (Figure 2.17), broken hairs, yellow dots, and short vellus hairs.

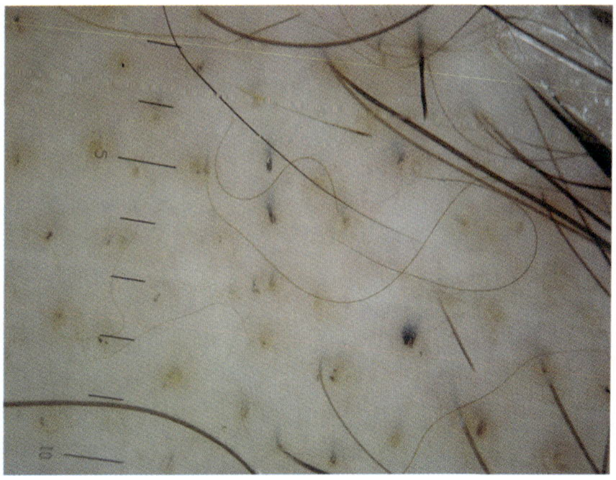

Figure 2.17 **Trichoscopy aspect of an alopecia areata. (Courtesy of Dr. Y. Bourezane.)**

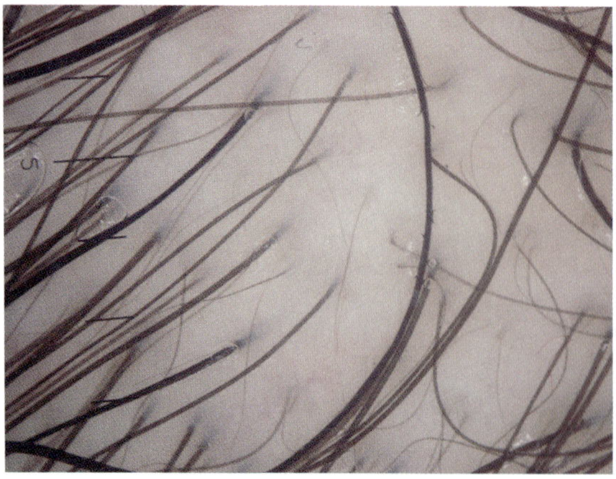

Figure 2.18 **Trichoscopy aspect of an androgenetic alopecia. (Courtesy of Dr. Y. Bourezane.)**

2. *Androgenetic alopecia (AGA):* In AGA (Figure 2.18), hair diameter diversity (HDD), perifollicular pigmentation/peripilar sign, and yellow dots are observed. In all cases of AGA, HDD is more than 20%, which corresponds to vellus transformation.
3. *Telogen effluvium (Figure 2.19):* In telogen effluvium, the clinical examination may reveal the fact but dermoscopy shows <20% variability in hair diameter.
4. *Cicatricial alopecia (see Figure 2.20):* In cicatricial alopecia, the loss of orifices and the associated changes including erythema or scale and hair tufting are observed. Tosti et al. have recently reported that the follicular red dot pattern is a specific feature of active lupus erythematosus of the scalp.[11]

An algorithmic method for trichoscopic diagnosis of common hair loss disease has been recently proposed (see Figure 2.21). The algorithmic method is for trichoscopic diagnosis of common hair loss diseases featuring black dots, broken hairs, discoid lupus erythematosus, short vellus hairs, and tapering hairs.[12]

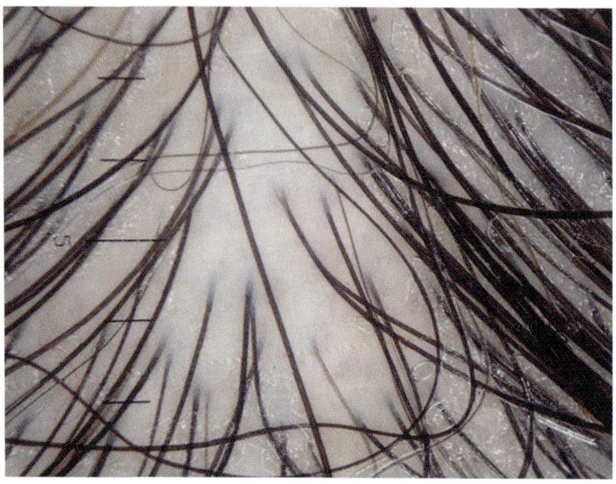

Figure 2.19 **Trichoscopy aspect of a telogen effluvium. (Courtesy of Dr. Y. Bourezane.)**

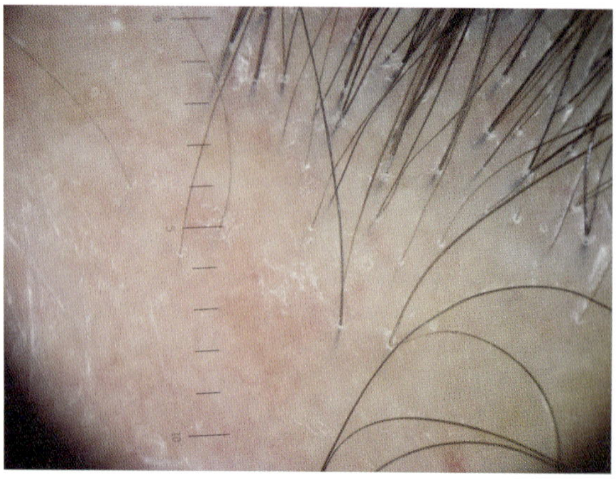

Figure 2.20 **Cicatricial alopecia due to lichen planopilaris with perpilar casts, white dots and absence of follicular openings. (Courtesy of Dr. Y. Bourezane.)**

The digital phototrichogram (DP)

The phototrichogram developed by Bouhanna in 1983 has many applications in clinical practice and in scalp surgery[13,14] (Figure 2.22a–c).

The area to be monitored is selected on the least visible site possible:

- An area of 1 cm^2 is then clipped with a minishaver and the peripheral hairs are separated by gel.
- The shaved area is then cleaned of all hair debris and all scales, using a jet of compressed air, marked by one or two semipermanent tattoos, and photographed at high magnification.
- The photographs are made under immersion—a slide of glass smooths the surface, and a drop of oil placed between the skin surface and the slide improves the contrast and sharpness of the image.
- The hair is then counted in a circular area of 7-mm diameter centered on the marker.

Software for digital image and statistical analysis is as follows[15]:

- A specially developed software program allows these parameters to be automatically measured.
- The digital phototrichogram (DP) is able to analyze the biological parameters of hair growth:
  - Hair density (n/cm^2)
  - Hair diameter (μm)
  - Hair growth rate (mm/day)
  - Anagen/telogen ratio if two photographs are done at 2–3 day interval.
- The hair area needs to be shaved, dyed, and digitally documented at a ×30 magnification.

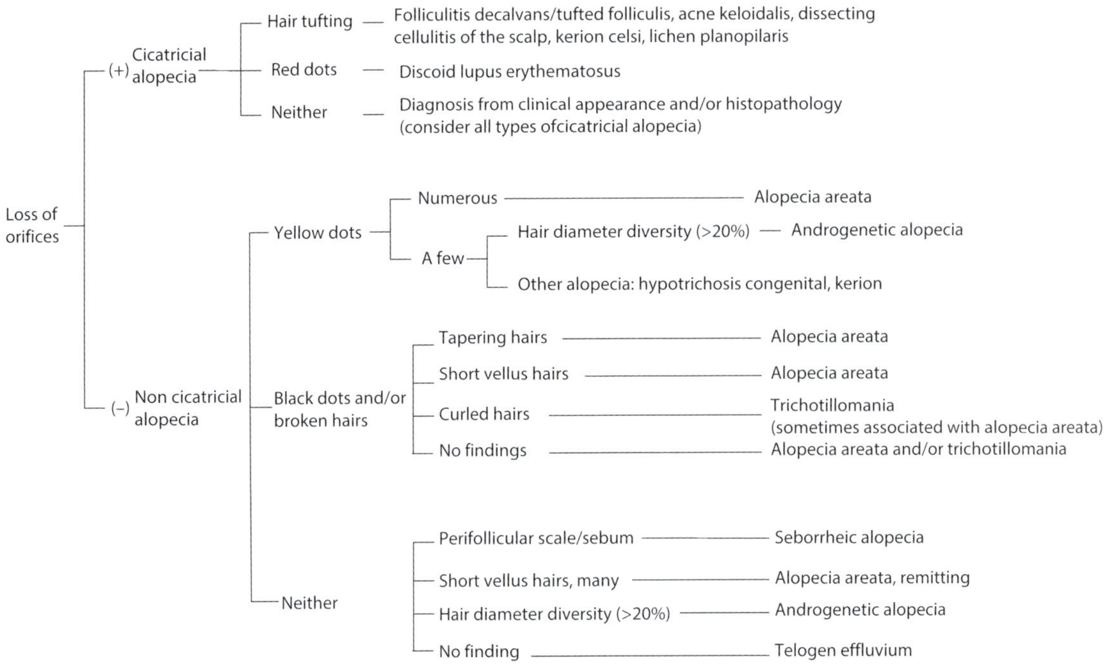

Figure 2.21 An Algorithmic Method for Trichoscopic Diagnosis of Common Hair Loss Disease. (Adapted from Inui S. *J Dermatol.* 2011;38:71–75.)

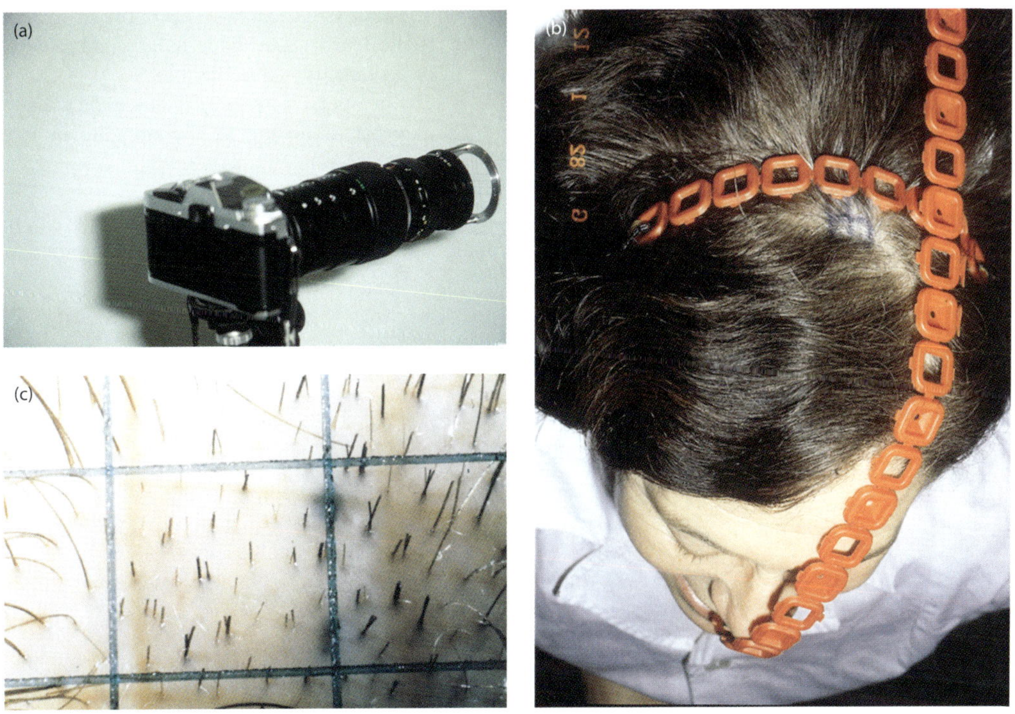

Figure 2.22 Conventional phototrichogram in the 1980s with (a) the macrophotographic camera, (b) the location system, and (c) the located macrophotographic view for hair counting.

- This procedure is painless and reproducible and allows for digital documentation.

Results

The total "hands-on" time for the digital phototrichogram operator is 15–20 minutes.

Effect of the hair dye

Analysis of white or gray hair produced only little contrast. Coloring the hairs increased hair detectability. The dye must be applied for 10 minutes.

Precision and sensitivity

Air bubbles, dust, scales, etc., are excluded. In doing so, only hairs are counted. Until now the analysis of the images has been a tedious and time-consuming process.

With the digital phototrichogram (DP), the images are taken with a video system.

The digital phototrichogram (DP) is highly validated with correlation between the same and different investigators.

The DP can be used for clinical studies for all hair colors to compare different capacities of different hair growth-promoting molecules.

The DP is able to measure significant changes in hair parameters even after 6 months of treatment (Figure 2.23). Therefore, it can be used for clinical studies for all hair to compare placebo versus active drugs or to compare different capacities of different hair growth-promoting molecules.

It can be used to evaluate AGA and diffuse hair loss and to study the effects of drugs (minoxidil, finasteride, cyproteron, spironolacton) or platelet-rich plasma treatment (Figures 2.24a–c and 2.25a and b).

It is used for the hair checkup before hair transplantation for a precise evaluation of the donor and the recipient area.

The tractiophototrichogram (TPTG)

The tractiophototrichogram is a variant of the phototrichogram.[16]

The goal is to evaluate with only one type of photography the rate of hair loss:

- An area of 1 cm^2 is located with two semipermanent tattoos. The scalp is unshaved for 3 days and is not combed before the examination.
- A pull-test is done on all the hair inside the delimited area of 1 cm^2, and the hairs are then counted.
- The same area is then clipped with a minishaver and the hairs are automatically counted in the same manner as with digital phototrichogram.

Multifactorial classification developed by Bouhanna

In contrast to existing static classifications such as the Hamilton–Norwood male androgenetic alopecia classification and the Ludwig female androgenetic alopecia classification (see Chapter 5),[17] this classification is dynamic and multifactorial. It allows the practitioner to combine measurable constants with the greatest accuracy, the better to define the medical, surgical, and cosmetic signs. It takes into account:

- The extent of bald and hairy surfaces (Figure 2.26).
- The degree of laxity of the scalp.
- The thickness of the scalp.
- The ability of the hair to cover the scalp according to the density, size, shape, length, and growth speed of the hair, as well as the color.
- The prospective evaluation of a male androgenetic alopecia according to the drawing of two axes (Figure 2.27).

This classification is useful in evaluating development of male and female androgenetic alopecia, under medical

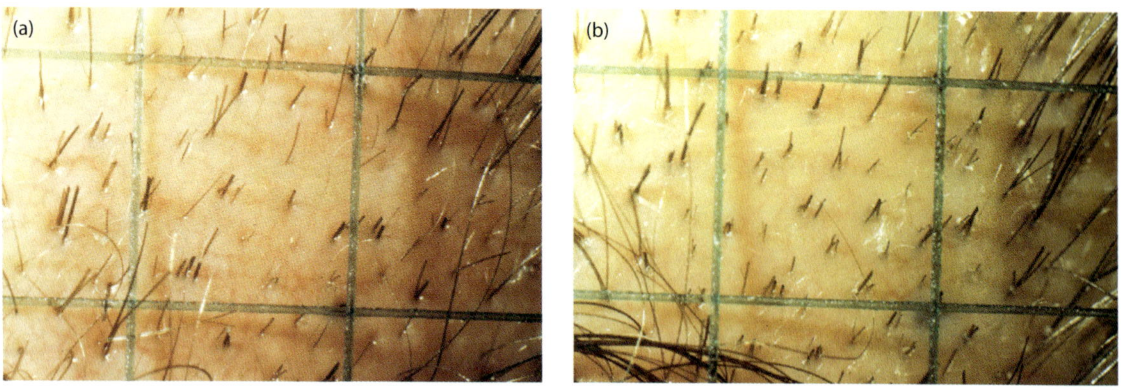

Figure 2.23 **(a) Phototrichogram of the same patient in Figure 2.6, before treatment, (b) phototrichogram of the same patient after 6 months of 2% minoxidil treatment. (The increase in the number and caliber of hair confirms with more precision the effect already visible clinically.)**

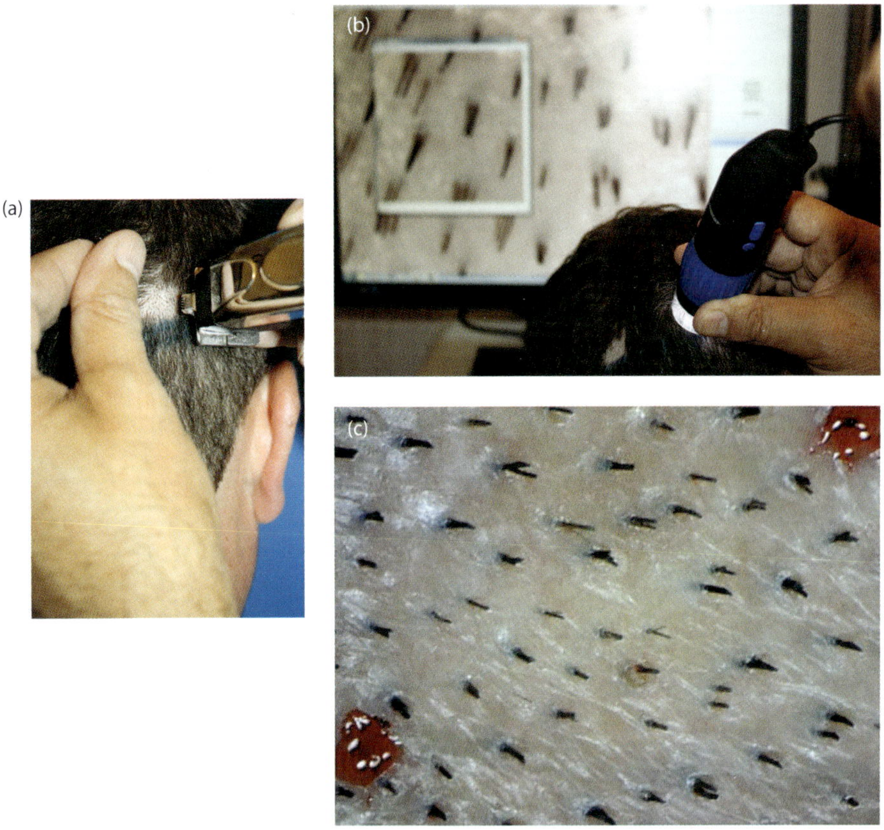

Figure 2.24 (a) An area of 1 cm^2 is clipped with a minishaver and (b) the photograph is made. (c) Detail of the photograph of the area located with two red tattoos.

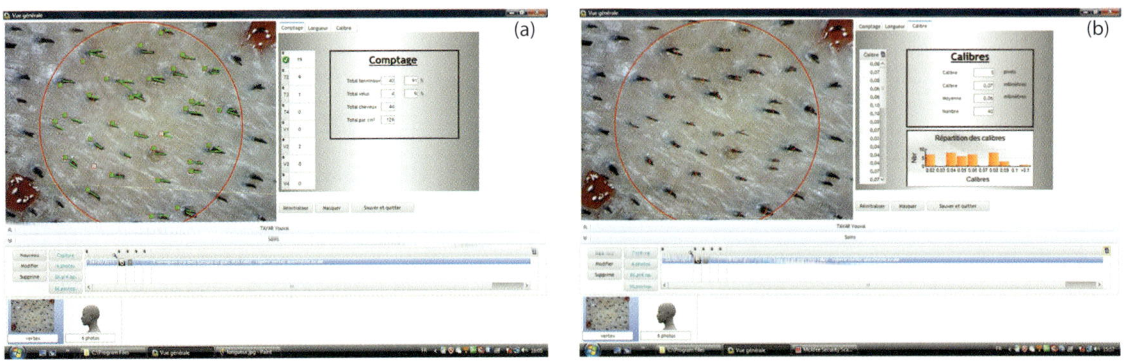

Figure 2.25 (a) Hair density counting. (b) Hair diameter evaluation.

treatment (minoxidil, hormones, finasteride) after hair transplantation and for the follow-up of evolutive cicatricial alopecia.

Examinations in special cases

Other tests are used to detect abnormalities of the hair or underlying pathologies for hair loss.[1]

Biopsy of the scalp

The histological study of combined vertical and transverse section is essential for the diagnosis of scarring alopecia (Figures 2.28 and 2.29).

This test will make the differential diagnosis between nonscarring alopecia (such as alopecia areata, androgenetic alopecia, diffuse alopecia etc.) and scarring alopecia

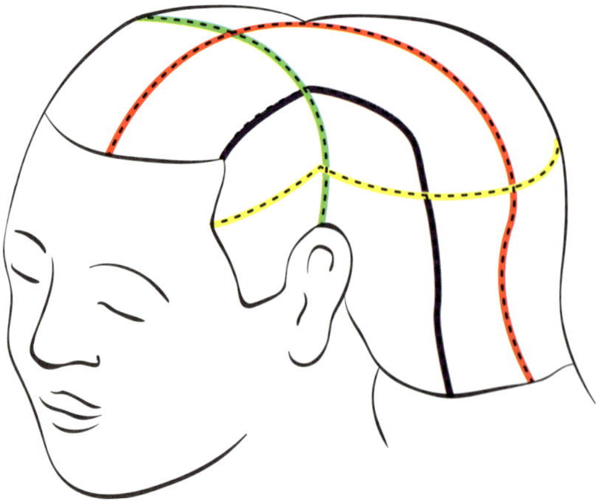

Figure 2.26 Four fixed parameters that allow an evaluation of the extent of the bald and hairy surfaces: median sagittal distance (red); left and right paramedian sagittal distances (blue); transverse subauricular distance (green); anterior intertemporal distance (yellow).

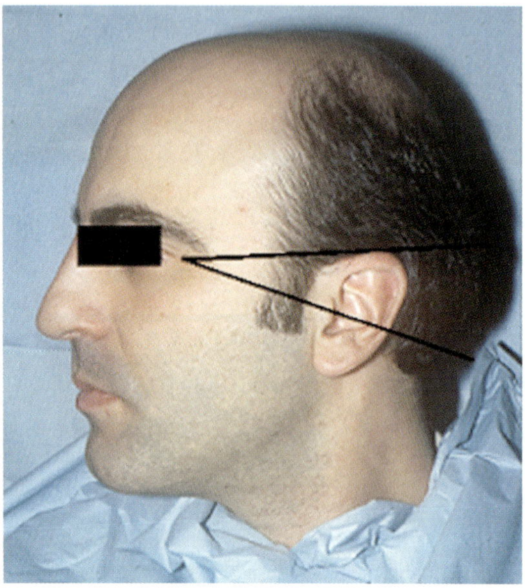

Figure 2.27 Prospective evaluation of a maximum male baldness evolution through the drawing of two axes. (From Bouhanna P. *Dermatol Surg*, 2000;26:555–561. With permission.)

(such as peripilar fibrosis, follicular transformations, lichenoid infiltration, hair atrophy, etc.).

In males, a biopsy is hepful when the pattern is diffuse or resembles female AGA or when there are changes suggestive of cicatricial alopecia.

In females, a biopsy may be helpful when trying to exclude cicatricial alopecia, diffuse alopecia areata (cf chapter on cicatricial alopecia), and telogen effluvium (see Chapter 8).

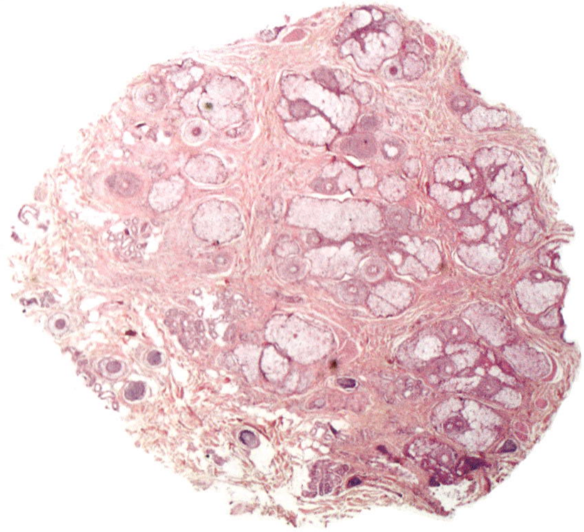

Figure 2.28 Histological section observed under an optical microscope. (Courtesy of Dr. B. Cavelier.)

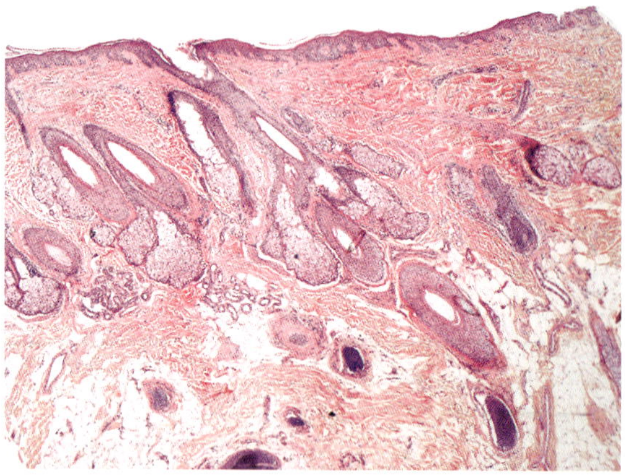

Figure 2.29 Histological vertical section observed under an optical microscope. (Courtesy of Dr. B. Cavelier.)

The diagnostic specimens of choice are paired 4-mm punch biopsies from both involved (e.g., vertex or frontal) and uninvolved (usually occipital) regions of the scalp. A comparison of follicular size and number in two specimens will allow for a definitive diagnosis.

The study of horizontal (Figure 2.28) and vertical (Figure 2.29) sections of scalp allows the assessment of all follicles at several levels of the scalp.[18–20]

A biopsy will reveal a mix of hairs with various bulb depths and shaft diameters. Terminal follicles produce a hair shaft greater than 0.06 mm in diameter and thicker than the follicle's inner root sheath. Besides the

Table 2.4 Normal Scalp Horizontal Section (4-mm punch = 12.56 mm²)

	Caucasian	Afro-Caribbean	Asian
Follicular unit	12–14 (*Headington*) 8 (*Jimenez*)	8–10	5–9
Hair follicles	20–30	20	13–20

Notes: Normal microanatomy of a horizontal cut with punch 4 mm (12.56 mm 2): Each follicular unit contains 2–4 follicles, sebaceous glands, and pilosebaceous arrector muscle attached to each follicle.[18,21,22] One follicular unit/mm². Shaft diameter: vellus <0.03 mm; intermediate: 0.03–0.06 mm; terminal 0.06–0.08 mm.

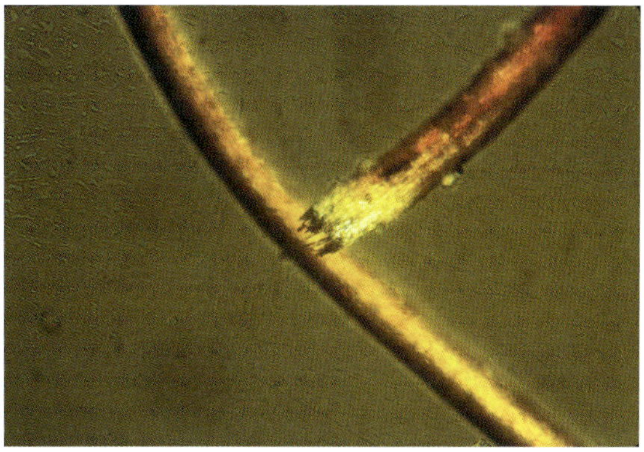

Figure 2.31 **Examination of the hair shaft under polarized light microscopy showing the split distal end of the peladic hair.**

narrowing of the shaft diameter and the diminished time spent lengthening, the hair becomes progressively less pigmented, appearing nearly invisible.

Histologically, follicular miniaturization can be identified by follicular bulbs present in the mid-to-deep dermis and shafts narrower than 0.06 mm. Hair shafts less than the 0.06-mm diameter of terminal hairs, but greater than the 0.03-mm diameter of vellus hairs are termed *intermediate* hairs (Table 2.4).

- *Microscopic examination of the hair shaft in polarized light*: This technique observes the hair shaft using a polarized light, turning the incident light into red, yellow, and blue monochromatic beams to give a three-dimensional image (Figure 2.30). Study of the hair shaft in polarized light is essential in the diagnosis of hair dysplasia. With examination of the distal end of the hair shaft, one can detect split hairs (trichoptilosis) in trichorrhexis nodosa (Figure 2.31) (see Chapter 4).
- *Mycological examination*: Direct examination is most commonly used to identify the offending organism with a drop of potassium hydroxide (10%–30%), cultured on Sabouraud medium (Figure 2.32). Examination with a Wood lamp is used primarily for the diagnosis of ringworm due to the characteristic fluorescence produced by the ultraviolet (UV) light on hair infected by some dermatophytes.
- *Scanning electron microscopy*: Usually electron microscopy is not necessary in clinical practice. However, it is indicated in certain abnormalities of the hair shaft, which can go undetected in optical light. Scanning electron microscopy provides three-dimensional images of the hair so that its shape and surface can be studied. This technique is very useful to confirm the diagnosis of pilar dysplasia (monilethrix, trichorrhexis nodosa, invaginated trichorrhexis, and trichonodosis), congenital hair loss syndromes, ectodermal dysplasia, and adverse reactions to cosmetic agents.

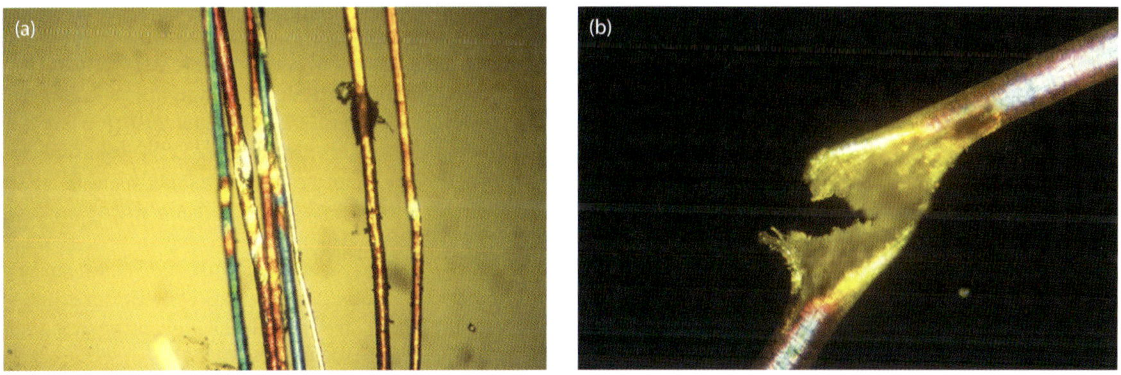

Figure 2.30 **Examination of the hair shaft under polarized light microscopy: (a) normal hair stems and (b) broken hair shaft.**

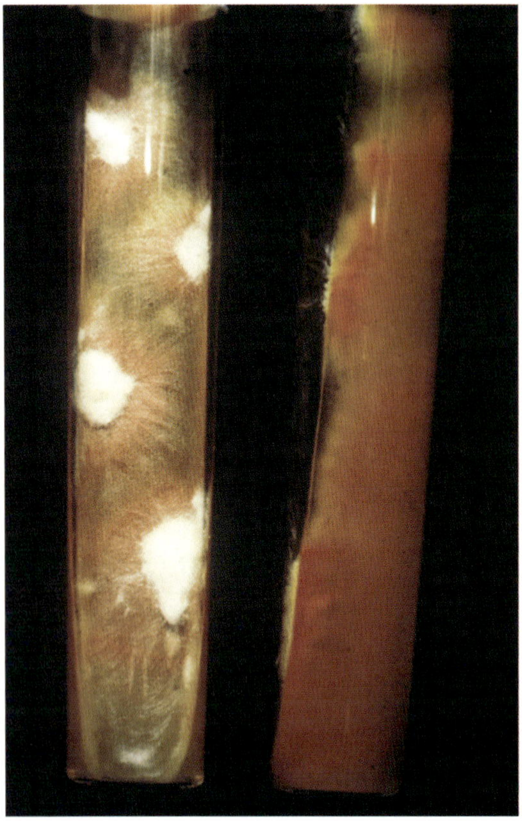

Figure 2.32 **Mycological examination by culture on Sabouraud medium.**

CONCLUSION

Hair loss is an intense psychological development generating several consultations with the hair and scalp specialist. A good clinical history, a thorough clinical examination of the scalp, and the use of different methods of exploration of the hair and scalp make it possible to establish the precise diagnosis of hair loss and eliminate the underlying causes. These different methods of testing will allow the scalp specialist to establish a medical or surgical treatment for every case of hair loss. In addition, they can be used to assess the effectiveness of medical or surgical treatment of the hair loss and the baldness.

REFERENCES

1. Blume-Peytavi U. *Hair Growth and Disorders: With 85 Tables*. Berlin Heidelberg: Springer; 2008.
2. Bouhanna P, Reygagne P. *Pathologie du cheveu et du cuir chevelu*. Paris: Masson; 1999.
3. Bouhanna P. *Les alopécies—de la clinique au traitement. Collection Guide Pratique de Dermatologie*. Paris: MED'COM; 2004.
4. Camacho F, Tosti A. *Montagna tricologia. Enfermedades del foliculo pilosebaceo*. 3rd edn. Madrid, Spain: Aula medica; 2013.
5. Bouhanna P. Les différentes méthodes d'appréciation objective d'une chute de cheveux et d'une alopécie. *Praxis*. 1997;86:1000–1003.
6. Assouly P. Dermatoscopie des cheveux et du cuir chevelu. *Ann Dermatol Venereol*. 2012;139:652–667.
7. Van Scott EJ, Reinerton RP, Steinmuller R. The growing hair roots of the human scalp and morphologic changes therein following amethopterin therapy. *J Invest Dermatol*. 1957;29:197–204.
8. Tosti A. *Dermoscopy of Hair and Scalp Disorders*. London: Informa Healthcare; 2007.
9. Rudnicka L, Olszewska M, Rakowska A et al. Trichoscopy: A new method for diagnosing hair loss. *J Drugs Dermatol*. 2008;7:651–654.
10. Bourezane Y. *Atlas pratique de tichoscopie*. Paris: Med'Com; 2014.
11. Tosti A, Torres F, Misciali C et al. Follicular red dots: A novel dermoscopic pattern observed in scalp discoid lupus erythematosus. *Arch Dermatol*. 2009;145: 1406–1409.
12. Inui S. Trichoscopy for common hair loss diseases: Algorithmic method for diagnosis. *J Dermatol*. 2011; 38:71–75.
13. Bouhanna P. The phototrichogram and a macrophotographic study of the scalp. *Bioeng Skin*. 1985; 1(3):265.
14. Bouhanna P. The phototrichogram: An objective technique used in hair replacement surgery evaluation. In: Unger WP, ed. *Hair Transplantation*. 3rd edn. rev, exp. New York, NY: Marcel Dekker Inc; 1995:2, 61–68.
15. Hoffmann R. Trichoscan: Results using 5% minoxidil in women with androgenetic alopecia. In: Van Neste D, ed. *Hair Science and Technology*; 2003: 331–341.
16. Bouhanna P. Le tractiophototrichogramme, méthode d'appréciation objective d'une chute de cheveux. *Ann Dermatol Vénéréol*. 1988;115:759–764.
17. Bouhanna P. Multifactorial classification of male and female androgenetic alopecia. *Dermatol Surg*. 2000;26:555–561.
18. Headington JT. Transverse microscopic anatomy of the human scalp. A basis for a morphometric approach to disorders of the hair follicle. *Arch. Dermatol*. 1984;120:449–456.
19. Garcia C, Poletti E. Scalp biopsy specimens: Transverse vs vertical sections. *Arch Dermatol*. 2007;143:268.
20. Whiting DA. Diagnostic and predictive value of horizontal sections of scalp biopsy specimens in male pattern androgenetic alopecia. *J Am Acad Dermatol*. 1993;28:755–763.
21. Jimenez F, Ruifernandez J. Distribution of human hair in follicular units. A mathematical model for estimating the donor size in follicular unit transplantation. *Dermatol Surg*. 1999;25(4):294–298.
22. Cavelier-Balloy B, Assouly P. Apport et limites de la biopsie cutanée dans le diagnostic des alopécies. *Ann Dermatol Venereol*. 2009;136:182–198.

3 Trichoscopy

Lidia Rudnicka

INTRODUCTION

Trichoscopy is dermoscopy of hair and scalp. The method is used for differential diagnosis of hair and scalp diseases but may be also applied for evaluation of other body hair.[1] Trichoscopy may be performed with a handheld dermoscope or a digital videodermoscopy system.[2] The technique is based on analysis of structures, which may be visualized with a dermoscope. These basic structures may be divided into four major groups: (1) hair shafts, (2) hair follicle openings (dots), (3) perifollicular epidermis, and (4) blood vessels.[3]

HAIR SHAFTS

A classification of hair shaft abnormalities, which may be visualized by trichoscopy, distinguishes the following groups of hair shaft abnormalities: (1) hair shafts with fractures, (2) hair narrowings, (3) hairs with node-like structures, (4) curls and twists, (5) bands, and (4) short hairs.[4]

HAIR FOLLICLE OPENINGS (DOTS)

"Dots" is a common trichoscopy term for hair follicle openings.[5] Black dots represent pigmented hairs broken or destroyed at scalp level.[5] Yellow dots are hair follicle openings that contain keratosebaceous material.[5,6] There are two types of white dots: the fibrotic white dots and the pinpoint white dots. The fibrotic white dots represent areas of perifollicular fibrosis and are observed most commonly in lichen planopilaris.[3,7] Pinpoint white dots correspond to hair follicle openings and eccrine gland openings, observed within pigmented background. They are present in patients with dark skin phototypes, regardless of hair loss.[8,9] Red dots were described in discoid lupus erythematosus and are considered a good prognostic finding, indicating possible hair regrowth.[10] It has also been shown that empty hair follicles may appear as red dots in patients with pigmentary disorders such as vitiligo.[11] Regularly distributed gray or brown-gray dots are a characteristic finding in the eyebrow area of patients with frontal fibrosing alopecia.[12]

PERIFOLLICULAR EPIDERMIS

Abnormalities of scalp skin color or structure that may be visualized by trichoscopy include scaling, changes in color, abnormalities in skin surface structure, and the presence of discharge. A classification of these abnormalities has been established recently.[13] Briefly, this classification is based on observation of scaling (diffuse or perifollicular), the color of the evaluated scalp area (brown, white, pink, yellow, red, and violaceous-blue) and discharge (yellow, white, or red), and skin surface structure abnormalities.[13]

BLOOD VESSELS

The appearance of cutaneous microvessels in trichoscopy may vary in type, arrangement, and number depending on disease. Analysis of blood vessel arrangement is of special importance in differential diagnosis of inflammatory scalp diseases such as scalp psoriasis, seborrheic dermatitis, or discoid lupus erythematosus.[2,12] Some authors indicate that the arrangement of blood vessels in trichoscopy may be indicative of systemic diseases, such as systemic lupus erythematosus, systemic sclerosis, or cutaneous T-cell lymphoma.[10]

TELOGEN EFFLUVIUM

Trichoscopy findings in telogen effluvium (Figure 3.1) include the presence of empty hair follicles, predominance of follicular units with only one hair, perifollicular discoloration (peripilar sign), and upright regrowing hairs. Trichoscopy results do not differ depending on the factor that induced telogen hair loss.[10]

ANDROGENETIC ALOPECIA

Male androgenetic alopecia and female androgenetic alopecia (Figure 3.2) share similar trichoscopy features.

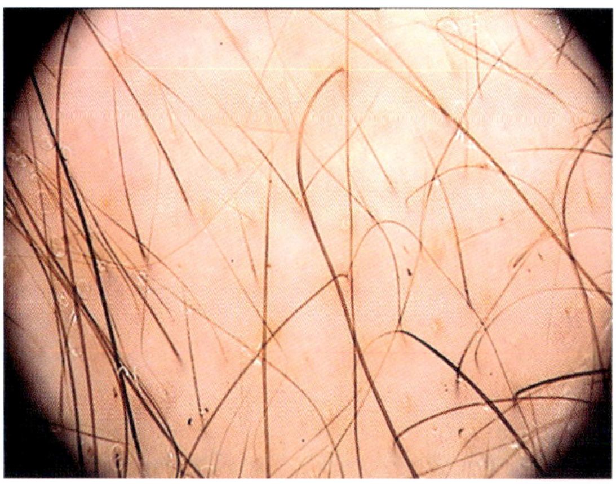

Figure 3.1 **Telogen effluvium. Multiple short regrowing hairs indicate a regrowth phase of telogen effluvium.**

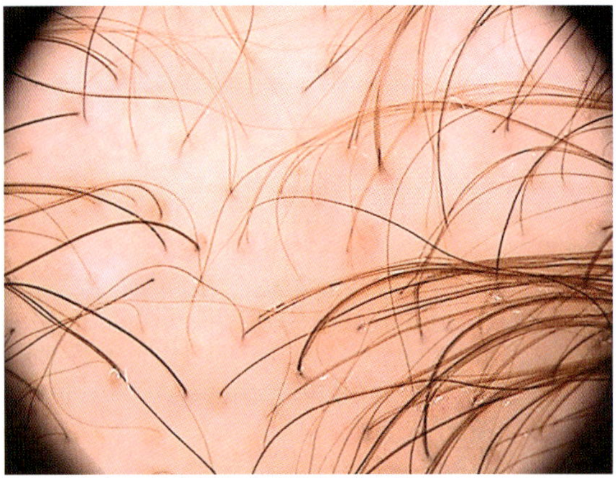

Figure 3.2 **Female androgenetic alopecia. Concomitant presence of thick, intermediate, and thin hair shafts is called hair shaft thickness heterogeneity. This is a trichoscopy manifestation of nonsimultaneous hair miniaturization.**

Hair shaft thickness heterogeneity, with simultaneous presence of thin, intermediate, and thick hairs, is the most characteristic feature of androgenetic alopecia. It has been shown that hair diameter diversity reflects follicle miniaturization in androgenetic alopecia.[14,15] Precise evaluation of hair shaft thickness in micrometers is not essential for clinical diagnosis but may be useful for monitoring treatment efficacy[16] and is indispensable for clinical trials.[10] Another trichoscopy feature of androgenetic alopecia is increased proportion of vellus hairs. The number of hairs in one follicular unit is decreased in androgenetic alopecia. Follicular units with only one hair predominate in these patients, especially in the frontal area.[17–19] The presence of yellow dots is a constant finding in androgenetic alopecia. These yellow dots mark mainly empty hair follicles with sebum.[17] These sebaceous yellow dots may be washed away by a vigorous hair wash. Thus, patients should not wash their hair directly preceding a trichoscopy examination. Brown perifollicular discoloration (peripilar sign)[20] is observed in 20%–66% of patients with androgenetic alopecia.[15,17] A proportion of about 30% of hair follicle openings is usually affected.[15,17]

Trichoscopy of senescent (senile, involutionary) alopecia shares with androgenetic alopecia a predominance of follicular units with only one hair, decreased hair shaft density with a honeycomb pattern pigmentation, and slight tendency to form brown perifollicular discoloration (peripilar sign).[12]

ALOPECIA AREATA

The most common trichoscopy features of alopecia areata (Figure 3.3) are regularly distributed yellow dots, exclamation mark hairs, tapered hairs, and black dots. Trichoscopy

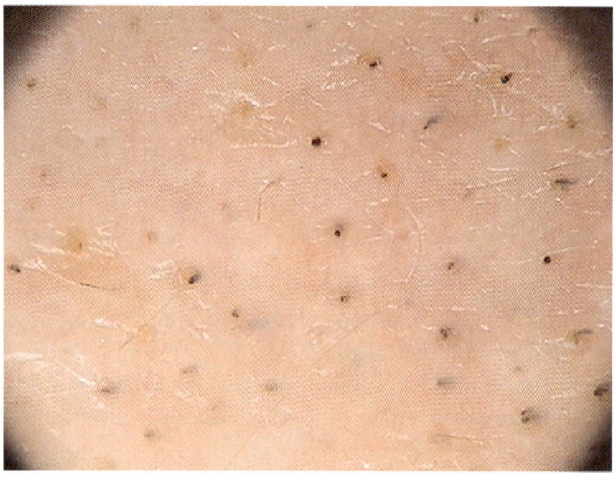

Figure 3.3 **Alopecia areata. Concomitant presence of regularly distributed yellow dots and black dots. The black dots reflect an active phase of disease.**

of alopecia areata may differ depending on disease activity, severity, and duration.[21] Lacarrubba et al.[6] identified three features of acute alopecia areata: micro-exclamation marks, black dots, and vellus hairs. Inui et al.[22] identified similar markers of disease activity (black dots, tapering hairs, and broken hairs) in another study. The experience of my team[3,23] shows that black dots and exclamation mark hairs are a constant marker of disease activity in alopecia areata.

Pohl-Pinkus constrictions and monilethrix-like hairs are observed in less than 5% of patients with alopecia areata.[24,25]

TRICHOTILLOMANIA

Trichotillomania (Figure 3.4) is a common and difficult differential diagnosis of alopecia areata.[26] Trichoscopy of

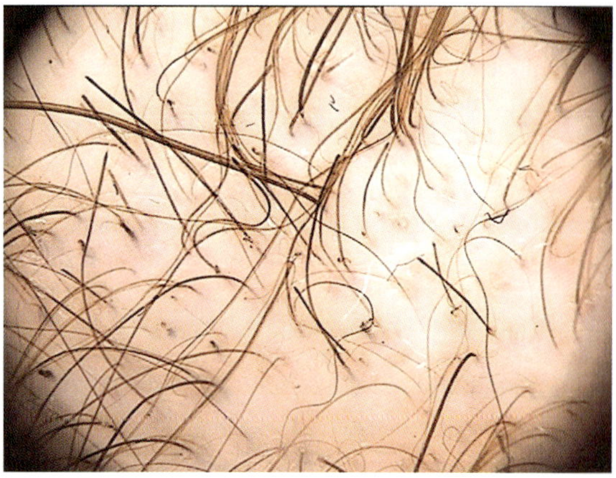

Figure 3.4 **Trichotillomania. The simultaneous presence of multiple hairs broken at different lengths (in the absence of exclamation mark hairs) may be indicative of trichotillomania.**

trichotillomania shows hairs broken at different lengths. Irregular coiled hairs[5] and flame hairs[23] are the most characteristic trichoscopy findings in trichotillomania. Other findings include short hairs with trichoptilosis ("split ends"), upright regrowing hairs, black dots, and the v-sign.[12,23,26–28] High-power trichoscopy (performed with a digital videodermoscope) may reveal the presence of hair residue particles, called "hair powder."[23] Exclamation mark hairs are rare in trichotillomania, but they may be a diagnostic pitfall and cause misdiagnosis of alopecia areata.[2,23]

TINEA CAPITIS

Slowinska et al. described comma hairs[29] as a characteristic feature of tinea capitis (Figure 3.5). Later, Hughes et al. identified corkscrew hairs[30] as another characteristic finding in patches of tinea capitis. Recent findings show also zigzag hairs and interrupted (Morse code–like) hairs are observed in these patients.[2,3] Ultraviolet (UV)-enhanced trichoscopy (UVET) (Figure 3.6), which is a combination of trichoscopy and Wood's light, may further aid in screening patients for tinea capitis.[3]

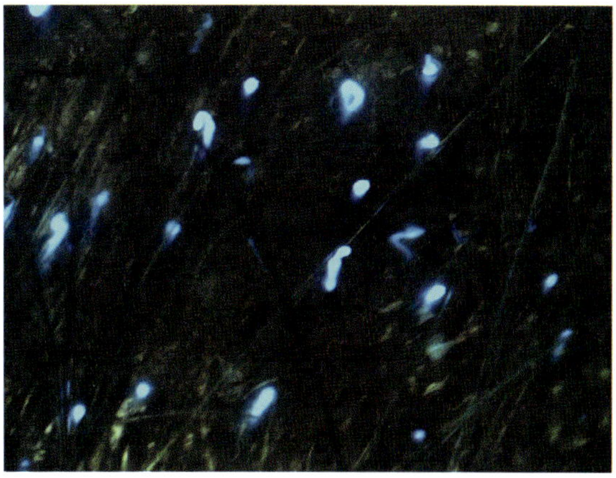

Figure 3.6 **UVET (UV-enhanced trichoscopy) is a combination of trichoscopy with Wood's light. The image shows fluorescence of multiple comma hairs infected with *Microsporum canis*.**

DISCOID LUPUS ERYTHEMATOSUS

The most characteristic trichoscopy features of discoid lupus erythematosus (Figure 3.7) localized on the scalp are thick arborizing vessels and large yellow dots.[2,25,31] Scattered brown discoloration of the skin may be observed in some patients.[2,25,31] Yellow dots with radial, thin arborizing vessels emerging from the dot are considered characteristic for discoid lupus erythematosus. This feature is sometimes referred to as "red spider in yellow dot."[32] Red dots, described by Tosti et al.,[10] are considered a good prognostic factor for hair regrowth. Long-lasting, inactive lesions with prominent fibrosis show structureless milky-red areas and lack of follicular openings in trichoscopy.[7]

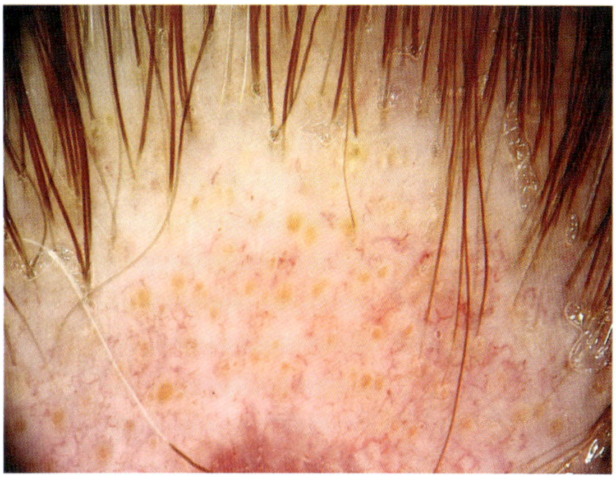

Figure 3.7 **Discoid lupus erythematosus. Trichoscopy shows arborizing vessels, large (keratotic) yellow dots at the hair-bearing margin of a scalp lesion.**

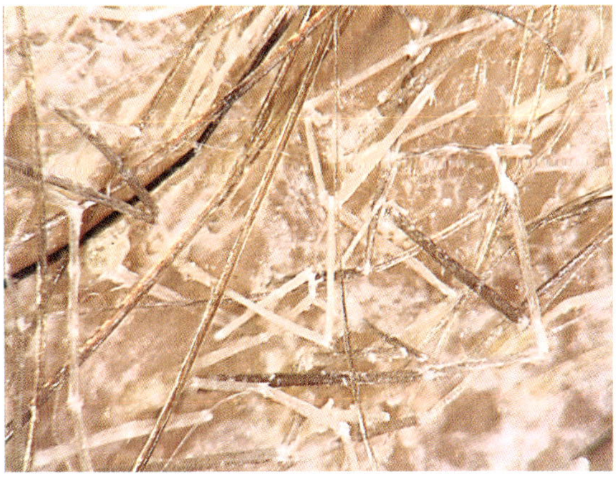

Figure 3.5 **Tinea capitis. The image shows multiple zigzag hairs in a patient with *Microsporum canis*–induced alopecia.**

LICHEN PLANOPILARIS AND FRONTAL FIBROSING ALOPECIA

The most characteristic trichoscopy feature of classic lichen planopilaris (Figure 3.8) is white perifollicular scaling with scales entangling hair shafts up to 2–3 mm above scalp surface. My team called this phenomenon "tubular scaling."[7] Other findings include perifollicular inflammation, elongated blood vessels, and violaceous-blue interfollicular areas.[7,33,34] In the late fibrotic stage of lichen planopilaris, the predominating features are fibrotic white dots, which merge into white and/or milky-red areas.[2,7]

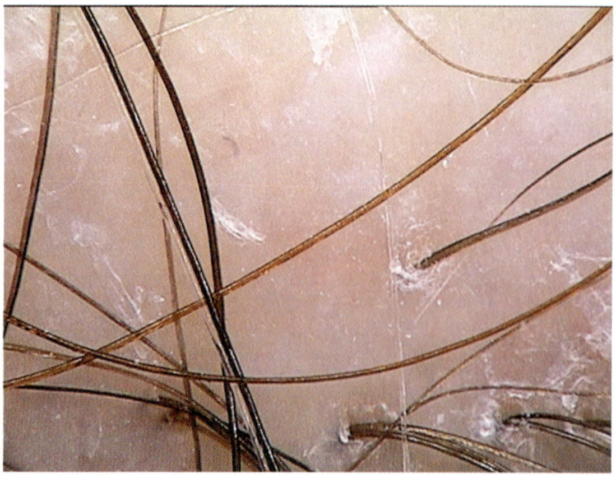

Figure 3.8 **Lichen planopilaris. Perifollicular scaling and a milky-red (strawberry ice cream color) area lacking follicular openings.**

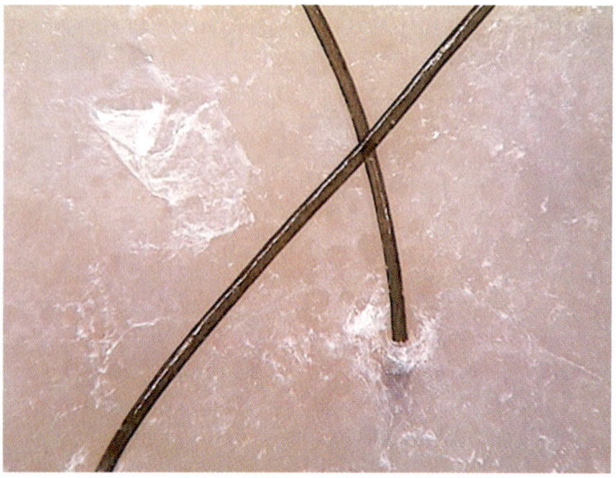

Figure 3.9 **Frontal fibrosing alopecia. A lonely hair surrounded by a fibrotic area.**

Trichoscopy findings in active frontal fibrosing alopecia (Figure 3.9) are similar but significantly less prominent. These features include minor perifollicular scaling and predominance of follicular openings with only one hair. The dark, terminal, "lonely hairs" surrounded by ivory-colored fibrotic areas may be seen both clinically as well as trichoscopically.[35]

DISSECTING CELLULITIS

In dissecting cellulitis (Figure 3.10) (dissecting folliculitis, perifolliculitis capitis abscedens et suffodiens), trichoscopy shows yellow, structureless areas. Characteristic trichoscopy findings include yellow "3D" dots imposed over dark hair shaft residues, pinpoint-like vessels with whitish halo, and confluent ivory-white areas lacking follicular openings in end-stage disease with prominent fibrosis.

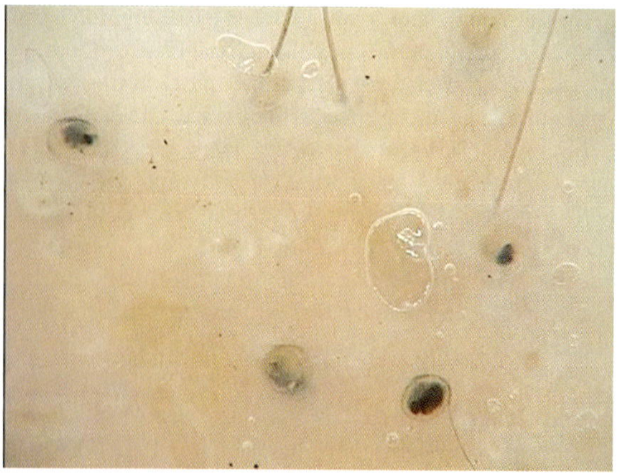

Figure 3.10 **Dissecting cellulitis. 3D yellow dots superimposed over black hair residues.**

FOLLICULITIS DECALVANS

Folliculitis decalvans (Figure 3.11) is characterized by the presence of multiple hairs in one follicular unit.[36] These follicular tufts usually consist of 5–20 hairs.[36] This feature may be observed both clinically and by trichoscopy. Additional trichoscopy findings include follicular pustules, perifollicular tubular scaling, and hyperplasia arranged in a starburst pattern.[37] The scales that entangle hair shafts in a tubular manner are characterized by a yellowish color and a tendency to fold away from the hair shafts in a collar-like fashion.[2] In end-stage fibrotic lesions, white or milky-red (strawberry ice cream color) areas lacking follicular openings predominate.[7]

GENETIC HAIR SHAFT ABNORMALITIES

Trichoscopy is a perfect tool for noninvasive evaluation of most genetic hair shaft abnormalities.[1,38,39] It has been

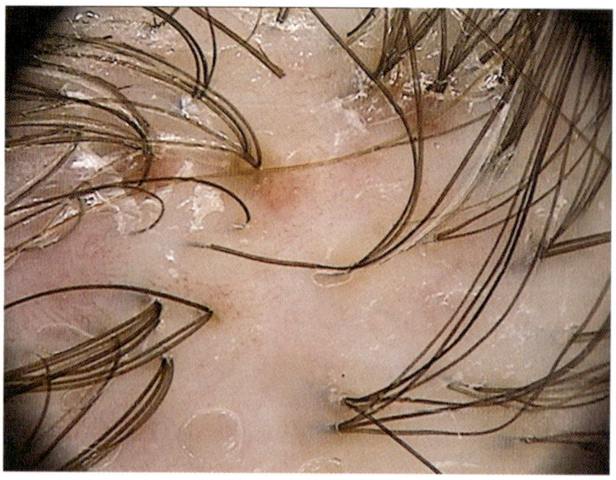

Figure 3.11 **Folliculitis decalvans. Hair tufts emerging from inflammatory areas. The milky-red area in the mid-part of the image indicates fibrosis of recent onset.**

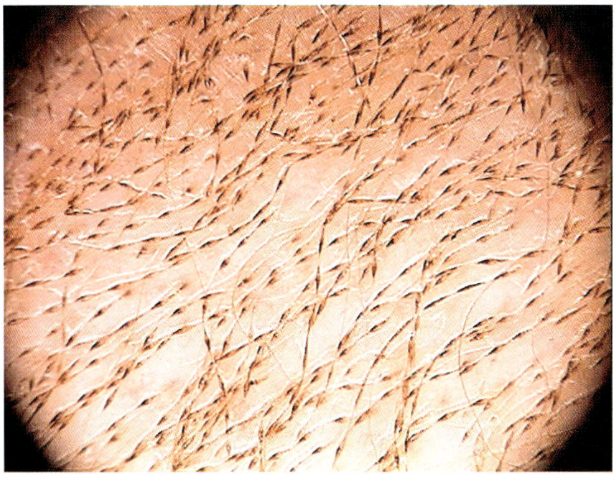

Figure 3.12 **Monilethrix. Trichoscopy easily replaces light microscopy in examination of hair shafts for genetic structure abnormalities.**

documented that trichoscopy allows for the detection of characteristic structural abnormalities of monilethrix,[40–44] (Figure 3.12) trichorrhexis invaginata,[43,45,46] trichorrhexis nodosa,[43] pili torti,[43] and pili annulati[43] without the need to pull hairs for light microscopy examination.[47]

APPLICATION OF TRICHOSCOPY IN CLINICAL TRIALS, RESEARCH, AND MONITORING TREATMENT EFFICACY

Trichoscopy is a precise, excellent tool for monitoring treatment efficacy in everyday practice and in clinical trials. This method allows quantitative evaluation of hair shaft thickness, number of hairs per follicular unit, number of empty hair follicles, and multiple other parameters. For the purpose of research and clinical trials, the examination should be performed in a standardized manner.[2,18]

REFERENCES

1. Rudnicka L, Olszewska M, Rakowska A, Kowalska-Oledzka E, Slowinska M. Trichoscopy: A new method for diagnosing hair loss. *J Drugs Dermatol.* 2008;7:651–654.
2. Atlas of trichoscopy. *Dermoscopy in Hair and Scalp Disease.* New York, NY: Springer; 2012.
3. Rudnicka L, Olszewska M, Rakowska A, Slowinska M. Trichoscopy update 2011. *J Dermatol Case Rep.* 2011;5:82–88.
4. Rudnicka L, Rakowska A, Kerzeja M, Olszewska M. Hair shafts in trichoscopy: Clues for diagnosis of hair and scalp diseases. *Dermatol Clin.* 2013;31:695–708.
5. Ross EK, Vincenzi C, Tosti A. Videodermoscopy in the evaluation of hair and scalp disorders. *J Am Acad Dermatol.* 2006;55:799–806.
6. Lacarrubba F, Dall'Oglio F, Rita Nasca M, Micali G. Videodermatoscopy enhances diagnostic capability in some forms of hair loss. *Am J Clin Dermatol.* 2004; 5:205–208.
7. Rakowska A, Slowinska M, Kowalska-Oledzka E et al. Trichoscopy of cicatricial alopecia. *J Drugs Dermatol.* 2012;11:753–758.
8. de Moura LH, Duque-Estrada B, Abraham LS, Barcaui CB, Sodre CT. Dermoscopy findings of alopecia areata in an African-American patient. *J Dermatol Case Rep.* 2008;2:52–54.
9. Abraham LS, Pineiro-Maceira J, Duque-Estrada B, Barcaui CB, Sodre CT. Pinpoint white dots in the scalp: Dermoscopic and histopathologic correlation. *J Am Acad Dermatol.* 2010;63:721–722.
10. Tosti A, Torres F, Misciali C et al. Follicular red dots: A novel dermoscopic pattern observed in scalp discoid lupus erythematosus. *Arch Dermatol.* 2009;145:1406–1409.
11. Pirmez R, Pineiro-Maceira J, Almeida BC, Sodre CT. Follicular red dots: A normal trichoscopy feature in patients with pigmentary disorders? *An Bras Dermatol.* 2013;88(3):459–461.
12. Rudnicka L OM, Rakowska A, eds. *Trichoscopy: Dermoscopy of Hair and Scalp.* Berlin, Germany: Springer-Verlag; 2012.
13. Rudnicka L, Rakowska A, Olszewska M. Trichoscopy: How it may help the clinician. *Dermatol Clin.* 2013;31:29–41.
14. de Lacharriere O, Deloche C, Misciali C et al. Hair diameter diversity: A clinical sign reflecting the follicle miniaturization. *Arch Dermatol.* 2001;137:641–646.
15. Inui S, Nakajima T, Itami S. Scalp dermoscopy of androgenetic alopecia in Asian people. *J Dermatol.* 2009;36:82–85.
16. Olszewska M, Rudnicka L. Effective treatment of female androgenic alopecia with dutasteride. *J Drugs Dermatol.* 2005;4:637–640.
17. Rakowska A, Slowinska M, Kowalska-Oledzka E, Olszewska M, Rudnicka L. Dermoscopy in female androgenic alopecia: Method standardization and diagnostic criteria. *Int J Trichology.* 2009;1:123–130.
18. Rakowska A. Trichoscopy (hair and scalp videodermoscopy) in the healthy female. Method standardization and norms for measurable parameters. *J Dermatol Case Rep.* 2009;3:14–19.
19. Slowinska M. *The Value of Videodermoscopy in Differential Diagnosis of Androgenetic Alopecia* [doctoral thesis]. Medical University of Warsaw, Poland.
20. Deloche C, de Lacharriere O, Misciali C et al. Histological features of peripilar signs associated with androgenetic alopecia. *Arch Dermatol Res.* 2004;295:422–428.
21. Karadağ Köse Ö, Güleç AT. Clinical evaluation of alopecias using a handheld dermatoscope. *J Am Acad Dermatol.* 2012 Aug;67(2):206–214.
22. Inui S, Nakajima T, Nakagawa K, Itami S. Clinical significance of dermoscopy in alopecia areata: Analysis of 300 cases. *Int J Dermatol.* 2008;47:688–693.

23. Rakowska A, Slowinska, M, Olszewska, M, Rudnicka, L. New trichoscopy findings in trichotillomania: Flame hairs, v-sign, hook hairs, hair powder, tulip hairs. *Acta Derm Venereol.* 2013;94:303–306.
24. Mane M, Nath AK, Thappa DM. Utility of dermoscopy in alopecia areata. *Indian J Dermatol.* 2011;56:407–411.
25. Rudnicka L, Olszewska, M, Rakowska, A. Hair shafts in trichoscopy. Clues for diagnosis of hair and scalp diseases. *Dermatol Clin.* 2013;31(4):695–708.
26. Abraham LS, Torres FN, Azulay-Abulafia L. Dermoscopic clues to distinguish trichotillomania from patchy alopecia areata. *An Bras Dermatol.* 2010;85:723–726.
27. Gallouj S, Rabhi S, Baybay H et al. Trichotemnomania associated to trichotillomania: A case report with emphasis on the diagnostic value of dermoscopy. *Ann Dermatol Venereol.* 2011;138:140–141.
28. Lee DY, Lee JH, Yang JM, Lee ES. The use of dermoscopy for the diagnosis of trichotillomania. *J Eur Acad Dermatol Venereol.* 2009;23:731–732.
29. Slowinska M, Rudnicka L, Schwartz RA, et al. Comma hairs: A dermatoscopic marker for tinea capitis: A rapid diagnostic method. *J Am Acad Dermatol.* 2008;59:S77–S79.
30. Hughes R, Chiaverini C, Bahadoran P, Lacour JP. Corkscrew hair: A new dermoscopic sign for diagnosis of tinea capitis in black children. *Arch Dermatol.* 2011;147:355–356.
31. Lanuti E, Miteva M, Romanelli P, Tosti A. Trichoscopy and histopathology of follicular keratotic plugs in scalp discoid lupus erythematosus. *Int J Trichology.* 2012;4:36–38.
32. Rakowska A SM, Kowalska-Oledzka E, Warszawik O, Czuwara J, Olszewska M, Rudnicka L. Trichoscopy of cicatricial alopecia. *J Drugs Dermatol.* 2012;11(6):753–758.
33. Duque-Estrada B, Tamler C, Sodre CT, Barcaui CB, Pereira FB. Dermoscopy patterns of cicatricial alopecia resulting from discoid lupus erythematosus and lichen planopilaris. *An Bras Dermatol.* 2010;85:179–183.
34. Assouly P. Dermatoscopy of hair and scalp. *Ann Dermatol Venereol.* 2012;139:652–667.
35. Tosti A. Lonely hair sign: Not specific for frontal fibrosing alopecia-reply. *Arch Dermatol.* 2012;148:1208–1209.
36. Otberg N, Kang H, Alzolibani AA, Shapiro J. Folliculitis decalvans. *Dermatol Ther.* 2008;21:238–244.
37. Trueb RM. Systematic approach to hair loss in women. *J Dtsch Dermatol Ges.* 2010;8:284–297, 284–298.
38. Olszewska M, Rudnicka L, Rakowska A, Kowalska-Oledzka E, Slowinska M. Trichoscopy. *Arch Dermatol.* 2008;144:1007.
39. Mirmirani P, Huang KP, Price VH. A practical, algorithmic approach to diagnosing hair shaft disorders. *Int J Dermatol.* 2011;50:1–12.
40. Rakowska A, Slowinska M, Czuwara J, Olszewska M, Rudnicka L. Dermoscopy as a tool for rapid diagnosis of monilethrix. *J Drugs Dermatol.* 2007;6:222–224.
41. Liu CI, Hsu CH. Rapid diagnosis of monilethrix using dermoscopy. *Br J Dermatol.* 2008;159:741–743.
42. Jain N, Khopkar U. Monilethrix in pattern distribution in siblings: Diagnosis by trichoscopy. *Int J Trichol.* 2010;2:56–59.
43. Rakowska A, Slowinska M, Kowalska-Oledzka E, Rudnicka L. Trichoscopy in genetic hair shaft abnormalities. *J Dermatol Case Rep.* 2008;2:14–20.
44. Wallace MP, de Berker DA. Hair diagnoses and signs: The use of dermatoscopy. *Clin Exp Dermatol.* 2010;35:41–46.
45. Rakowska A, Kowalska-Oledzka E, Slowinska M, Rosinska D, Rudnicka L. Hair shaft videodermoscopy in netherton syndrome. *Pediatr Dermatol.* 2009;26:320–322.
46. Burk C, Hu S, Lee C, Connelly EA. Netherton syndrome and trichorrhexis invaginata—A novel diagnostic approach. *Pediatr Dermatol.* 2008;25:287–288.
47. Haliasos EC, Kerner M, Jaimes-Lopez N et al. Dermoscopy for the pediatric dermatologist part I: Dermoscopy of pediatric infectious and inflammatory skin lesions and hair disorders. *Pediatr Dermatol.* 2013;30:163–171.

4 Hair dysplasias

Juan Ferrando, L. Alheli Niebla, and Gerardo A. Moreno-Arias

INTRODUCTION

Hair dysplasia means an alteration of the hair shaft. Most cases are congenital, some are hereditary, and others are acquired (e.g., bubble hair). It may involve a localized or generalized defect, but always follows a characteristic morphological pattern.[1,2] The defect may be restricted to the hair or constitute a diagnostic clue for a genodermatosis (e.g., Netherton syndrome and trichothiodystrophy). Classification of hair dysplasias is difficult, but in practical terms we accept the classification as presented in Table 4.1.[3–6] The main clinical and morphological diagnostic characteristics of hair dysplasias are discussed in this chapter.

MONILETHRIX

This is an AD (autosomal dominant) defect of the hair shaft. Hair is short, just a few millimeters long, and beaded. Breaking of the hair shaft occurs as soon as hair goes out of the *ostium*, due to narrowing segments of the shaft. Focal follicular hyperkeratosis and marked hypotrichosis may also be seen. It generally affects some individuals of different generations of the same family. The morphological defect is the periodical narrowing of the hair shaft, which may be seen deep in the hair follicle in biopsy specimens.[4,7,8]

Table 4.1 Classification of Hair Dysplasia

Hair dysplasia with hair fragility:
Monilethrix
Pseudomonilethrix
Pili torti
Menkes syndrome (kinky hair)
Trichorrhexis invaginata (Netherton syndrome)
Trichothiodystrophy
Trichonodosis
Distal trichorrhexis nodosa
Proximal trichorrhexis nodosa
Bubble hair
Loose anagen hair
Hair dysplasia with no or little hair fragility:
Pili annulati
Pseudopili annulati
Diffiuse woolly hair
Woolly hair nevus
Acquired progressive kinking of hair
Diffuse partial *woolly hair*
Acquired partial curly hair
Straight hair nevus
Pili canaliculi

Genetics. Monilethrix is an autosomal dominant hereditary defect caused by mutation of genes *hHb1*, *hHb3*, and *hHb6* localized in chromosome (cr) band 12q13 that encodes diverse trichokeratins. We reported a new family with a change in the nucleotide in heterozygosis of position 154 of exon1 of gen *KRT81* (154G > C). In the DNA sequence, this substitution involves a change of one amino acid in a protein (glycine for arginine in position 52). Interruption of keratin synthesis may be the cause of periodic variation of hair shaft diameter. Autosomal recessive (AR) cases have also been reported and are due to a gene mutation (18q) that encodes desmoglein 4 (*DSG4*), a situation that affects affinity for plakoglobin and alters hair shaft desmosomes.[9–12]

Clinical diagnosis. The clinical picture includes diffuse hypotrichosis and short, fragile, and beaded hairs. Localized (occipital region) or generalized marked follicular hyperkeratosis may also be seen (Figure 4.1).

Optical microscopy. Alternating periodical beading (defect) and knots (normal hair shaft diameter), is characteristic, may also be seen in dermoscopy (Figure 4.2).

Scanning electron microscopy. Microscopic images are similar to those observed in optical microscopy: hair shaft fracture is evidenced in narrowed segments.

Trichoscopy. Dermoscopy is a useful tool in order to see follicular hyperkeratosis in the proximal segment of the hair. The typical image of "pearl necklace" refers to elliptical beading, regularly separated by narrowing segments where hair shaft fracture is usually observed. The hair shaft diameter is normal in the beaded segment of the hair shaft, and medulla is observed, while this is not seen in the narrowed segments. These findings are easily identified by dermoscopy, a simple method for a quick diagnosis (Figure 4.3).[13–14]

Histology. Intrafollicular hair shaft narrowing is observed.

PSEUDOMONILETHRIX

Pseudomonilethrix is a rare AD defect characterized by hair fragility. Localized or diffuse hypotrichosis and fake knots (irregular hair shaft flattening) occur as the result of compulsive and frequent combing of the hair. Follicular

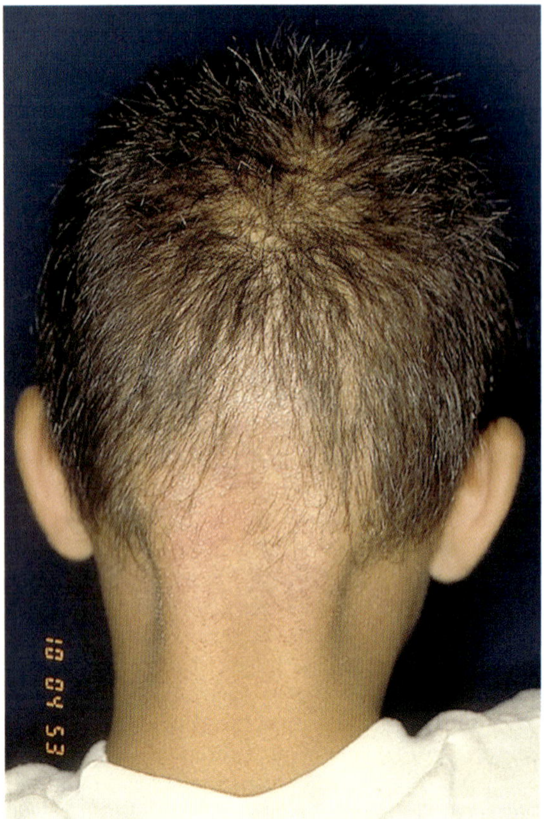

Figure 4.1 **Diffuse hypotrichosis with severe hyperkeratosis follicularis in the occipital region is characteristic.**

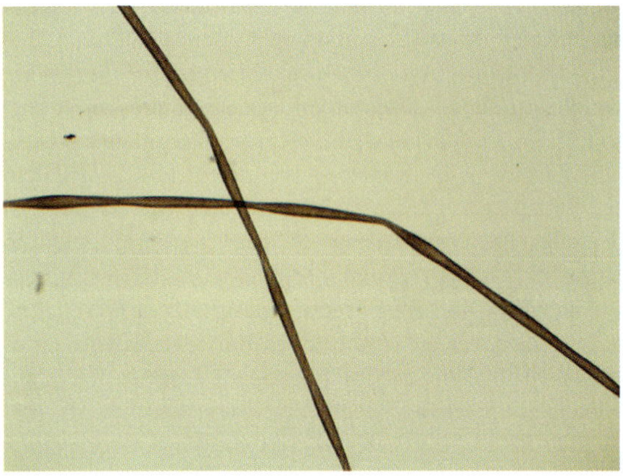

Figure 4.2 **Typical beading with alternating knots and narrowed segments.**

hyperkeratosis is not observed. Individuals of different generations may be affected in the same family.[15,16] It may be associated with *trichorrhexis nodosa* and *bubble hair*.

Genetics. It is an AD defect. Specific genetic alterations have not yet been reported.

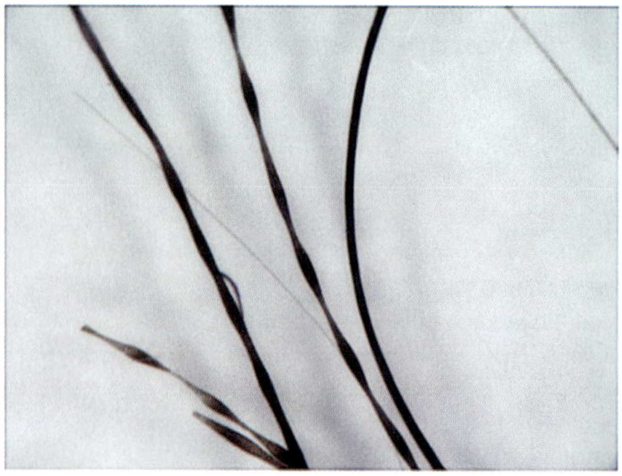

Figure 4.3 **Elliptical beading with narrowed segments are seen on trichoscopy.**

Clinical diagnosis. It is a familiar localized or diffuse hypotrichosis without follicular hyperkeratosis.

Optical microscopy. There are rounded, normal appearing hairs with scarce and irregular oval/round knots. Hair shaft narrowing is not observed (Figure 4.4).

Electron microscopy. "Knots" actually are flat segments of the hair shaft (Figure 4.5).

Trichoscopy. There are irregular oval/round nodules without hair shaft narrowing segments and alternating normal/wider segments of the hair shaft. No follicular hyperkeratosis is observed.

ACQUIRED OR IATROGENIC PSEUDOMONILETHRIX (PSEUDOPSEUDOMONILETHRIX)

This is a similar defect as *pseudomonilethrix* due to improper hair handling. It occurs when excessive pressure is applied to the hair shaft when collecting samples from patients with *monilethrix*, woolly hair, etc.[17–19]

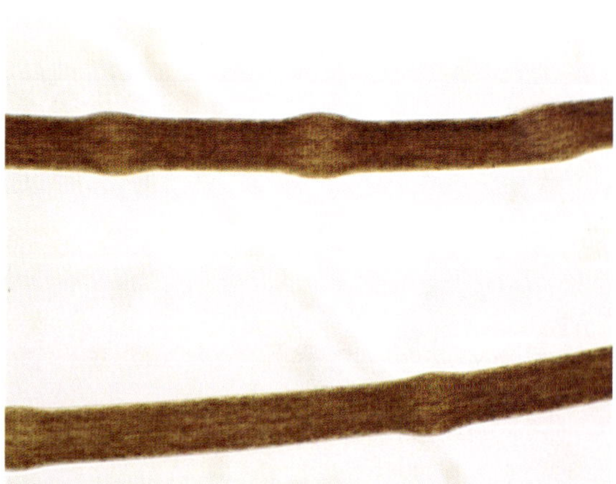

Figure 4.4 **There are round nodules without hair shaft narrowing.**

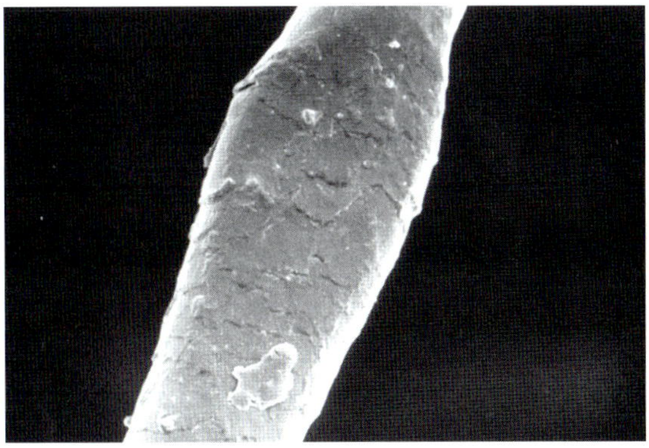

Figure 4.5 **Hair shaft flattening is observed with scanning electron microscopy (SEM).**

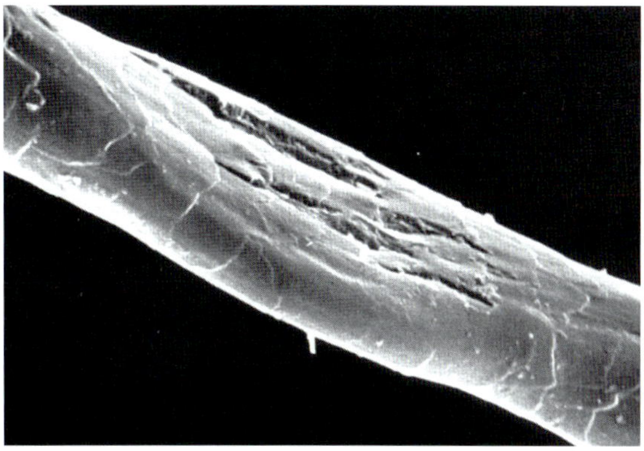

Figure 4.7 **Detail of Figure 4.6 under the SEM.**

(Figure 4.6). The same artifact is seen when the hair shaft is pressed between two slides (Figure 4.7).

Pili torti

This is a braided hair with periodic angles about its longitudinal axis. It is an AD/AR defect that may be found isolated or associated with other diseases such as Beare, Bazex, Crandall, and Björnstad syndromes, and type 2 congenital pachionychia. Atypical *pili torti* has also been observed associated with Menkes' syndrome (kinky hair) or other hair dysplasias such as *pili canaliculi* and woolly hair.[4,20] Hair appears unusually bright due to light reflection, and hypotrichosis may be observed due to an oblique fracture of the hair shaft (*trichoclasis*). Acquired and sporadic types are also recognized.[21,22]

Genetics. Mutation of *BSC1L* (Cr 2q34–36, 2q33) is responsible for the malfunctioning of ATPase that is involved in mitochondrial complex III synthesis, a situation that leads to oxygen reactive species that damage ear and hair follicle sensitive cells.[23] At least this is the case in Björnstad syndrome (AD), in which neurosensorial deafness and *pili torti* are observed.[24–27] More recently this gene has been identified in 2Mb region between *D2S2210* and *D2S2244*.

In those cases associated with type 2 congenital pachionychia, a structural alteration of keratin 17 has been observed.[28] Mutation of the *ST14* gene (Cr 11q24.3-q.25) that encodes a protease (type II transmembrane serine protease matriptase) has been identified in cases of *pili torti* associated with hypotrichosis and ichthyosis.[29] When associated with congenital hypotrichosis and juvenile macular dystrophy mutation has been identified in 16q22.1.[30,31] Other mutations have also been identified in *CDH3*.

Clinical diagnosis. Patients usually have much hair which appears irregularly bright like sequins, depending on incidence of light (Figure 4.8). It may be associated with localized hypotrichosis.

Optical microscopy. Braided hair with regular periodic angles is observed (Figure 4.9).

Electron microscopy. Images are similar to those observed in optical microscopy. Additionally, cuticle defects are found where steep angles occur.

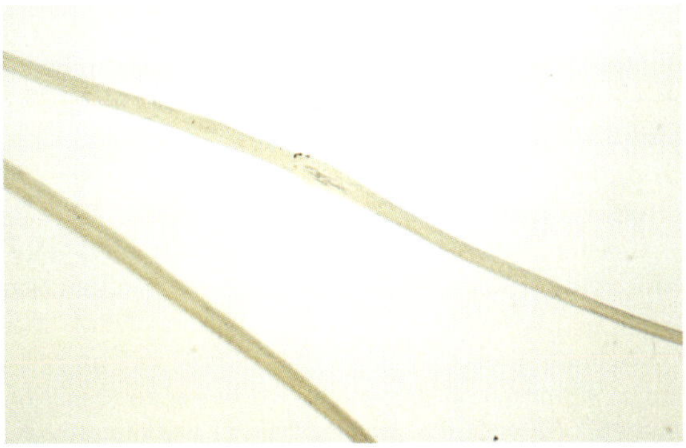

Figure 4.6 **Artifact occurs in dysplastic hair due to excessive pressure when removing it with fingers or forceps/tweezers.**

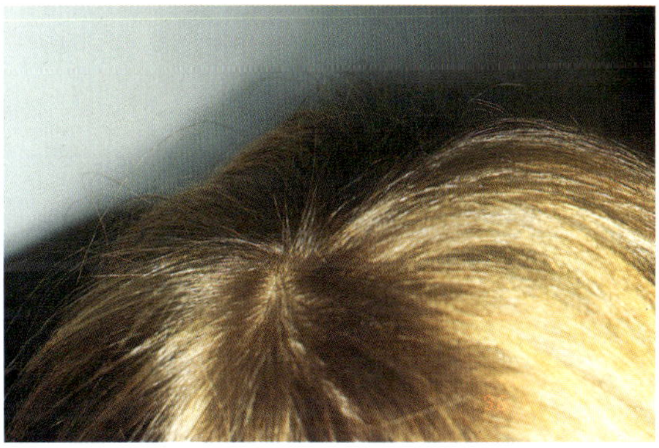

Figure 4.8 **Abundant hairs with variable bright areas appearing like sequins on *pili torti*.**

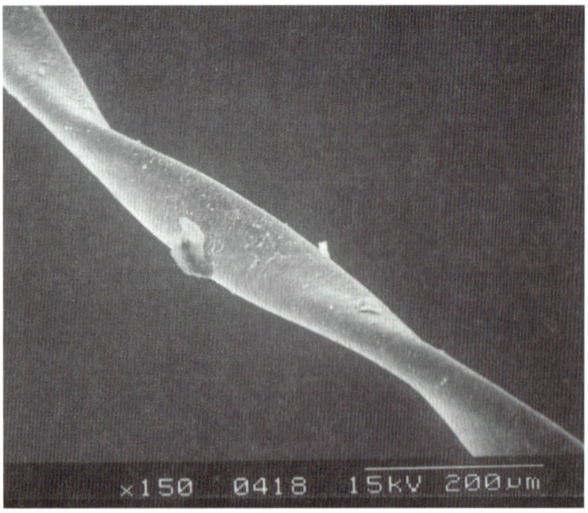

Figure 4.9 **Braided hair with cuticle defects are observed.**

Trichoscopy. A flattened hair shaft with turns at regular intervals is observed. In some cases the defect is restricted only to a segment of the hair shaft.[14] These findings are more easily observed at X70.

Biopsy. The same defect is observed intrafollicularly.

Associated conditions. Pili torti may be associated with nail dystrophy, ocular and teeth defects, follicular hyperkeratosis, and mental retardation.

Menkes, syndrome (kinky hair)

This is a recessive, sex-linked hereditary trait due to an alteration of the intracellular copper use and transfer, a condition that leads to intestinal malabsorption of this metal and consequently to a low level of copper and ceruloplasmin in plasma and organs (brain, liver, bone, elastin, hair, and skin). This syndrome is complex and involves neurological manifestations associated with hypothermia, delay in psychomotor development, limbs palsy, deafness, dwarfism, hernias, etc.[32–34] Affected children have distinctive facial features ("pudgy face," "partridge face"), scarce, fine, brittle, and light hair. Death takes place soon due to neurological complications. We reported a case of a newborn with Menkes syndrome (MS) and transitory neonatal erythroderma.[35]

Genetics. Gene *ATP7A* encodes a transmembrane protein that controls cellular exit of copper. A mutation of this gene is responsible for MS, among other conditions. The gene is located in chromosomes X (Xq21.1), 4, 9 (9q31–q32), 14, and 18 (18.26.0 cM).[36–39]

Clinical diagnosis. Characteristically, it is a newborn with a partridge profile of the face, convulsions, and fine, scarce, brittle, and light hair (Figure 4.10).

Optical microscopy. Kinky or polydysplastic hair displays atypical irregular *pili torti*, monilethrix, and/or trichorrhexis nodosa.

Electron microscopy. Images are similar to those observed under optical microscopy (Figure 4.11). Defects

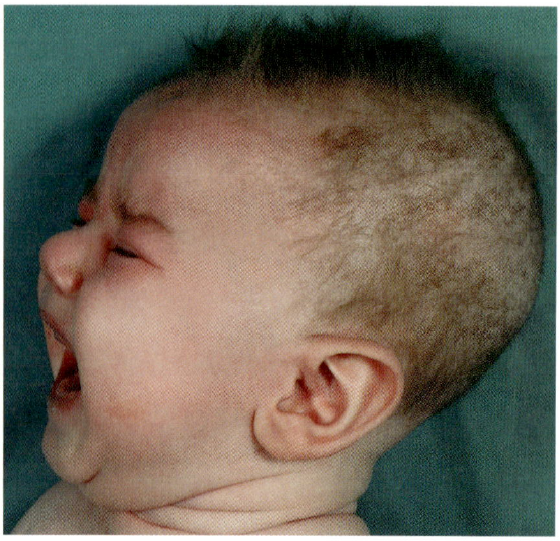

Figure 4.10 **Characteristic partridge face in a child with Menkes' syndrome. (From Galve J et al. *Pediatrics.* 2012;130:239–242. With permission.)**

of the hair cuticle are also observed, especially cuticle cells with saw aspect.

X-ray microanalysis. Low copper and sulfur content has been reported.

Trichoscopy. Hair diameter is variable. Some segments are narrow, while others look irregularly flat and twisted around the hair axis (atypical *pili torti*), a condition that may be like monilethrix. Frequently, irregular or atypical trichorrhexis may be found.

Trichorrhexis invaginata (Netherton disease)

Trichorrhexis invaginata includes both a ballooning distortion of the hair shaft as well as a chaliced deformation of the proximal hair shaft. This characteristic alteration gives the hair shaft a bamboo cane aspect; therefore, this hair dysplasia is also known as "bamboo hair," a specific hair anomaly that is considered a marker for Netherton disease.

Netherton syndrome is an autosomal recessive genodermatosis that is more frequently observed in females and may be associated with *trichorrhexis invaginata*, atopy, *ichthyosis linearis circumflexa*, *erythroderma ichthyosiformis*, and *ichthyosis vulgaris*.[4,40–42]

Genetics. Various gene mutations have been reported: kallikrein 5 (19q13.33)[43] and 7 (19q13.41), corneodesmosin (6p21.3),[44] desmochollin 1 and desmoglein 1 (18q12.1),[45] transglutaminase 1 (14q11.2) and 3 (20q11.2),[46] filaggrin (1q21), serine peptidase inhibitor (chromosomes 5 and 18, 21,5 cM), SPINK5 that encodes LEKTI a serine protease inhibitor (5q.32), and NETS (5q.32).[47,48]

Clinical diagnosis. Characteristically, the affected individual is a female with *ichthyosis linearis circumflexa* (plaques with doubled squamous border), atopy,

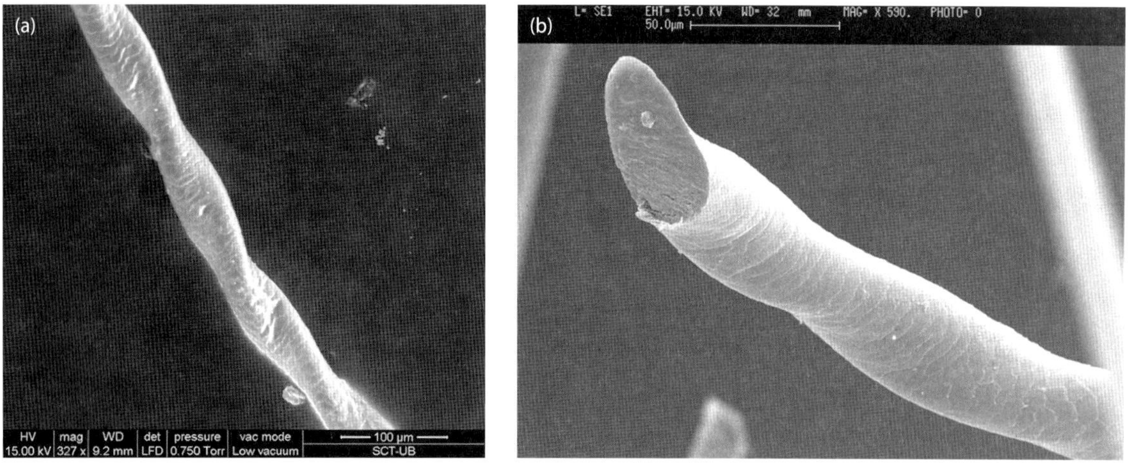

Figure 4.11 **(a,b) Atypical *pili torti* as seen under the SEM.**

and diffuse hypotrichosis (scarce and brittle hair). Other associated conditions are *ichthyosis vulgaris* and *congenital erythroderma ichthyosiformis*. Trichothiodystrophy may also be associated with ichthyosis, a condition that should be ruled out.

Optical microscopy. Bamboo hair or trichorrhexis invaginata is a typical image: the base of the hair shaft is chaliced shaped while the rest of the hair shaft shows a ballooning deformity. Eyebrows and eyelashes may also be affected.

Electron microscopy. The image is similar to that observed by the optical microscope (Figure 4.12). Hair shaft distal end may also appear as a golf tee due to hair fracture at the knot of trichorrhexis invaginata.

Trichoscopy Hairs are fractured at the nodule or knot where the shaft appears as a bamboo cane. The typical aspect includes a chalice shape of the proximal end and a ballooning distortion of the rest of the hair shaft. The distal end of the hair shaft shows a golf tee aspect due to local fracture.[49,50]

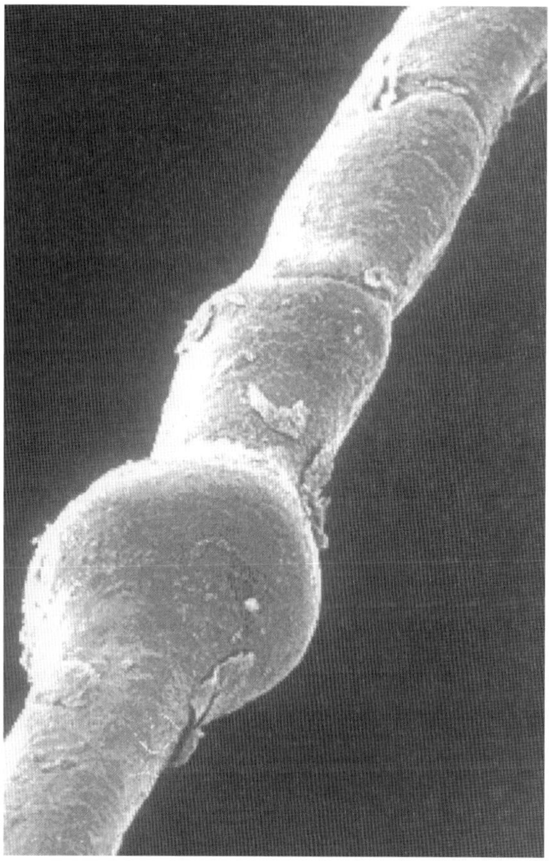

Figure 4.12 **Trichorrhexis invaginata (Netherton disease) with "bamboo hair." Proximal dilatation of the hair shaft is characteristic, with a chalice-shape distortion and a distal ballooning alteration.**

Trichothiodystrophy

Trichothiodystrophy is a complex syndrome due to a low content of sulfured compounds in the hair that leads to a specific hair dysplasia ("trichodystrofic hair")[1,4,51] in association with other clinical findings such as a delay in psychomotor development, ichthyosis, onychodystrophy, microdolichocephalia, photosensitivity, among other defects.[52,53] There are some variations of this syndrome: BIDS, IBIDS, PIBIDS, SIBIDS, ONMRS, or syndromes of Pollitt, Tay, and Sabinas, and Amish brittle hair.[54,55]

Genetics. Mutations of *TTD, ERCC2, C7orf11, ERCC3, GTF2H5, XPC,* and *GTF2H4* genes have been reported which were localized in 19q13.2-q13.3, 19q13.3, 7p14.1, 2q21, 6q25.3, 3p25, and 6p21.3, respectively.[56–61]

Clinical diagnosis. The affected individual is a newborn with congenital ichthyosis, scarce, short, and brittle hair,

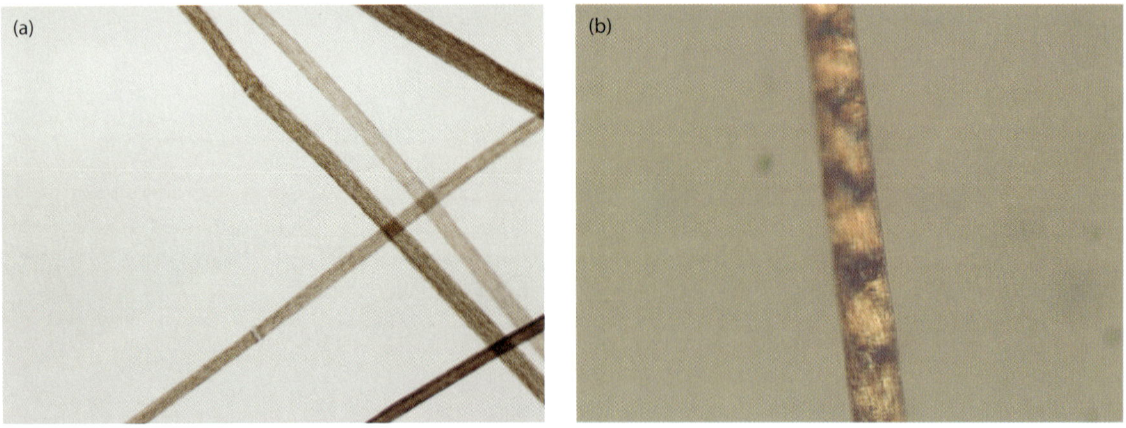

Figure 4.13 **(a) Flat hair with a typical transverse fracture. (b) Spotted and tiger-like hair surface.**

characteristic facial features, microdolichocephalia, and pleasant attitude. Other clinical findings may include mental retardation, growth delay, onychodystrophy (nail striae), and photosensitivity.[52]

Optical microscopy. Flat hair appears with typical transverse and clean transversal fractures (trichoschisis) (Figure 4.13a).

Polarized light. Alternating light and dark bands in the hair are observed, with a typical spotted tiger-like surface (Figure 4.13b).

Scanning electron microscopy. Completely rigid flat hairs like tapes are observed. Trichoschisis with a clean fracture is pathognomonic. The hair surface shows longitudinal crests and cuticle defects (Figure 4.14).

X-rays microanalysis. Sulfur content is lower than 50%.

Hair amino acid chromatography. Sulfured amino acids are clearly lowered.

Trichoscopy. Dermoscopy is not characteristic except for the trichoschisis.[62] This hair shaft may show a weaving contour and nonhomogenous structures appearing as grains of sand, alternating dark and light bands, and spotted tiger-like surface.

Trichonodosis

This is a frequent but rarely diagnosed hair dysplasia in which true knots are observed along the hair shaft. It may be suspected when the hair shaft shows an angle and changes abruptly its direction.[4,63,64] This condition is more frequently observed in individuals with curly hair in association with local trauma, scraping maneuvers, and ticks.[65] It may be found in the axillae and genitalia in association with pediculosis and acarophobia. It is not yet completely understood how double or even more complex knots are originated.

Clinical diagnosis. It usually occurs as an isolated finding. Suspicious arises when a hair changes abruptly its direction due to a true knot.

Optical microscopy. A simple, double, or even a complex true knot ("tie knot") is observed (Figure 4.15).

Scanning electron microscopy. Similar images to those observed by optical microscopy are seen. Amplification may reveal cuticle defects in the true knot area (Figure 4.16).

Trichoscopy. A simple, double or complex true knot is observed. Sometimes a "tie knot" or a "sailor knot" is observed in dermoscopy.

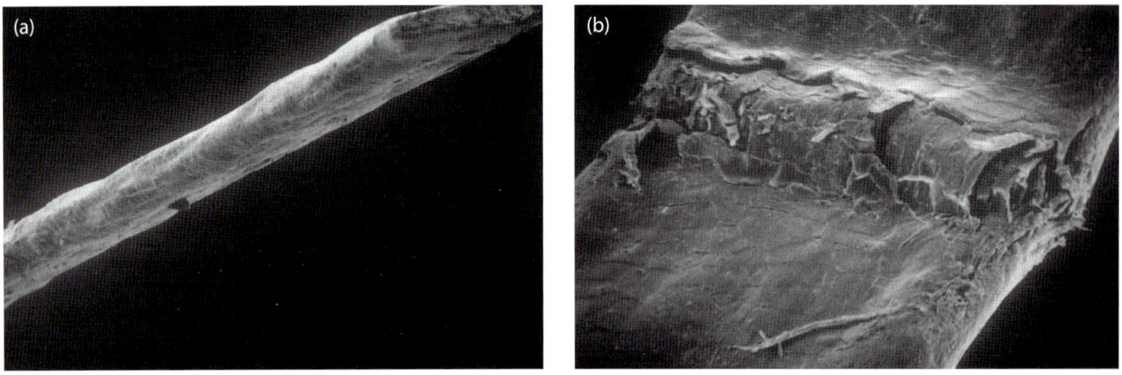

Figure 4.14 **(a) Flat hair like a tape. (b) Inicial trichoschisis at the SEM.**

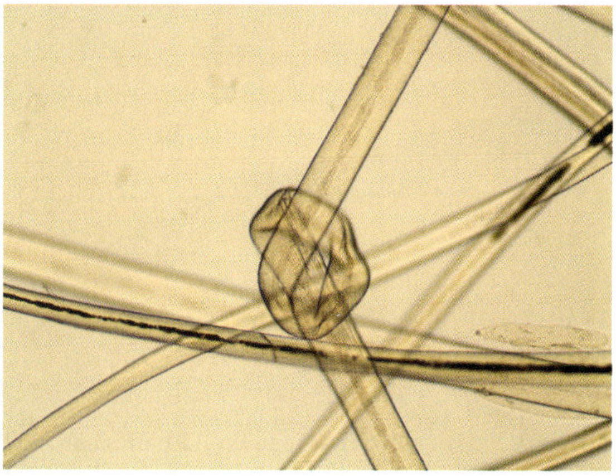

Figure 4.15 **True knot in the hair shaft. It may be simple, double, or more complex.**

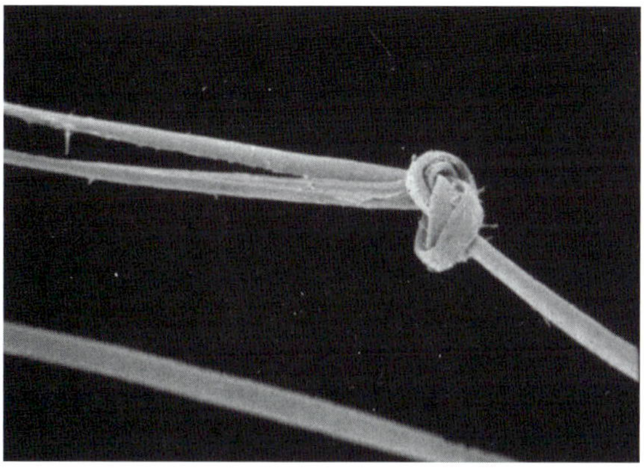

Figure 4.16 **True knot with cuticle defects in the area is observed using SEM.**

Distal trichorrhexis nodosa

This hair dysplasia is defined as a sharp fracture of the hair shaft due to a node. Clinical findings are different depending if the fracture occurs proximally or distally in the hair shaft.[66] In the former case, but not in the latter, alopecia is observed.

Distal trichorrhexis nodosa is an acquired diffuse condition, more frequently observed in long hair, and is caused by external physical–chemical factors and weathering in predisposed individuals.

Clinical diagnosis. This disorder is more frequently seen in young, long-haired women subjected to physical–chemical factors related to esthetic procedures. Hair usually shows some little balls in the distal end. The more distal, the closer the little balls appear. The hair shaft breaks at these little balls and final end of the hair shaft bifurcates; consequently, the hair of the affected individuals shows trichoptilosis and trichorrhexis nodosa.

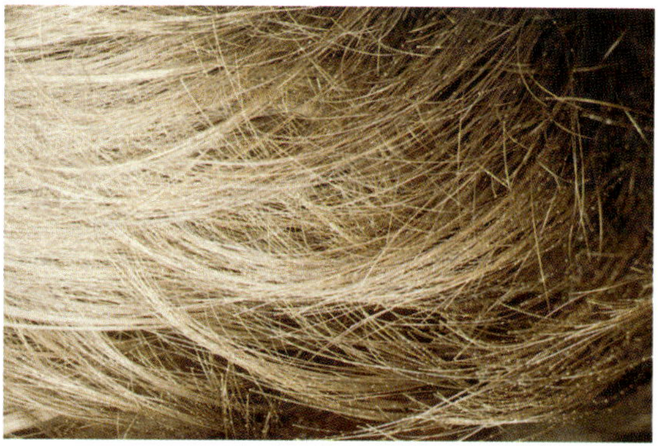

Figure 4.17 **Long-haired individuals are more frequently affected by distal trichorrhexis nodosa. Hair shows little balls that appear as dust spots and bifurcated hair endings (trichoptilosis).**

Patients normally complain of no hair growth and that a haircut is not needed due to easy breaking off of hair when minimally manipulated (Figure 4.17).

The pull test is positive (Saboureaud sign) and hair easily breaks off at the point where little balls appear. The examiner usually gets short segments of distal broken hair shafts.

Optical microscopy. Fracture at a nodule is clearly seen, and both sides of the nodule show a chipping aspect of the cortex (Figure 4.18). When pulling apart two segments of the hair shaft, both ends look like a brush. Bifurcated hair endings (trichoptilosis) as a result of external factors are also seen.

Trichorrhexis nodosa may also be observed in other hair dysplasias, mainly in Menkes syndrome.

Electron microscopy. Absence or altered cuticle is observed along with typical images of trichorrhexis

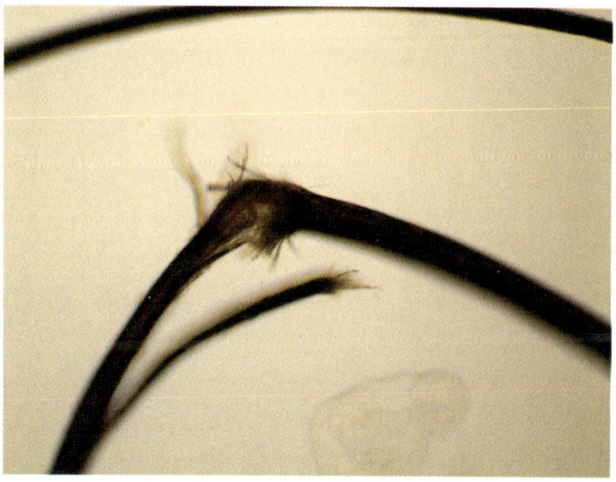

Figure 4.18 **Fracture of the hair shaft at the nodule, with both sides of the nodule showing open spalling of the cortex.**

nodosa and trichoptilosis. The cuticle and cortex show small spalling areas close to the fracture zone at the nodule in both electron and scanning electron microscopy.[67]

Trichoscopy. Nodules where the fracture takes place are easily seen. At higher magnification, cortex fibers are also seen at the fracture point. At lower magnification, lighter nodules and slits along the hair shaft are observed. Hair endings look like brushes. Dermoscopy is a useful and fast tool to diagnose trichorrhexis nodosa.[14,62]

Treatment. It is mandatory to avoid compulsive hair treatments such as obsessive combing and brushing, as well as exposure to heat, dust, wind, salt, or other physical–chemical repetitive and intense cosmetic treatments. Finally, haircut, just some centimeters long, is advisable.

Proximal trichorrhexis nodosa

The morphological defect is the same as that observed in the distal variant; however, it is a more complex condition because trichorrhexis nodosa and trichoptilosis repetitively alternate in the same hair. It is more frequently observed in black people, who may show hypotrichosis in the scalp, beard, mustache, and other anatomical regions. It may be a hereditary hair disorder.[68,69] Proximal trichorrhexis nodosa can be a hair marker of congenital arginosuccinuria and the trichohepatoenteric syndrome.

Genetics. Trichorrhexis nodosa associated with the syndrome of Pollitt is a variant of trichothiodystrophy without photosensitivity. Gene mutations have been reported in *C7orf11* and *TFIIH*.

Clinical diagnosis. There may be alopecic areas in the scalp, beard, mustache, axillae, and mons pubis. Hairs look short and broken, with endings that show little balls appearing like dust spots (Figure 4.19). It may be easily confused with trichotillomania and "bubble hair."

Optical microscopy. Typical images of trichorrhexis nodosa and trichoptilosis are observed (Figure 4.20).

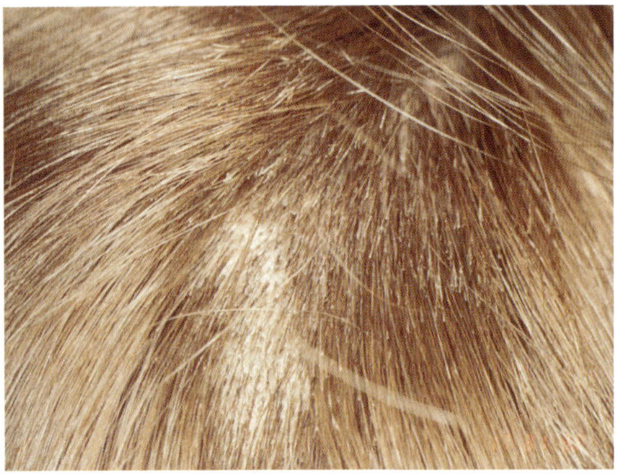

Figure 4.19 **Proximal trichorrhexis nodosa is seen as a hypotrichotic area with short, broken hairs.**

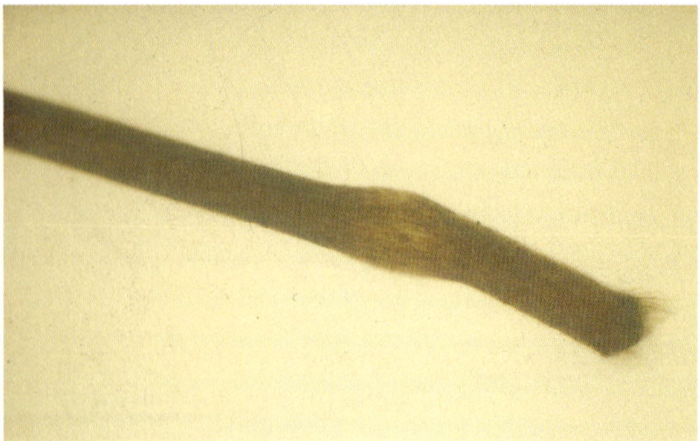

Figure 4.20 **Trichorrhexis nodosa and hair shaft fracture at the nodule with spalling of the cortex distally is seen.**

Electron microscopy. Complex images of trichorrhexis nodosa and trichoptilosis are observed in the same area and associated with cuticle defects in both electron microscopy (EM) and scanning electron microscopy (SEM) (Figure 4.21).

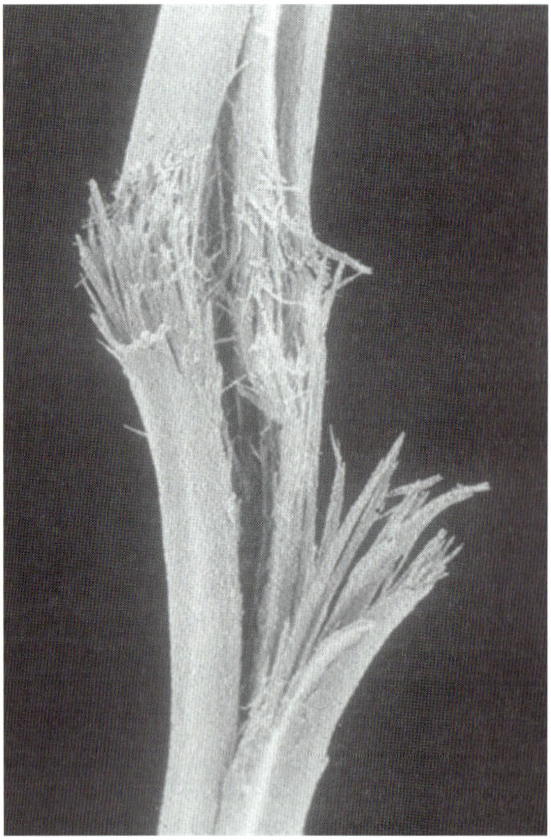

Figure 4.21 **Complex images of trichorrhexis nodosa and trichoptilosis are frequently seen.**

Trichoscopy. As stated in the previous section, dermoscopy shows complex images of some nodules and fractures in the same hair shaft, but always proximally.

Bubble hair

This acquired hair dysplasia is caused by air bubbles trapped within the hair—a situation that may be due to intense hair drying in predisposed individuals.[70–72] It is more common in women who show a localized hypotrichotic plaque. Dry heating may widen hair medulla and cause cortex dilatations, which appear as bubbles in the hair shaft surface. The hair shaft may break off in its widest ballooning portion.

Clinical diagnosis. This condition may be suspected in women with a sudden hypotrichotic plaque with short, broken hair without little balls in the hair endings. Predisposed individuals usually admit intense and close hair drying.

Optical microscopy. The typical image is that of a ballooning hair shaft surface with trapped air bubbles.

Scanning electron microscopy. A swollen or ballooning aspect of the hair shaft due to cortex dilatation is seen. Superficial orifices and fissures may also be present. The hair ending shows an image of "Gruyère cheese" due to bubbles or cavitations. Bubbles may also be found between cuticle layers.[73]

Trichoscopy. Either confluent or ballooning at different points of the hair shaft is observed (Figure 4.22).

Treatment. It is necessary for patients to avoid the cause—intense and frequent hair drying.

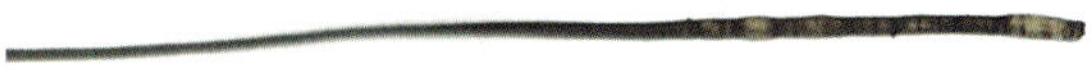

Figure 4.22 **In *bubble hair*, either confluent or ballooning at different points of the hair shaft is observed.**

Loose anagen hair

Loose anagen hair is a hair dysplasia due to lack of adhesion of the hair shaft to the hair follicle. It is more frequently observed in young blonde girls in whom hair is lost easily and with no pain when pulled.[74–76] Affected hair shows a ruffling aspect in its intrafollicular portion.

Genetics. Gene mutations have been reported in *SHOC2* and *KRT75*.[77,78] The former encodes leucine-rich repeat-containing protein, which participates in protein–protein interaction during cascade activation of kinases (RAS/ERK MAP). This mutation is responsible for Noonan like syndrome with loose anagen hair. *KRT75* encodes a family of type 2 keratins that participate in the formation of hair and nails. Its mutation causes *pseudofolliculitis barbae* and loose anagen hair. Genes have been identified in 10q.25 and 12q.13, respectively.

Clinical diagnosis. It is more frequently observed in 3- to 6-year-old blonde girls. Hair is lost easily and without pain when pulling. Parents describe spontaneous, diffuse hair loss, especially when it is minimally pulled, and a haircut is not necessary because hair seems not to be growing farther than a certain length (Figure 4.23). Familiar cases have been seldom reported and may be associated to ectodermic dysplasias.[79]

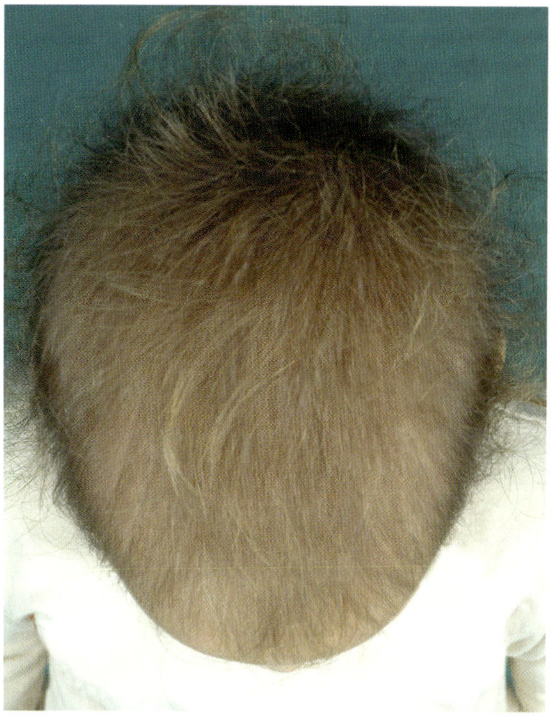

Figure 4.23 **This hair dysplasia is observed in 3- to 6-year-old blonde girls who show spontaneous, easy, and painless hair loss, especially when minimally pulled. The condition improves with time.**

Optical microscopy. Twisted anagen roots and proximal cuticle ruffling are observed (Figure 4.24).

Scanning electron microscopy. Twisted anagen roots with cuticle ruffling limited to the intrafollicular portion are observed. *Pili canaliculi* may also be seen.

Trichoscopy. Twisted anagen roots with cuticle ruffling may be observed.

Prognosis. No treatment has been reported. However, the condition may improve spontaneously with time.

Pili annulati (ringed hair)

Pili annulati or "morse alphabet" hair is perhaps the only condition that affects the hair medulla, which shows alternating dilatations that give the hair shaft a ringed appearance. Alternating dark and bright bands are observed in the hair shaft due to trapped air in the cortex and medulla (dark bands) and keratin distortions that diffuse incident light (bright bands).[1,4] This is either an autosomal dominant trait or a sporadic condition that affects individuals

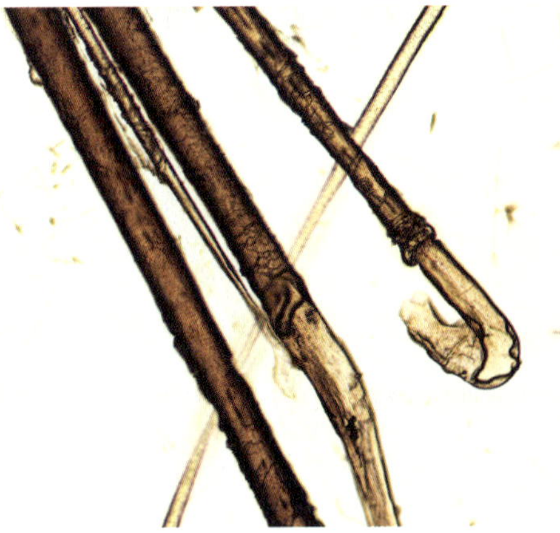

Figure 4.24 **Twisted anagen hair with cuticle ruffling is observed.**

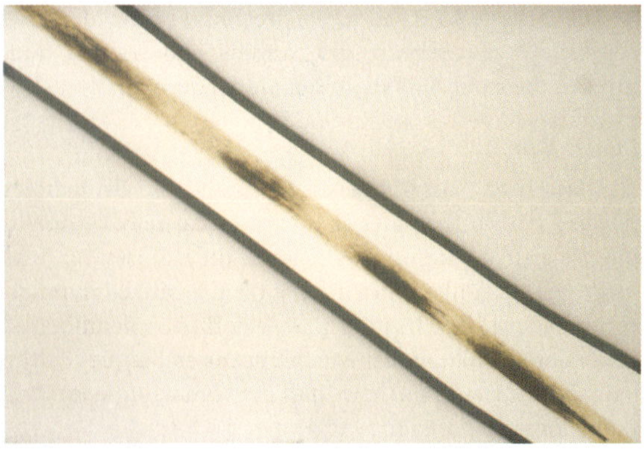

Figure 4.26 **Regular alternating dark and light bands are clearly seen.**

with thick and apparently normal hair. In either case, this is an esthetic condition that may be well accepted by the affected individual. A delay in hair growth and a low cystine content that may lead to an alteration of the formation of the microfibrils complex have been reported.

Genetics. The gene responsible for this hair dysplasia has been reported to be in the region 9.2 cM of chromosome arm 12q between D12S367 and D12S1723.[80]

Clinical diagnosis. This hair condition affects young females with thick, normal appearing hair that shows alternating dark and bright bands that may appear as sequins, like in pili torti, but without using any light source (Figure 4.25).

Optical microscopy. Regular alternating dark (cavitations with trapped air in the medulla) and bright bands are seen. Polarized light clearly reveals these bands (Figure 4.26).

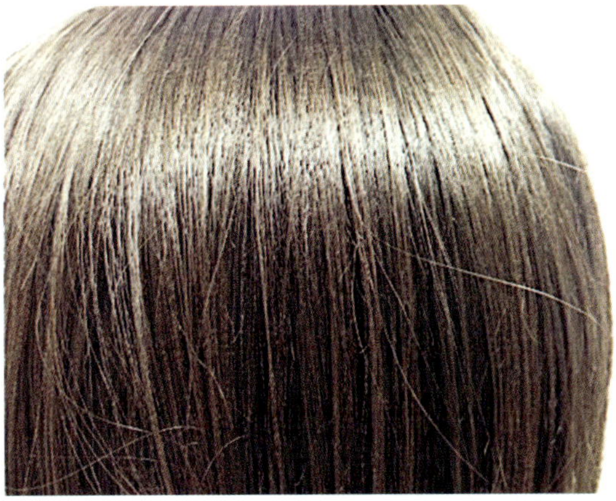

Figure 4.25 **Alternating dark and light bands are seen in ringed hair in females with thick and bright normal appearing hair.**

Electron microscopy. Alternating dark and bright bands are observed in electron microscopy and scanning electron microscopy. As in optical microscopy, dark bands correspond to cavitations in the medulla and a thinner cortex. The cuticle shows little cavitations that lead to an increased permeability and trapped air within the hair.[81–83]

Trichoscopy. Light bands correspond to trapped air in cavitations in contrast to what is seen in optical microscopy in which they appear as dark bands. Individuals with normal, thick hair may show light bands, pseudopili annulati, that correspond to less than 50% of the hair width.[14]

Pseudopili annulati

This is considered a variation of normal hair in which an optical/physical defect leads to the presence of bands, as those observed in *pili annulati*, but with no hair fragility. Bands are the consequence of light that is reflected in a straight angle by flat and twisted segments of the hair shaft that act as little mirrors.[40,84]

Clinical diagnosis. Dark- or golden-haired children show alternating dark and bright bands. So far no hereditary cases have been reported.

Optical microscopy. Bands are observed only if light shines perpendicularly on the longitudinal axis of the hair.

Polarized light microscopy. This tool reveals only variability in hair shaft diameter without alternating bands, a finding that contrasts with true *pili annulati*.

Scanning electron microscopy. The hair shaft cross section is elliptical, while the long axis shows wider and narrower segments. Moreover, alternating 30°–40° twisting in two different directions is observed.[85]

Trichoscopy. A variation in hair shaft diameter is observed. No alternating bands are present as in true *pili annulati*.

Generalized woolly hair

Woolly hair is defined as the presence of curly, flat, and thinner than normal hair in Caucasians in contrast to black individuals in whom hair is normally flat and curly. Three different groups of woolly hair are recognized: (a) generalized or diffuse woolly hair (congenital and AD or AR), (b) woolly hair nevus (congenital and sporadic, localized or multifocal, associated or not), and (c) acquired woolly hair (progressive curly hair, partial and diffuse, mainly). The generalized or diffuse variant rarely occurs and may affect the entire scalp. It may be associated with alteration of keratinization, and eye, teeth, and bone defects, among others.[86–88]

Genetics. Autosomal dominant variants are due to a mutation of *KTR75* (12q13, 20.91 MB between D12S1301 and D12S1610).[89] Autosomal recessive variants are caused by mutations in *P2RY5* (13q14.2-q14.3), *LIPH* (3q27-q28), and *LAH2* (3q27-q28).[90] In Naxos disease, woolly hair is associated with cardiomyopathy and keratoderma of the palms and soles and is caused by the mutation of the plakoglobin gene (17q.21).[91,92]

Clinical diagnosis. Children normally present with very thin, soft, and curly hair that resembles wool. Hair density is low, and the scalp can be seen very easily (Figure 4.27). Hair fragility may lead to some hypotrichotic areas. This condition should be differentiated from uncombable hair, a distinctive hair dysplasia with which this has been confused in the medical literature.

Optical microscopy. Thin and curly hairs form small balls.

Histopathology. Groups of miniaturized anagen hair follicles that appear in normal quantity are observed.

Scanning electron microscopy. Very flat, tagliatelle-like, curly hair with an oval cross section is revealed by SEM (Figure 4.28). It may also been found isolated twisting and *pili canaliculi.*

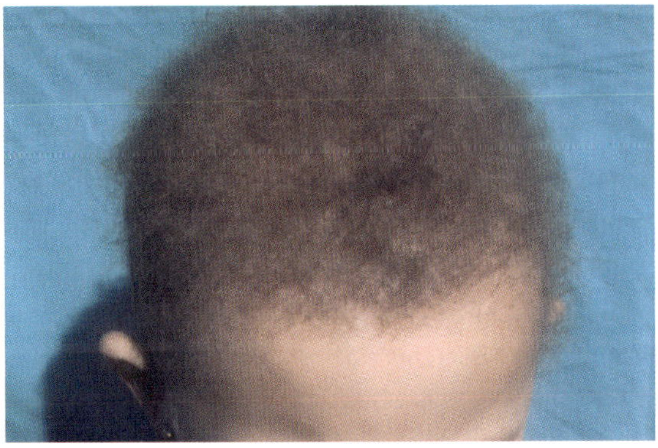

Figure 4.27 **Characteristically diffuse woolly hair is presented in a child with soft, curly hair that leads to scarce density that enables the examiner to easily see the scalp.**

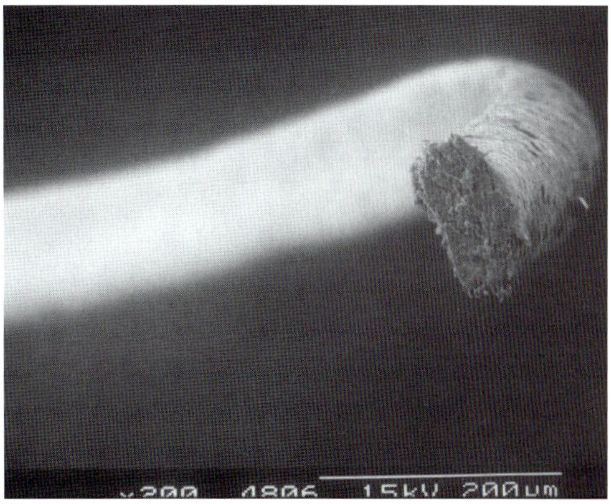

Figure 4.28 **In woolly hair the hair shaft is very flat, tagliatelle-like, with an oval cross section.**

Trichoscopy. Rudnicka et al.[62] have reported cyclical short, wavy hair that recalls a characteristic "moving snake" image. Broken hairs are also seen due to fragility caused by longitudinal twisting (Figure 4.29).

Woolly hair nevus

This is a localized, congenital, nonfamilial variant of woolly hair. It can be isolated or multifocal. This is the most frequently seen clinical form of curly/kinky hair syndromes.[93] Approximately 50% of cases are associated with melanocytic nevus or epidermal nevus in the same affected area or in the head.[94] Other alterations may include ocular (cataracts, retinal dysplasia, persistent pupillary membrane), and teeth defects, as well

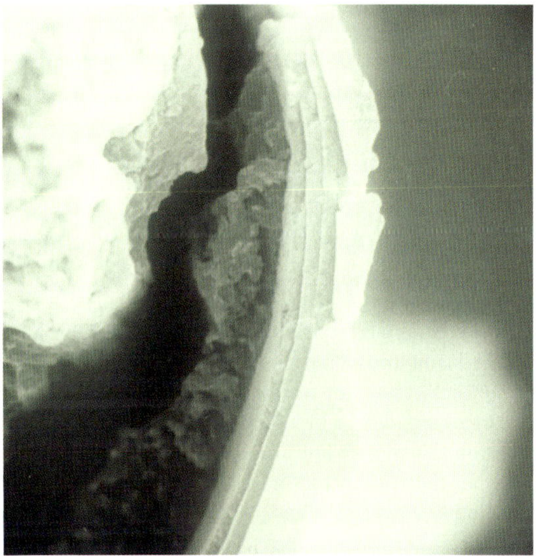

Figure 4.29 **Woolly hair at the SEM present also a thinkiness of hair cuticle.**

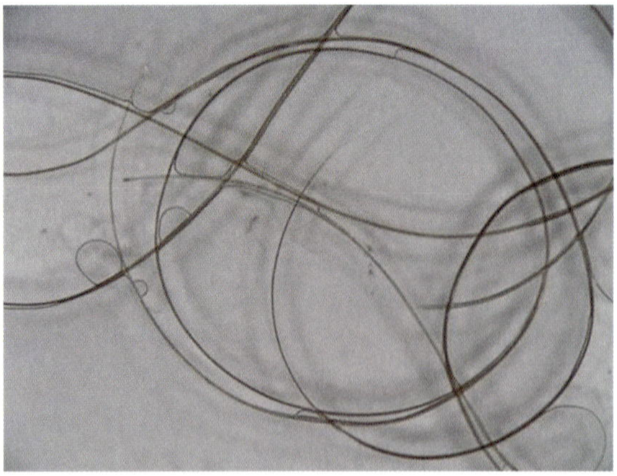

Figure 4.30 **At the trichoscopy, woolly hair is observed as a cyclical short, wavy hair that recalls a characteristic "moving snake" image; longitudinal twisting increases hair fragility and leads to broken hair.**

as gingivitis, growth and speaking delay, and congenital triangular alopecia.[95] No genetic findings have been reported.

Clinical diagnosis. One or some areas of woolly, curly, thin, and light hair are observed, surrounded by normal hair. An isolated plaque is the most frequent presentation, but multifocality is occasionally reported (Figure 4.30). Melanocytic and epidermal nevi may be present in the same affected area or other areas of the head.

Optical microscopy. Under optical microscopy, hair looks very thin, flat, light, and as forming a ball. The cross section is oval.

Histopathology. An area of grouped miniaturized anagen follicles are observed.

Scanning electron microscopy. The hair appears flat and curly, and the cross section is oval. Longitudinal twisting and channels along the axis are also observed. Fewer cells in cuticle layers may be found.

Trichoscopy. Similar findings to those found in generalized woolly hair are observed, but in a circumscribed area.

Treatment. Being a localized hair dysplasia, surgery is a therapeutic alternative to be considered.

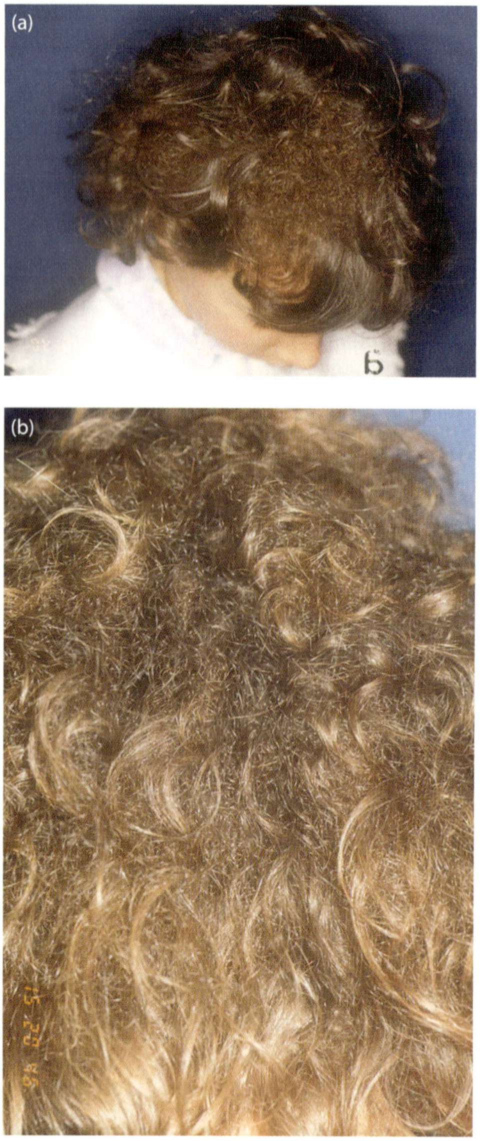

Figure 4.31 **(a) In woolly hair nevus an area of woolly, fine, thin, and curly hair surrounded by normal appearing hair is observed. (b) In acquired progressive kinking of hair multiple locks of hair acquire a curly and kinky features.**

Acquired and progressive kinking hair

Acquired and progressive kinking hair is an acquired nonfamilial variant of woolly hair. It frequently affects male teenagers. Locks of hair become curly and kinky, a condition that slowly but progressively affects the entire scalp. No external factors have been identified, and the condition slowly progresses to androgenetic alopecia.[96–98] A localized variant has also been reported; it is whisker hair nevus or circumscribed symmetric allotrichia. Systemic retinoids have been reported as a possible cause of acquired and progressive kinky hair. No genetic findings have yet been reported.

Clinical diagnosis. Typically it is a male teenager that shows locks of acquired thin, kinky hair (Figure 4.31).

Optical microscopy. Curly, flat hair that appears oval in the cross section is observed.

Histopathology. The cross section of the specimen shows oval hair follicles (Figure 4.32).

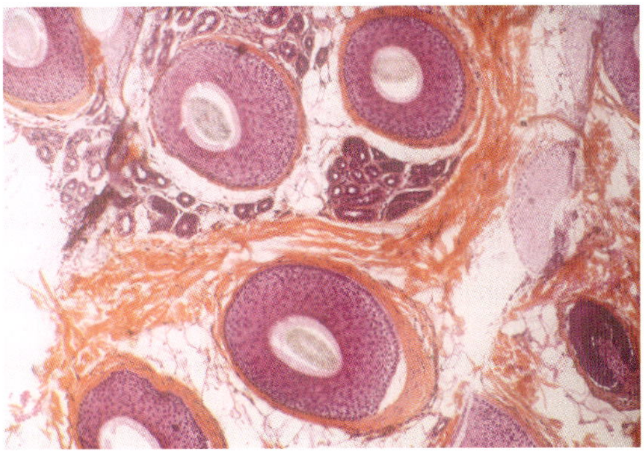

Figure 4.32 **In those cases, a cross section shows oval hair follicles.**

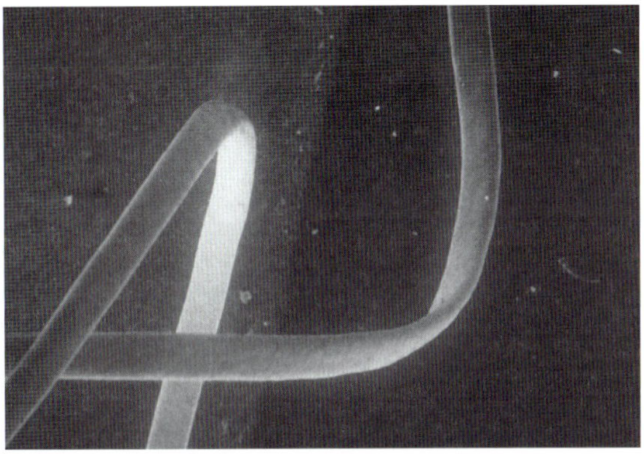

Figure 4.33 **Affected hairs are flat, like a tagliatelle, thinner, curly, and oval in the cross section.**

Scanning electron microscopy. Affected hair looks very flat like tagliatelles, thinner, and curly; the cross section reveals an oval hair as in congenital woolly hair, either diffuse or localized (Figure 4.33).

Trichoscopy. The same findings as in generalized or diffuse woolly hair are observed.

Diffuse partial *woolly hair*

This is a new variant of acquired kinky hair. In this condition, individual and isolated kinking occurs; consequently, only one curly kinky hair is observed amid 10–12 normal hairs. The disorder may be sporadic or familial. No external factors have been identified, and most affected individuals are children or teenagers.[99–100]

Genetics. Autosomal dominance may be related to mutation of *KRT74* (12q.13) as discussed previously.

Clinical diagnosis. It is observed in children or teenagers with isolated curly and kinky hair that stands out from normal hair.

Optical microscopy. Affected hair looks flat, curly, and oval in the cross section.

Histopathology. Anagen curved hair follicles are observed amid normal appearing follicles.

Scanning electron microscopy. Affected hair is thinner and flatter than normal hair, and oval at cross section. Twisting and longitudinal channels may also be present.

Trichoscopy. Affected hair is less curly, but findings parallel those described above for woolly hair nevus.

Acquired partial curly hair

This is a partial and acquired variant of kinky hair that affects isolated hair in the scalp and may be confused with diffuse partial woolly hair. This is a nonfamilial condition that affects only the distal part of the hair shaft; it improves with time and may be a response to external factors, either environmental factors or cosmetic procedures.[101]

Clinical diagnosis. The typical case is a young woman with isolated curly hairs surrounded by normal hair (Figure 4.34). This is a sporadic and acquired condition, which differentiates it from diffuse partial woolly hair.

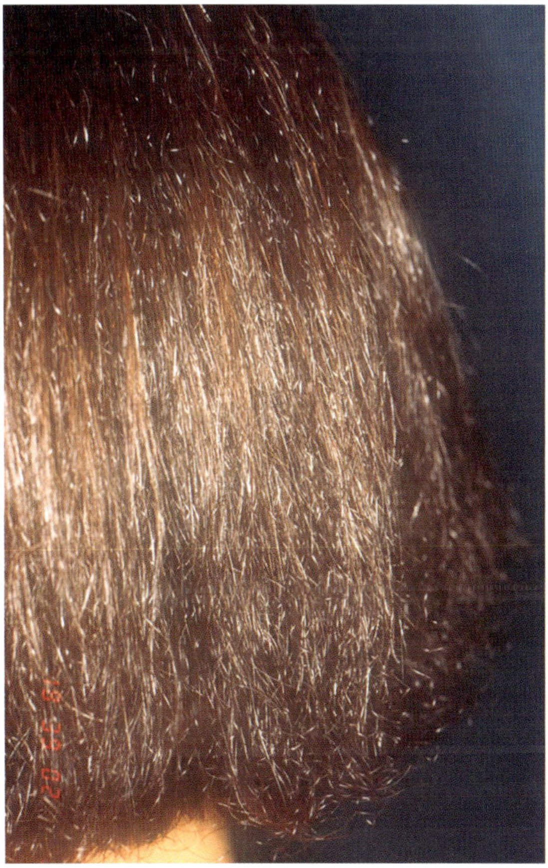

Figure 4.34 **A child or teenager is affected by acquired partial curly hair.**

Optical microscopy. Affected hair is thinner, flatter, and curly only distally.

Scanning electron microscopy. Affected hair is flatter, thinner, and oval in cross section. Characteristically, hair is normal in its proximal portion, but acquires a thinner and curly aspect in the distal half of the hair shaft.

Trichoscopy. The same findings as seen in woolly hair nevus are observed, but only in isolated affected hairs, which appear less curly.

Treatment. Hair conditioners may help. Avoidance of weathering and aggressive cosmetic treatments is mandatory.

Straight hair nevus

Similar to woolly hair nevus, straight hair nevus has been described, which corresponds to the inverse image of the former. It is the presence of a delimited area with straight hair locks surrounded by curly hairs.[102] In the few cases that have been reported, the condition is linked to a local keratinization disorder associated with ichthyosis or epidermal nevus,[103] and it has also been reported in a patient with straight hair.[104] No genetic changes have been reported.

Clinical diagnosis. One or more locks of straight hair are observed, and characteristically they are surrounded by curly hair. However, some cases have been reported to occur in individuals who have straight hair but variable hair diameter, and associated local epidermal defects.

Histopathology. In the only case that we reported, hyperplasia of the sebaceous glands was reported, which gave a yellowish discoloration to the affected skin in an 8-year-old child.

Optical and electron microscopy. We observed minimal channels along the longitudinal axis.

X-ray microanalysis. No findings have been reported.

Trichoscopy. It is the inverse image of woolly hair; affected hair in this case appears straight.

Comment. Straight hair nevus has been reported to be associated with *ichthyosis hystrix* and warty plaques of the affected skin, independent of ethnic origin. Another plausible theory is that this condition corresponds to either hair mosaicism or a hair follicle disorder induced by the affected skin, instead of an individual and distinctive hair disease.

Uncombable hair (pili canaliculi)

This syndrome is characterized by dry, light, and slurred hair in children or teenagers with thick hair but with locks of hair in different directions that makes it impossible to comb or style.[104,105] It is also known as "fiberglass hair." This is a sporadic or familial autosomal dominant or recessive condition.[106] It is generally described in a child with straight uncombable hair, but it has also been reported to occur in curly haired young individuals. Localized variants have also been reported. In all cases, the common finding of this hair dysplasia is the presence of *pili canaliculi*. However, *pili canaliculi* may also be found in ectodermal dysplasias, other hair dysplasias, and in almost all cases of loose anagen hair.

Genetics. No genetic changes have been reported. However, in Rapp–Hodgkin syndrome (anhydrotic ectodermal dysplasia and cleft lip/palate) the mutation has been identified in *TP63* (3q.27).[107]

Clinical diagnosis. It is seen in children or teenagers who present with dry, lusterless hair that cannot be combed. This disorder can be familial (Figure 4.35).

Optical microscopy. A channel alongside the hair shaft is easily observed when adjusting the micrometer (Figure 4.36). If the hair has medulla, it is impossible to see the channel.

Histopathology. The biopsy is seldom required. Inner sheaths adhesions are observed as well as hair shaft twisting.

Scanning electron microscopy. One or more channels are observed along the longitudinal axis of the hair shaft, and this is definitive for the diagnosis (Figure 4.37).[108] Depending on the number of channels, the cross section

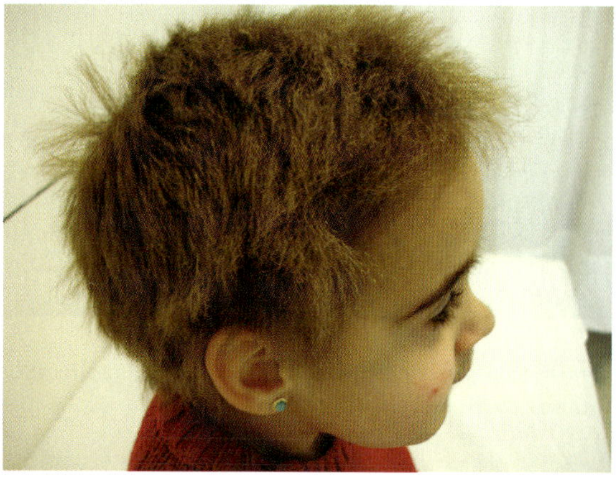

Figure 4.35 **Pili canaliculi affects a child or young individual with dry, lusterless, and uncombable hair.**

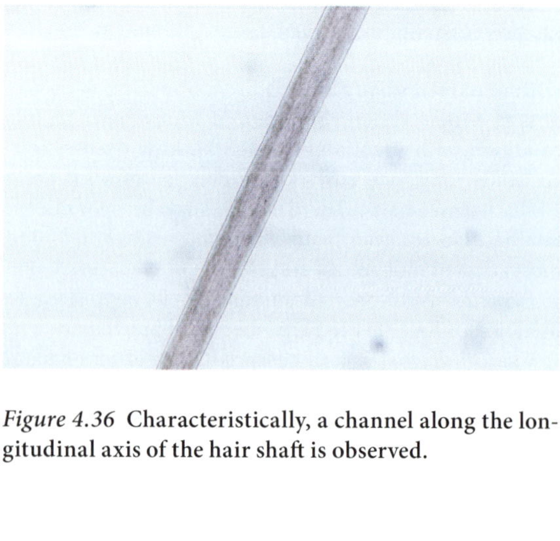

Figure 4.36 **Characteristically, a channel along the longitudinal axis of the hair shaft is observed.**

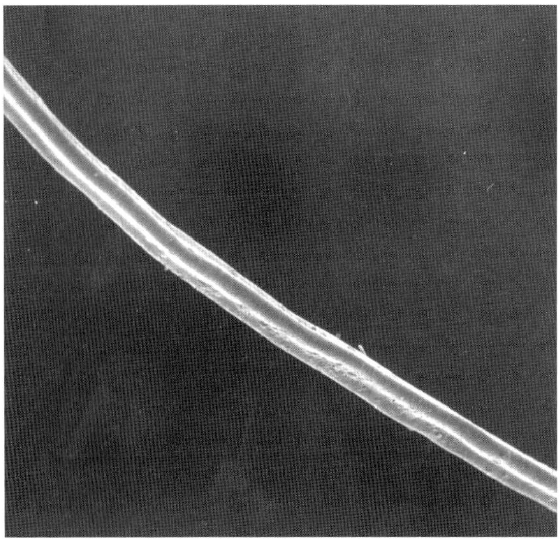

Figure 4.37 **Deep channels are clearly observed along the hair shaft.**

of the hair shaft may show a kidney-like, triangular, square, or irregular shape.[109]

Trichoscopy. More recently, this dermoscopy was demonstrated to be a useful, simple, and fast diagnostic tool. Flattening and longitudinal channels are observed along the hair shaft axis, while the cross section of the hair shows a kidney-like or triangular shape.

Treatment. Spontaneous improvement with time has been reported. Zinc pyrithione shampoo may improve hair due to the rebound fat effect.

REFERENCES

1. Camacho-Martínez F, Ferrando J. Hair shaft dysplasias. *Int J Dermatol.* 1988;27:71–80.
2. Dupré A, Bonafé JL. *Les Dysplasies Pilaires.* Paris, France: Lab. Lutsia; 1979.
3. Ferrando J, Fontarnau R, Mascaró JM. Aplicación de la microscopía electrónica de barrido al estudio de las distrofias pilosas. In: Camacho F, Montagna W, eds. *Tricología, Trichology, Trichologie.* Madrid, Spain: Garsi Eds; 1982.
4. Ferrando J, Grimalt R. *Atlas of Diagnosis in Pediatric Dermatology.* Madrid, Spain: IM&C Eds; 2000.
5. Navarra R, Ferrando J. Displasias pilosas. *Piel.* 1991;6:177–182.
6. Van Neste D. Dysplasies pilaires congénitales: Conduite á tenir et intérét de diverses méthodes de diagnostic. *Ann Dermatol Venereol.* 1989;116:251–263.
7. De Berker DAR, Ferguson DJP, Dawber RPR. Monilethrix: A clinicopathological illustration of a cortical defect. *Br J Dermatol.* 1993;128:327–331.
8. Ferrando J, Fontarnau R, Castells Mas A et al. Sequential study of the transversal fracture formation of the hair in monilethrix and trichorrhexis nodosa. *J Cutan Pathol.* 1981;8:165.
9. Ferrando J, Galve J, Torres-Puente M et al. Monilethrix: A new family with the novel mutation in KRT81 gene. *Int J Trichol.* 2012;4:53–55.
10. Gummer CL, Dawber RPR, Swift JA. Monilethrix: An electron microscopic and electron histochemical study. *Br J Dermatol.* 1981;105:529–541.
11. Redler S, Pasternack SM, Wolf S, Stienen D, Wenzel J, Nöthen MM, Betz RC. A novel KRT86 mutation in a Turkish family with monilethrix, and identification of maternal mosaicism. *Clin Exp Dermatol.* 2015 Mar 21. doi: 10.1111/ced.12631.
12. Zlotogorski A, Marek D, Horev L et al. An autosomal recessive form of monilethrix is caused by mutations in DSG4: Clinical overlap with localized autosomal recessive hypotrichosis. *J Invest Dermatol.* 2006;126:1292–1296.
13. Ferrándiz L, Moreno D, Peral-Rubio F, Camacho Martinez F. Tricoscopia. *Piel.* 2011;296:1–7
14. Miteva M Tosti A. Dermatoscopy of hair shaft disorders. *J Am Acad Dermatol.* 2013;68:473–481.
15. Bentley-Phillips B, Bayles MAH. A previously undescribed hereditary hair anomaly (pseudomonilethrix). *Br J Dermatol.* 1973;89:159–167.
16. Bentley-Phillips B, Bayliss MA. Letter: Pseudomonilethrix. *Br J Dermatol.* 1975;92:113–114.
17. Ferrando J, Fontarnau R, Hausmann G. Is pseudomonilethrix an artifact? *Int J Dermatol.* 1990;29: 380–381.
18. Phillips BB, Bayles MA, Grace HJ. Pseudomonilethrix: Further family studies. *Humangenetik.* 1974; 25:331–337.
19. Zitelli JA. Pseudomonilethrix. An artifact. *Arch Dermatol.* 1986;122:688–690.
20. Marayuma T, Toyoda M, Kanei A et al. Pathogenesis in pili torti: Morphological study. *J Dermatol Sci.* 1994;(suppl.):S5–S12.
21. Kurwa AR, Abdel-Aziz AHM. Pili torti-congenital and acquired. *Acta Dermatovenereol.* 1973;53: 585–588.
22. Lyon JB, Dawber RPR. A sporadic case of dystrophic pili torti. *Br J Dermatol.* 1977;96.197–201.
23. Hinson JT, Fantin VR, Schönberger J et al. Missense mutations in the BCS1L gene as a cause of the Björnstad syndrome. *N Engl J Med.* 2007; 356:809–819.
24. BJS Bjornstad syndrome (pili torti and deafness) [*Homo sapiens* (human)]. Gene ID: 7856, discontinued April 26, 2007. http://www.ncbi.nlm.nih.gov/gene/7856.
25. Petit A, Dontenwille MM, Bardon CB et al. Pili torti with congenital deafness (Bjornstad's syndrome)—Report of three cases in one family, suggesting autosomal dominant transmission. *Clin Exp Dermatol.* 1993;18:94–95.

26. Lubianca Neto JF, Lu L, Eavey RD et al. The Bjornstad syndrome (sensorineural hearing loss and pili torti) disease gene maps to chromosome 2q34–36. *Am J Hum Genet*. 1998;62:1107–1112.
27. Hinson JT, Fantin VR, Schönberger J et al. Missense mutations in the BCS1L gene as a cause of the Björnstad syndrome. *N Engl J Med*. 2007;356:809–819.
28. McGowan KM, Coulombe PA. Keratin 17 expression in the hard epithelial context of the hair and nail, and its relevance for the pachyonychia congenita phenotype. *J Invest Dermatol*. 2000;114:1101–1107.
29. Basel-Vanagaite L, Attia R, Ishida-Yamamoto A et al. Autosomal recessive ichthyosis with hypotrichosis caused by a mutation in ST14, encoding type II transmembrane serine protease matriptase. *Am J Hum Genet*. 2007;80:467–477.
30. Indelman M, Bergman R, Lurie R et al. A missense mutation in CDH3, encoding P-cadherin, causes hypotrichosis with juvenile macular dystrophy. *J Invest Dermatol*. 2001;119:1210–1213.
31. Sprecher E, Bergman R, Richard G et al. A hypotrichosis with juvenile macular dystrophy is caused by a mutation in CDH3, encoding P-cadherin. *Nature Genet*. 2001;29:134–136.
32. Danks DM, Cartwright E, Stevens BJ et al. Menkes' kinky hair disease: Future definition of the defect in cooper transport. *Science*. 1973;179:1140–1142.
33. Díaz Pérez JL, Rúa MJ, Prats J et al. Enfermedad de Menkes. Estudio anatomo-clínico. *Med Cutan Iber Lat Am*. 1980;2:23–32.
34. Jeremías Torruella FJ, Pou Serradell A, Giménez Camarasa JM. Enfermedad de Menkes. *Piel*. 1992;7:397, 401.
35. Galve J, Vicente A, González-Enseñat MA et al. Neonatal erythroderma as a first manifestation of Menkes disease. *Pediatrics*. 2012;130:239–242.
36. Kaler SG. Translational research investigations on ATP7A: An important human copper ATPase. *Ann N Y Acad Sci*. 2014;1314:64–68.
37. Wada T, Haddad MR, Yi L et al. A novel two-nucleotide deletion in the ATP7A gene associated with delayed infantile onset of Menkes disease. *Pediatr Neurol*. 2014;50:417–420.
38. Steveson TC, Ciccotosto GD, Ma XM et al. Menkes protein contributes to the function of peptidylglycine alpha-amidating monooxygenase. *Endocrinology*. 2003;144:188–200.
39. Wee NK, Weinstein DC, Fraser ST et al. The mammalian copper transporters CTR1 and CTR2 and their roles in development and disease. *Int J Biochem Cell Biol*. 2013;45:960–963.
40. Guillén B, Valencia A, Toledo M et al. Las displasias pilosas. *Dermatol CMQ*. 2012;10:115–122.
41. Dupré A, Bonafé JL, Carrère S. Ichthyose linéare circonflexe de Comel et sindrome de Netherton. *Ann Dermatol Venereol*. 1978;105:49–54.
42. Furio L, de Veer S, Jaillet M et al. Transgenic kallikrein 5 mice reproduce major cutaneous and systemic hallmarks of Netherton syndrome. *J Exp Med*. 2014;211:499–513.
43. Wang S, Olt S, Schoefmann N et al. SPINK5 knockdown in organotypic human skin culture as a model system for Netherton syndrome: effect of genetic inhibition of serine proteases kallikrein 5 and kallikrein 7. *Exp Dermatol*. 2014;23:524–526.
44. Ishida-Yamamoto A, Igawa S. Genetic skin diseases related to desmosomes and corneodesmosomes. *J Dermatol Sci*. 2014;74:99–105.
45. Wang S, Olt S, Schoefmann N et al. SPINK5 knockdown in organotypic human skin culture as a model system for Netherton syndrome: Effect of genetic inhibition of serine proteases kallikrein 5 and kallikrein 7. *Exp Dermatol*. 2014;23:524–526.
46. Raghunath M, Tontsidou L, Oji V et al. SPINK5 and Netherton syndrome: Novel mutations, demonstration of missing LEKTI, and differential expression of transglutaminases. *J Invest Dermatol*. 2004;123:474–483.
47. Magert HJ, Standker L, Kreutzmann P et al. LEKTI, a novel 15-domain type of human serine proteinase inhibitor. *J Biol Chem*. 1999;274:21499–21502.
48. Spink5 serine peptidase inhibitor, Kazal type 5 [*Mus musculus* (house mouse)]. Gene ID: 72432, updated on November 13, 2010. http://www.ncbi.nlm.nih.gov/gene/72432.
49. Ito M, Ito K, Hashimoto K. Pathogenesis in trichorrhexis invaginata (bamboo hair). *J Invest Dermatol*. 1984;83:1–6.
50. De Berker DAR, Paige DG, Ferguson DJP et al. Golf tee hairs in Netherton disease. *Pediatr Dermatol*. 1995;12:7–11.
51. Price VH, Odom RB, Ward WH et al. Trichothiodystrophy. *Arch Dermatol*. 1980;116:1375–1384.
52. Ferrando J, Mir-Bonafé JM, Cepeda-Valdés R et al. Further insights in trichothiodistrophy: A clinical, microscopic, and ultrastructural study of 20 cases and literature review. *Int J Trichology*. 2012;4:158–163.
53. Malvehy J, Ferrando J, Soler J et al. Trichothiodystrophy associated with urological malformation and primary hypercalciuria. *Pediatr Dermatol*. 1997;14:441–445.
54. Itin PH, Pittelkow MR. Trichothiodystrophy: Review of sulfur-deficient brittle hair syndromes and association with the ectodermal dysplasias. *J Am Acad Dermatol*. 1990;22:705–717.
55. Tolmie JL, Berker D, Dawber R et al. Syndromes associated with trichothiodystrophy. *Clin Dysmorphol*. 1994;3:1–4.
56. C7orf11 chromosome 7 open reading frame 11 [*Homo sapiens* (human)]. Gene ID: 136647, updated November 29, 2010. http://www.ncbi.nlm.nih.gov/gene/136647.

57. Kralund HH, Ousager L, Jaspers NG et al. Xeroderma Pigmentosum-Trichothiodystrophy overlap patient with novel XPD/ERCC2mutation. *Rare Dis.* 2013; 1:e24932.
58. Kiyohara C, Yoshimasu K. Genetic polymorphisms in the nucleotide excision repair pathway and lung cancer risk: A meta-analysis. *Int J Med Sci.* 2007;4:59–71.
59. Giglia-Mari G, Miquel C, Theil AF et al. Dynamic interaction of TTDA with TFIIH is stabilized by nucleotide excision repair in living cells. *PLoS Biol.* 2006;4:e156.
60. Briggs FB, Goldstein BA, McCauley JL et al. Variation within DNA repair pathway genes and risk of multiple sclerosis. *Am J Epidemiol.* 2010;172:217–224.
61. Singh A, Compe E, Le May N, Egly JM. TFIIH subunit alterations causing xeroderma pigmentosum and trichothiodystrophyspecifically disturb several steps during transcription. *Am J Hum Genet.* 2015; 96:194–207.
62. Rudnicka L, Rakowska E, Kerzeja M et al. Hair shafts in trichoscopy. Clues for diagnosis of hair and scalp diseases. *Dermatol Clin.* 2013;31:695–708.
63. Itin PH, Bircher AJ, Lautenschlager S et al. A new clinical disorder of twisted and rolled body hairs with multiple large knots. *J Am Acad Dermatol.* 1994; 30:31–35.
64. Zhu W-Y, Xia M-Y. Trichonodosis. *Pediatr Dermatol.* 1993;10:392–393.
65. Trüeb RM. Trichonodosis neurotica and familial trichonodosis. *J Am Acad Dermatol.* 1994;31:1077.
66. Leonard JM, Gummer CL, Dawber RPR. Generalized trichorrhexis nodosa. *Br J Dermatol.* 1980;103:85–90.
67. Ferrando J, Fontarnau R, Bassas S et al. Expresividad clínica y morfológica de la tricorrexis nodosa. *Dermatol Cosmética.* 1990;1:7–9.
68. Camacho F. Localized trichorrhexis nodosa. *J Am Acad Dermatol.* 1989;20:696–697.
69. Pollitt RJ, Jenner FA, Davies M. Sibs with mental and physical retardation and trichorrhexis nodosa with abnormal amino acid composition of the hair. *Arch Dis Child.* 1968;43:211–216.
70. Brown VM, Crounse RG, Abele DC. An unusual new hair shaft abnormality: "Bubble hair." *J Am Acad Dermatol.* 1986;15:1113–1117.
71. Elston DM, Bergfeld WF, Whiting DA et al. Bubble hair. *J Cutan Pathol.* 1992;19:439–444.
72. Detwiler SP, Carson JL, Woosley JT. Bubble hair. Case caused by an overheating hair dryer and reproducibility in normal hair with heat. *J Am Acad Dermatol.* 1994;30:54–60.
73. Ferrando J, Solé T, Grimalt R. Scanning electron microscopy details in bubble hair. In: de Van Neste DJJ, Randall VA, eds. *Hair Research for the Next Millenium.* Elsevier Science BV; 1996.
74. Price VH, Gummer CL. Loose anagen hair. *J Am Acad Dermatol.* 1989;20:249–256.
75. Grimalt R, Barbareschi M, Menni S. Loose anagen hair of chilhood: Report of a case and review of the literature. *Eur J Dermatol.* 1992;2:570–572.
76. Baden HP, Kvedar JC, Magro CM. Loose anagen hair as a cause of hereditary hair loss in children. *Arch Dermatol.* 1992;128:1349–1353.
77. Chen J, Jaeger K, Den Z, Koch PJ, Sundberg JP, Roop DR. Mice expressing a mutant Krt75 (K6hf) allele develop hair and nail defects resembling pachyonychia congenita. *J Invest Dermatol.* 2008; 128:270–279.
78. Baldassarre G, Mussa A, Banaudi E et al. Phenotypic variability associated with the invariant SHOC2 c. 4A > G (p.Ser2Gly) missense mutation. Am *J Med Genet A.* 2014;164A:3120–3125.
79. Azón-Masoliver A, Ferrando J. Loose anagen hair in hypohidrotic ectodermal dysplasia. *Pediatr Dermatol.* 1996;13:29–32.
80. Green J, Fitzpatrick E, de Berker D et al. A gene for pili annulati maps to the telomeric region of chromosome 12q. *J Invest Dermatol.* 2004;123:1070–1072.
81. Ferrando J, Fontarnau R, Hausmann G. Pili annulati. Estudio ultrastructural. *Dermatol Cosmética.* 1990;1:10–11.
82. Gummer CL, Dawber RPR. Pili Annulati: Electron, histochemical studies on affected hairs. *Br J Dermatol.* 1981;105:303–309.
83. Lalevié-Basié B, Polié DJ. Pili annulati. Etude en microscope électronique à balayage. *Ann Dermatol Venereol.* 1988;115:433–440.
84. Price VH, Thomas RS, Jones FT. Pseudopili annulati: An unusual variant of normal hair. *Arch Dermatol.* 1970;102:354–358.
85. Lee SS, J, Lee YS, Giam YC. Pseudopili annulati in a dark-haired individual: A light and electron microscopic study. *Pediatr Dermatol.* 2001;18:27–30.
86. Rodríguez-Pichardo A, Moreno Giménez JC, Camacho F et al. "Woolly hair." A propósito de 5 observaciones. *Med Cutan Iber Lar Am.* 1983;11:393–398.
87. Ferrando J, Gratacós R, Fontarnau R. "Woolly hair." Estudio histológico y ultraestructural en cuatro casos. *Actas Dermosifiliogr.* 1979;70:203–214.
88. Taylor AEM. Hereditary woolly hair with ocular involvement. *Br J Dermatol.* 1990;123:523–525.
89. Shimomura Y, Wajid M, Petukhova L et al. Autosomal-dominant woolly hair resulting from disruption of keratin 74 (KRT74), a potential determinant of human hair texture. *Am J Hum Genet.* 2010;86:632–638.
90. Shimomura Y, Wajid M, Ishii Y et al. Disruption of P2RY5, an orphan G protein-coupled receptor, underlies autosomal recessive woolly hair. *Nature Genet.* 2008;40:335–339.
91. Tosti A, Misciali C, Barbareschi W. Woolly hair, palmoplantar keratoderma and cardiac abnormalities: Report of a family. *Arch Dermatol.* 1994;130:522–524.
92. McKoy G, Protonotarios N, Crosby A et al. Identification of a deletion in plakoglobin in

arrhythmogenic right ventricular cardiomyopathy with palmoplantar keratoderma and woolly hair (Naxos disease). *Lancet.* 2000;355:2119–2124.
93. Lantis SDH, Pepper MC. Woolly hair nevus. Two cases reports and discussion of unruly hair forms. *Arch Dermatol.* 1978;114:233–238.
94. Peteiro C, Oliva NP, Zulaica A. Woolly hair nevus: Report of a case associated with a verrocous epidermal nevus in the same area. *Pediatr Dermatol.* 1989;6:188–190.
95. Soler-Carrillo J, Azón-Masoliver A, Malvehy J et al. Nevus de cabello lanoso asociado a alopecia triangular congénita. *Actas Dermosifiliogr.* 1995;86:89–95.
96. Cullen ST, Fulghum DD. Acquired progressive kinking of the hair. *Arch Dermatol.* 1989;125:252–255.
97. Ferrando J, Salas J, Vicente A et al. Ensortijamiento adquirido y progresivo del cabello: Una forma adquirida de cabello lanoso. *Actas Dermosifiliogr.* 1993;84:235–240.
98. Rebora A, Chiappara GM, Guarrera M et al. Cheveux crépus acquis un cas fémenin avec revue de la litérature. *Ann Dermatol Venéreol.* 1990;117:29–31.
99. Ormerod AD, Main RA, Ryder ML et al. A family with diffuse partial woolly hair. *Br J Dermatol.* 1987;116:401–405.
100. Guidetti MS, Fanti BM, Piraccini M et al. Diffuse partial woolly hair. *Acta Derm Venereol.* 1995;75:141–142.
101. Ferrando J, Grimalt R. Acquired partial curly hair. *Eur J Dermatol.* 1999;9:544–547.
102. Gibbs RC, Berger RA. The straight-hair nevus. *Int J Dermatol.* 1970;9:47–50.
103. Day TL. Straight-hair nevus, icththyosis hystrix. *Arch Dermatol.* 1967;96:606.
104. Dupré A, Bonafé JL, Litoux F et al. Le syndrome des cheveux incoiffables: Pili trianguli et canaliculi. *Ann Dermatol Venerol.* 1978;105:627–630
105. Mallon E, Dawber RPR, De Berker D et al. Cheveux incoiffables. Diagnostic, clinical and hair microscopic findings, and pathogenic studies. *Br J Dermatol.* 1994;131:608–614.
106. Ferrándiz C, Henkes J, Peyrí J et al. Pili canaliculi familiar. *Actas Dermosifiliogr.* 1980;7(1):225–228.
107. Salinas CF, Montes-G GM. Rapp-Hodgkin syndrome: Observations on ten cases and characteristic hair changes (pili canaliculi). *Birth Defects Orig Art Ser.* 1988;24:149–168.
108. Ferrando J, Gratacós MR, Fontarnau R et al. Síndrome de los cabellos impeinables. *Med Cutan Iber Lat Am.* 1977;5:39–46.
109. Ferrando J, Fontarnau R, Gratacós R et al. Pili canaliculi ("Cheveux incoiffables" ou "Cheveux en fibre de verre"). Dix nouveaux cas avec étude au microscope électronique á balayage. *Ann Dermatol Venerol.* 1980;107:243–248.

5 Alopecia classifications

Pierre Bouhanna

ALOPECIA CLASSIFICATIONS

Alopecia classifications allow accurate diagnosis, a targeted therapy and a precise prognosis. The most common types of alopecia are androgenetic alopecia, telogen effluvium, alopecia areata, and cicatricial alopecia. Hair loss can occur through a variety of mechanisms. If hair shafts are defective or traumatized, they can be prone to breakage or premature loss. Intentionally or unintentionally, people may subject their hair follicles to physical trauma that can result in alopecia. Traction alopecia, postoperative pressure-induced alopecia, and trichotillomania are a few examples. The remaining types of alopecia are due to failure of the follicular epithelium. This can be due to inflammation, infection, senescence, hormonal influences, medications, genetics, combinations of these, and other unknown causes.

For these reasons, various classifications are useful guides.

Cicatricial versus noncicatricial alopecia

The most common classification system divides the diseases into cicatricial versus noncicatricial forms of alopecia. Cicatricial means that follicular epithelium has been replaced by connective tissue. However, in some cases of alopecia, the follicles seem to simply "disappear" without any noticeable alteration (Figure 5.1). The definition of cicatricial alopecia might include all forms of alopecia in which hair follicles are permanently lost. In contrast, noncicatricial forms of alopecia preserve the follicular epithelial apparatus and are potentially reversible.

Some hair diseases demonstrate a biphasic pattern, where noncicatricial hair loss is seen early in the course of the disease, and permanent hair loss becomes apparent in the later stages of disease. Examples of diseases demonstrating this biphasic pattern include androgenetic alopecia, alopecia areata, and traction alopecia.

Classification of cicatricial alopecia

Clinically, cicatricial alopecia is defined by the loss of follicular ostia (Figure 5.2). Histologically, cicatricial alopecia can be subdivided into two categories.[1,2] The first is primary cicatricial alopecia, where the target of inflammation appears to be the follicle, more specifically, the noncycling portion of the follicle and/or the bulge zone (the location of follicular stem cell).[3] Most of the primary cicatricial alopecias do not have a well-defined cause (Figure 5.3a–c).

In secondary cicatricial alopecia, the follicle is destroyed in a nonspecific manner.[3,4] Examples are burns, radiation dermatitis, cutaneous malignancies, cutaneous sarcoidosis, sclerosing dermatoses, necrobiosis lipoidica, and cutaneous tuberculosis.

The primary cicatricial alopecias result in "naked" hair shafts suggesting that the follicular epithelium is quickly destroyed around terminal anagen shafts. Any inflammatory process is to destroy the follicular stem cells in the bulge zone.

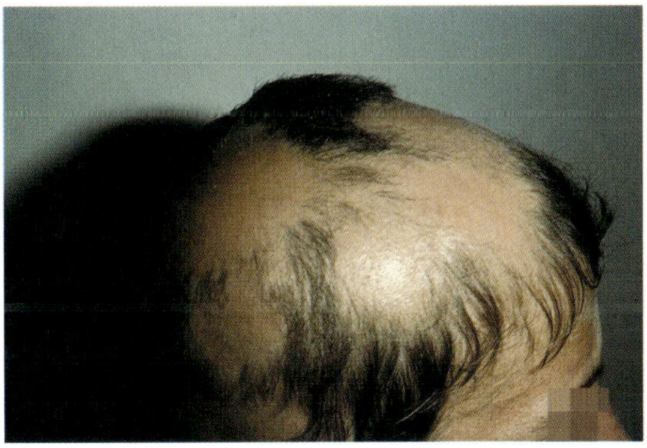

Figure 5.1 **Noncicatricial alopecia with regular and round patches of alopecia areata where all the hair has disappeared; the skin surface has a normal aspect.**

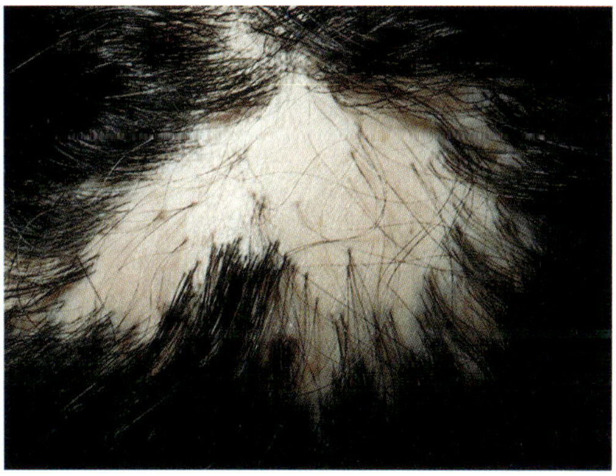

Figure 5.2 **Cicatricial alopecia with irregular bald patches; note the presence of normal-looking hair within the balding patch.**

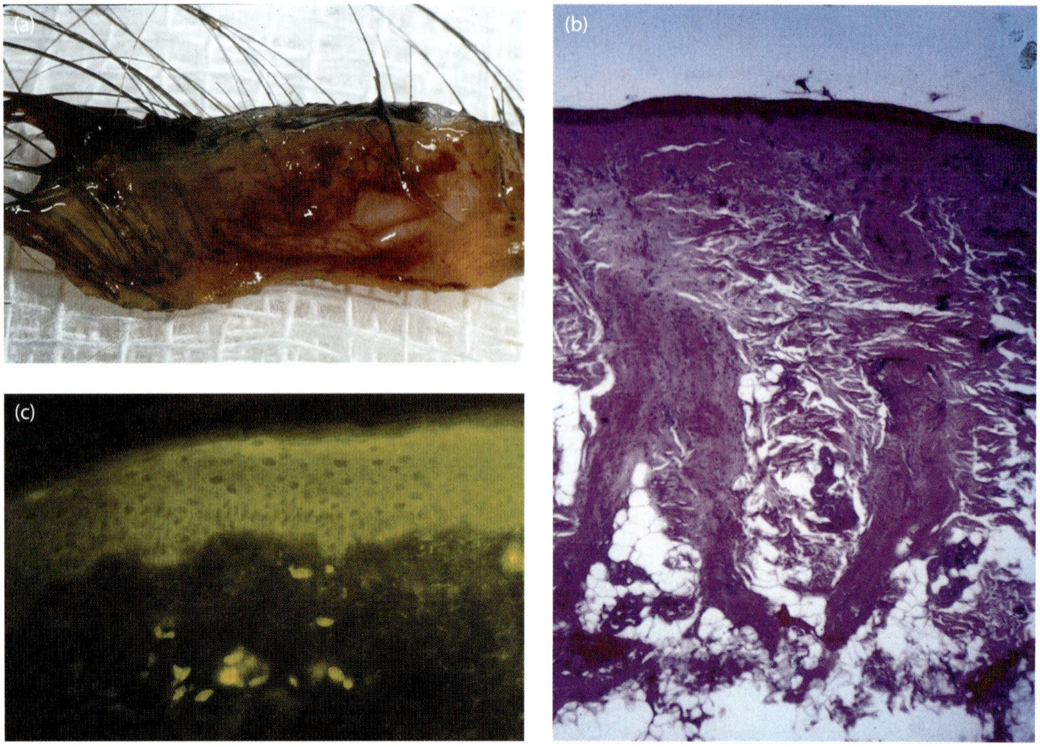

Figure 5.3 **(a) Macroscopic view and (b) histological aspect of skin and follicular lesions of irreversible cicatricial alopecia, (c) histological aspect on direct immunofluorescence of lichenoid cicatricial alopecia.**

Classification based on the primary inflammatory cell present in the biopsy specimen is subdivided as follows: lymphocytic, neutrophilic, mixed, and nonspecific (Table 5.1).

Classifications of male and female androgenetic alopecia

Various classifications of male androgenetic alopecia have been described (Figures 5.4 and 5.5). In fact, all the classification schemes proposed so far are only topographic. A multifactorial classification[5] has been developed to study parameters such as fixed distances of the face, scalp laxity and thickness, and hair coverage. This includes density, caliber, shape, length, growth rate, and hair color. This approach will lead to a better evaluation of the evolution of androgenetic alopecia in both sexes, either spontaneously or under treatment.

Male or female androgenetic alopecia induces a relatively early hair loss phenomenon of varying incidence and extent. Several intermediate evolutive stages exist between minimal thinning due to a decrease in hair density (frontotemporal recessions, crown or vertex) and the stage where only a narrow, horseshoe-shaped band remains. Classifications of baldness require a more objective, precise, and detailed approach for the different modifications determined by the evolutive process. This is equally true for all the experimental, medical, and surgical approaches of alopecia.

Table 5.1 Classification of Primary Cicatricial Alopecia

Lymphocytic
Chronic cutaneous lupus erythematosus
Lichen planopilaris (LPP)
Classic LPP
Frontal fibrosing alopecia
Graham-Little syndrome
Classic pseudopelade (Brocq)
Central centrifugal cicatricial alopecia
Alopecia mucinosa
Keratosis follicularis spinulosa decalvans
Neutrophilic
Folliculitis decalvans
Dissecting cellulitis/folliculitis (perifolliculitis abscedens et suffodiens)
Mixed
Folliculitis (acne) keloidalis
Folliculitis (acne) necrotica
Erosive pustular dermatosis
Nonspecific

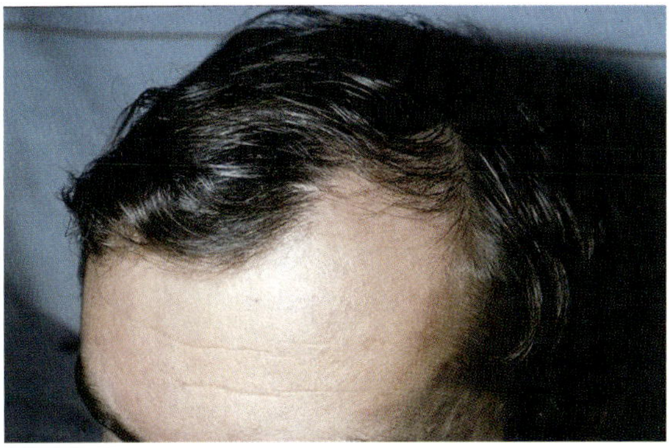

Figure 5.4 **Typical frontotemporal recessions of a male androgenetic alopecia.**

History of classifications

Various classifications have been proposed, since the study of Beek[6] in 1950, and Ogata[7] in 1953.

In 1951, Hamilton[8] established a classification modified by Norwood[9] based on the description of eight evolutive aspects and three subgroups. He also made a comparison between the incidence of baldness in Caucasians and in Chinese.

In 1976, Bouhanna[10] proposed a simplified classification of alopecia in three evolutive stages and two subgroups.

In 1977, Ludwig[11] classified female androgenetic alopecia in three evolutive stages. In women, there is a diffuse alopecia of the top of scalp with a preserved frontal fringe.

In 2000, Bouhanna[5] developed the multifactorial classification for a better assessment of male and female androgenetic alopecia evolution with or without medical and surgical treatments.[12,13]

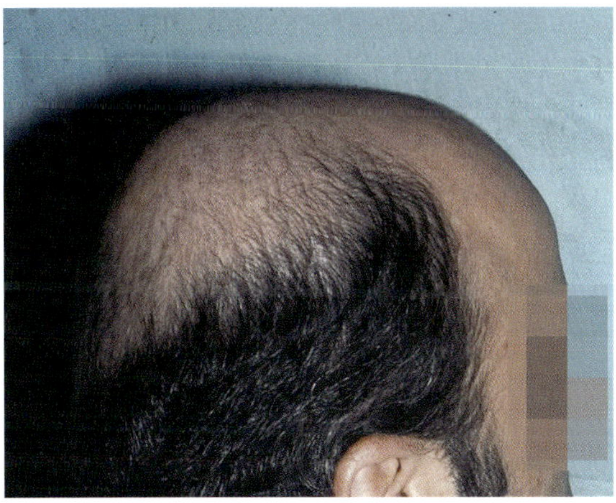

Figure 5.5 **Typical male androgenetic alopecia.**

Hamilton-Norwood classification for male pattern baldness

Schematically, male androgenetic alopecia is graded according to the topography:

Type I: Minimal recession is seen along the anterior border of the frontotemporal hairline.
Type II: Frontotemporal triangular areas of recession are more or less symmetrical.
Type III: Deep frontotemporal recessions are usually symmetrical.
Type III vertex: In this type, the hair is lost also in the vertex.
Type IV: The frontal and frontotemporal recession is more severe.
Type V: The vertex region of alopecia remains separated from the frontotemporal region of alopecia.
Type VI: The frontotemporal and vertex regions of alopecia are confluent.
Type VII: The most severe form in which remains a narrow, horseshoe-shaped band of hair (Figure 5.6).[8,9]

Other types of androgenetic alopecia include the following:

- Diffuse, unpatterned alopecia in which there is a general decrease in the density of hair, without any definite pattern.
- Diffuse, patterned alopecia which is essentially the same as in the more common male pattern

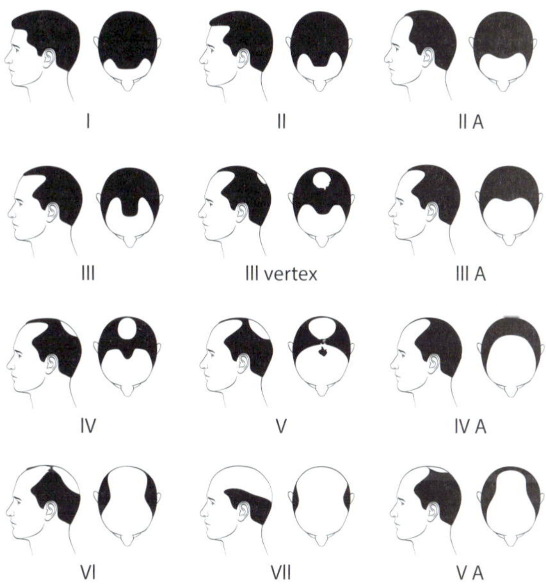

Figure 5.6 **Seven stages of evolution of male androgenetic alopecia. (Adapted from Hamilton JB. *Ann NY Acad Sci.* 1951;53:708–728.)**

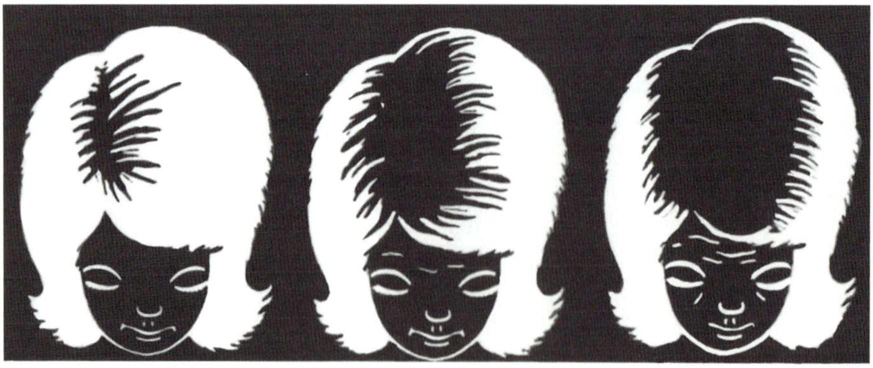

Figure 5.7 **Three stages of evolution of the female androgenetic alopecia classification. (Adapted from Ludwig E. *Br J Dermatol*. 1977;97:247–254.)**

baldness, but the areas involved do not become totally bald; the hair decreases only in density.

- Male pattern alopecia with persistent midfrontal forelock.
- Persistent anterior fringe almost totally preserved frontal hairline, but with a baldness posterior to this.

Ludwig classification for female pattern baldness

Schematically, female androgenetic alopecia is graded according to the topography:

Stage 1: Moderate oval vertex alopecia with long axis anteroposterior, located 2 cm behind the frontal fringe, which is preserved.

Stage 2: Clear alopecia located 1 cm from the frontal fringe.

Stage 3: Complete alopecia of the vertex, with persistence of a very light fringe (Figure 5.7).[11]

Bouhanna multifactorial classification. The multifactorial classification allows a better assessment of male or female androgenetic alopecia.[5]

Precise evaluation of various objective parameters helps to determine the medical and surgical indications, through the evaluation of the extent of bald and hairy areas, the degree of laxity and thickness of the scalp, and the ability of the hair to cover according to hair density, caliber, shape, length, growth rate, and hair color.

Bald and hairy areas measurements. The extent of bald and hairy areas is measured with precision with a ruler (Figure 5.8a) according to various parameters (Figure 5.8b). In men the values of the fixed measurements corresponding to the stage of a normal head of hair are:

- *Median Sagittal Distance (MS):* 34–37 cm (mean 35 cm); the distance between the edge of the frontal hairline and the lower occipital line (——).

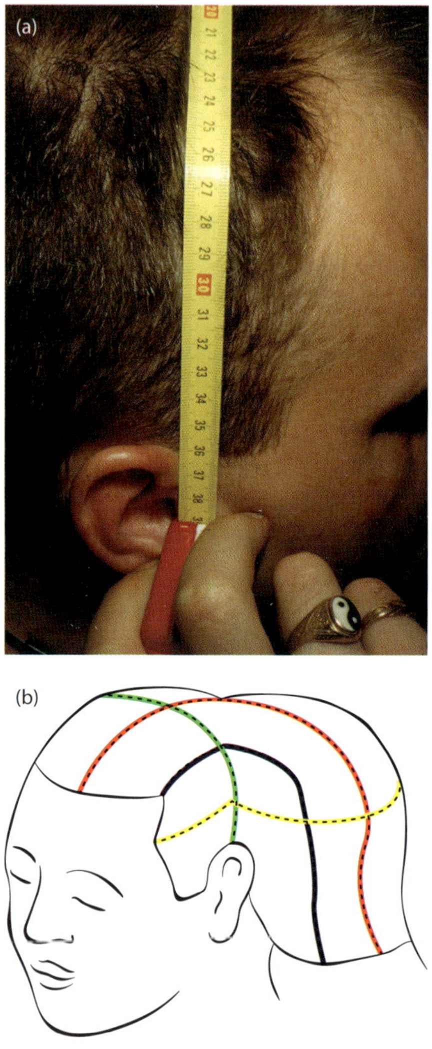

Figure 5.8 **(a) Male profile and measurement with a ruler. (b) The four schematic axes to be calculated.**

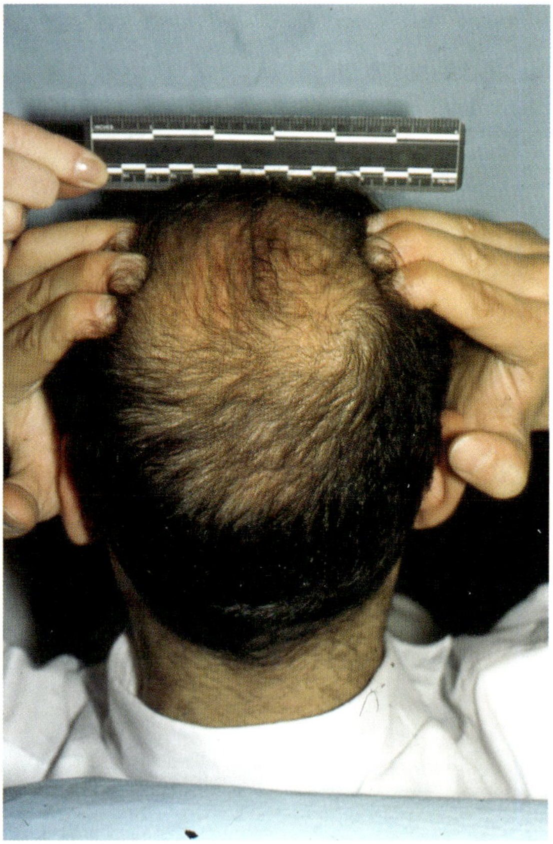

Figure 5.9 **Evaluation of the laxity by counting the number of folds after bimanual compression.**

- *Left and Right Sagittal Paramedian Distances (LSPM and RSPM):* 33–36 cm (mean 34 cm); the distances between the bottom of the left or right frontal recession and the lower occipital line (——).
- *Transverse Supra-Auricular Distance (TSA):* 30–34 cm (mean 32 cm); the distance between the two left and right supra-auricular hairlines (——).
- *Temporal Anterior Spacing Distance (TAS):* 34–40 cm (mean 37 cm); the distance between the two most proximal anterior temporal lines (——).
- *Stage of Maximal Balding (SMB):* Median occipital height.

MS = 30–34 cm (mean = 32 cm)
LSPM and RSPM = 30–33 cm (mean = 32 cm)
TSA = 28–32 cm (mean = 30 cm)
TAS = 30–36 cm (mean = 34 cm)

The stage of maximal baldness cannot be measured as the female androgenetic alopecia is diffuse.

Laxity of the scalp

Laxity of the scalp is measured on a scale, according to Norwood,[14] and graded:

0 = 0 folds
1 = 1 to 2 folds
2 = 3 to 4 folds
3 = Folds >5

It depends on the folds resulting from the bimanual compression of the scalp to determine degree of laxity (Figure 5.9).

Thickness of the scalp

In order to measure scalp thickness, we set up a simple method. A disposable subcutaneous needle is inserted vertically until it reaches the galea. The emerging portion of the needle is extracted with a Kocher forceps (Figure 5.10a). The sunken portion is then measured with a micrometer measuring device (Figure 5.10b). Scalp thickness is graded on a scale:

0 = Very thin (<2 mm)
1 = Thin (2–5 mm)

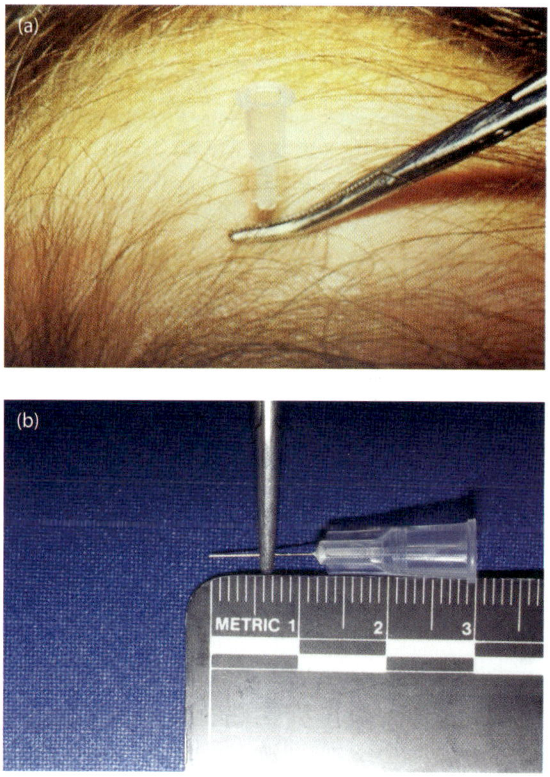

Figure 5.10 **(a,b) Evaluation of the scalp thickness by measurement of the sunken portion of a needle inserted vertically deep to the galea and extracted with a Kocher forceps.**

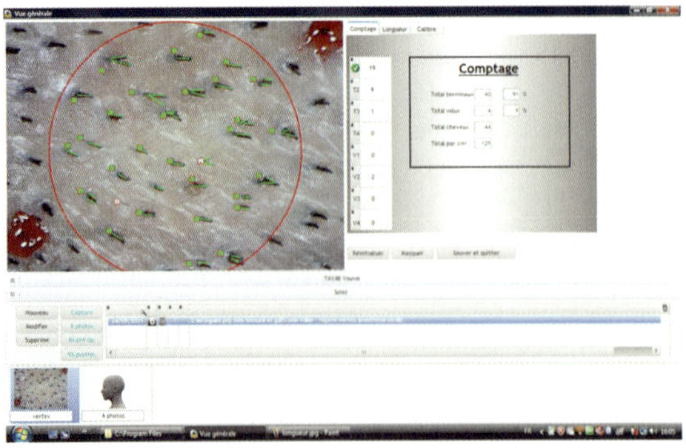

Figure 5.11 Digital phototrichogram for hair density evaluation.

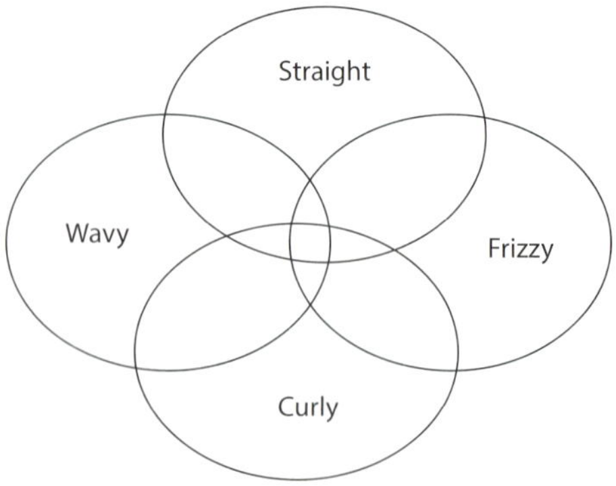

Figure 5.13 Various hair shaft shapes.

2 = Medium (5–8 mm)
3 = Thick (>8 mm)

Ability for hair to cover

Hair density. This is measured with great precision with the digital phototrichogram[15] (Figure 5.11) and graded:

0 = Poor (< 50 hairs/cm^2)
1 = Medium (50–100 hairs/cm^2)
2 = Good (100–200 hairs/cm^2)
3 = Very good (>200 hairs/cm^2)

The digital phototrichogram allows a precise evaluation of hair caliber less or more than 40 μmn (Figure 5.12).

Shape of hair shaft. This variable classifies the shape of the hair shaft as straight, wavy, curly, or frizzy (Figure 5.13).

Hair length (L). This is graded on a scale:

0: L < 1 cm
1: L = 1–2 cm
2: L = 3 to 5 cm
3: L > 5 cm

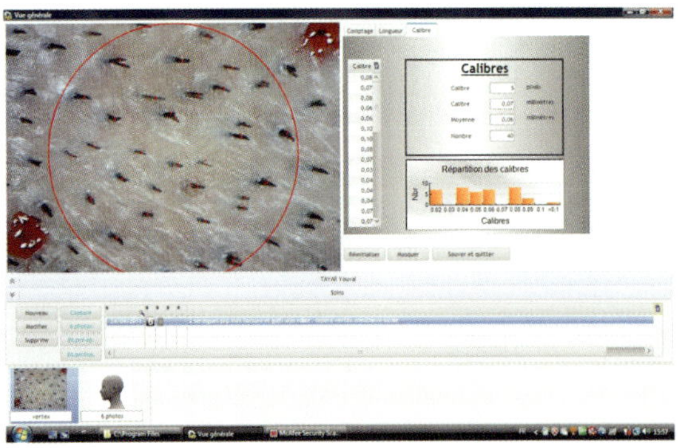

Figure 5.12 Digital phototrichogram for hair caliber evaluation.

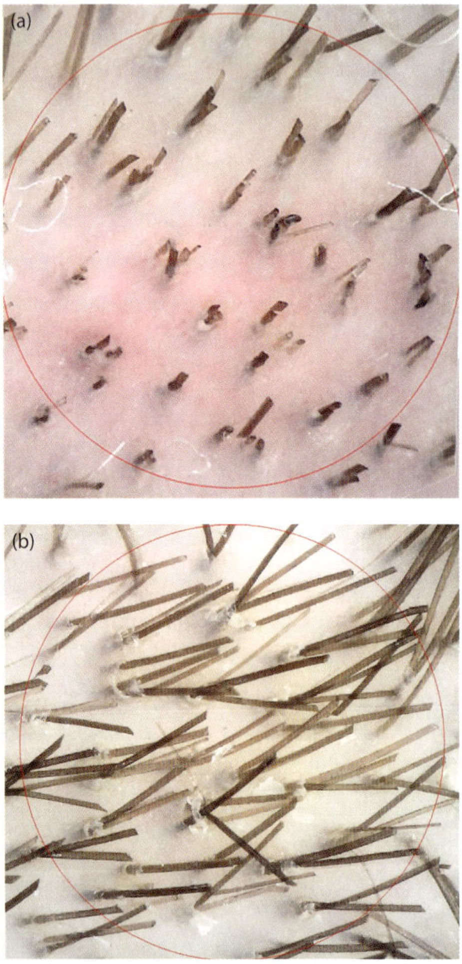

Figure 5.14 Two successive digital macrophotographs, 3 days apart, allow one to evaluate the hair growth rate (phototrichogram). (a) At day 0 the circle locates the area for the hair count. (b) At day 3 on the same area, the anagen hair are still growing. The telogen have stopped their hair growth.

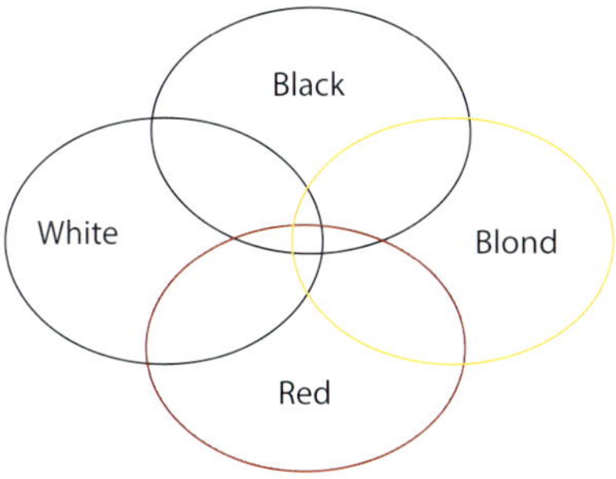

Figure 5.15 **Various hair shaft colors.**

Growth rate of hair. The growth rate of hair can be evaluated through a digital phototrichogram, which measures the growth rate of hair on two successive macrophotographs at a three days' interval (Figure 5.14).

Hair color. For practical classification purposes, we propose four basic tones: black (Bk), blond (B), red (R), and white (W). These are mixed together according to the natural appearance of hair (e.g., gray hair = Bk + W) (Figure 5.15).

CONCLUSION

The use in current practice of hair and scalp classifications helps in making an accurate diagnosis in the case of cicatricial alopecia. The various classifications for male and female androgenetic alopecia allow for a precise prognosis with or without targeted therapy.

REFERENCES

1. Ross EK, Tan E, Shapiro J. Update on primary cicatricial alopecias. *J Am Acad Dermatol.* 2005;53:1–37; quiz 38–40.
2. Sperling LC, Solomon AR, Whiting DA. A new look at scarring alopecia. *Arch Dermatol.* 2000;136:235–242.
3. Olsen E, Stenn K, Bergfeld W et al. Update on cicatricial alopecia. *J Investig Dermatol Symp Proc.* 2003;8:18–19.
4. Olsen EA, Bergfeld WF, Cotsarelis G, et al. Summary of North American Hair Research Society (NAHRS)-sponsored Workshop on Cicatricial Alopecia, Duke University Medical Center, February 10 and 11, 2001. *J Am Acad Dermatol.* 2003;48:103–110.
5. Bouhanna P. Multifactorial classification of male and female androgenetic alopecia. *Dermatol Surg.* 2000;26:555–561.
6. Beek CH. A study on extension and distribution of the human body hair. *Dermatologica.* 1950;101:317–331.
7. Ogata T. Development of patterned alopecia. *Sogo Rinsho.* 1953;2:101–106.
8. Hamilton JB. Patterned loss of hair in man: Types and incidence. *Ann NY Acad Sci.* 1951;53:708–728.
9. Norwood OT. Male pattern baldness: Classification and incidence. *Southern Med J.* 1975;68:1359–1365.
10. Bouhanna P, Nataf J. A propos des transplantations de cuir chevelu: Critiques et propositions. *Rev Chir Esth.* 1976;7(2):17–23.
11. Ludwig E. Classification of the types of androgenetic alopecia (common baldness) arising in female sex. *Br J Dermatol.* 1977;97:247–254.
12. Bouhanna P. Les différentes méthodes d'appréciation objective d'une chute de cheveux et d'une alopécie. *Praxis.* 1997;86:1000–1003.
13. Bouhanna P. Androgenetic alopecia: Combining medical and surgical treatments. *Dermatol Surg.* 2003;29:1130–1134.
14. Norwood OT, Shiell RC. *Hair Transplant Surgery.* 2nd edn. Springfield, IL: Charles C Thomas; 1984.
15. Bouhanna P. The phototrichogram and a macrophotographic study of the scalp. *Bioeng Skin.* 1985; 1(3):265.

6 Management of male androgenetic alopecia

Ralph M. Trüeb

WEEDING OUT THE MYTHS

Alopecia is a common complaint in clinical practice, with androgenetic alopecia, also referred to as male-pattern hair loss or common baldness, representing by far the most frequent cause of hair loss in men. The first signs may occur in adolescence, leading to an age-dependent progressive, patterned, nonscarring, loss of scalp hair. Due to the frequency and the often significant impairment of life quality perceived by affected individuals, hair loss cures have been experimented on for centuries. What is remarkable about their history is that despite the more recent genuine advances in effective medical treatments, hair cosmetics, and surgical procedures, phony hair loss solutions continue to be marketed today with an amazing success. For prevention or treatment of hair loss, countless herbal solutions, oils, lotions, magic pills, and even spiritual invocations have been advanced with questionable result. With the advance of medical technologies, ultraviolet light-emitting lamps, electrical scalp simulators, and vacuum-cap machines have all been alleged to help stimulate the follicles to grow hair. Despite their outrageous claims, most lack scientifically measurable efficacy in preventing hair loss or promoting hair growth. But people are so concerned about their hair loss, they want to believe some miracle cure or some charismatic healer will help them. Therefore, competent diagnosis and treatment are particularly important in dealing with hair loss.

Exactly as the fixation on treating hair loss is not a new phenomenon, age-old myths regarding hair growth and shedding continue to exist up to this day. In the effort to find ways to prevent hair loss or to promote hair growth, many people have fallen victim to these myths. In dealing with the fear or complaint of hair loss, it is important to weed out these myths from the facts (Table 6.1).

Table 6.1 Most Frequent Layman's Myths Regarding Hair Loss in Men

- Wearing hats causes hair loss
- Frequent washing and blow drying can lead to hair loss
- Hairstyling products and dyes cause hair loss
- Brushing your hair can make it stronger and more resistant to hair loss
- Cutting your hair will make it grow back thicker
- Hair loss cannot be stopped or helped

In a community-based survey of men conducted in Switzerland in 1998 to characterize the significance of scalp hair and self-perception of hair loss, and to evaluate treatment of hair loss, of 508 men, aged 15–74 years (27% age 15–27 years, 41% age 30–49 years, and 32% age 50–74 years), 43% reported hair loss. Of these, 26% admitted to the use of hair growth-promoting agents, while 31% rejected use of hair growth-promoting agents because of no need, and 27% because they did not believe that they worked.[1]

PREREQUISITES FOR SUCCESSFUL MANAGEMENT OF HAIR LOSS

Prerequisites for a successful management of hair loss are twofold: on the psychological and on the technical levels. These require on the part of the attending physician a genuine interest in the patient's complaint on the emotional level, and a genuine interest in the problem of hair loss on the scientific level.[2]

On the psychological level, for a successful encounter at an office visit, one must be sure that the patient's key concerns have been directly and specifically solicited and addressed: acknowledge the patient's perspective on the hair loss problem, explore the patient's expectations from treatment, and educate patients in the basics of the hair cycle, and why patience is required for effective cosmetic recovery. One must recognize the psychological impact of hair loss. Physicians should recognize that alopecia goes well beyond the simple physical aspects of hair loss. Patients' psychological reactions to hair loss are less related to physicians' ratings than to patients' own perceptions. Some patients have difficulties adjusting to hair loss. The best way to alleviate the emotional distress is to eliminate the hair disorder that is causing it. Only a minority of patients suffer from true imaginary hair loss. These have varied underlying mental disorders ranging from overvalued ideas to delusional disorder. In these cases, one must aim at making a specific psychopathologic diagnosis.

On the technical level, prerequisites for success are a specific diagnosis, a profound understanding of the underlying pathophysiology, the best available evidence gained from the scientific method for clinical decision making, and regular follow-up of the patient combining standardized global photographic assessments and epiluminescence microscopic photography with or without computer-assisted image analysis.

METHOD OF RIGHTLY CONDUCTING THE REASON, AND SEEKING TRUTH IN THE SCIENCES

As with any medical problem, the patient complaining of hair loss requires a comprehensive medical and drug history, physical examination of the hair and scalp, and appropriate laboratory evaluation to identify the cause. The clinician also has a host of diagnostic techniques that enable classification of the patient's disorder as a shedding disorder or a decreased density disease, and documentation of true pathology or only perceived pathology.

With respect to the diagnosis and treatment, one must remain open minded for the possibility of a multitude of cause-relationships underlying hair loss, and therefore also for the possibility of combined treatments and multitargeted approaches to hair loss.

The diagnosis of male androgenetic alopecia is usually quite straightforward and easy. Challenges in male androgenetic alopecia are listed in Table 6.2.

By approaching the hair loss patient in a methodical way, commencing with objects the simplest and easiest to recognize, ascending step by step to the knowledge of the more complex, and making enumerations so complete and reviews so general that nothing is omitted, an individualized treatment plan can be designed that usually results in success.[3]

PATHOPHYSIOLOGICAL UNDERSTANDING OF MALE ANDROGENETIC ALOPECIA

Androgenetic alopecia affects at least 50% of men by the age of 50 years, and up to 70% of all males in later life.[4] The hair loss is heritable, androgen dependent, and occurs in a defined pattern. It is assumed that the genetically predisposed hair follicles are the target for androgen-stimulated hair follicle miniaturization, leading to gradual replacement of large, pigmented hairs (terminal hairs) by barely visible, depigmented hairs (vellus hairs) in affected areas.[5] The result is a progressive decline in visible scalp hair density. Male-pattern androgenetic alopecia is characterized by its typical bitemporal recession of hair and balding vertex, while diffuse thinning of the crown area with an intact hairline is referred to as female-pattern androgenetic alopecia. Although the majority of men present with the male pattern, the female pattern is observed in children with premature alopecia, and in an estimated 4% of adult men with androgenetic alopecia.

Table 6.2 Challenges in Male Androgenetic Alopecia

- Premature alopecia
- Unusual patterns of androgenetic alopecia
- Androgenetic alopecia with comorbidities
- Androgenetic alopecia with follicular microinflammation and fibrosis

Although the genetic involvement is pronounced but poorly understood, major advances have been achieved in understanding principal elements of the androgen metabolism involved.[6] Androgen-dependent processes are predominantly due to the binding of dihydrotestosterone (DHT) to the androgen receptor (AR). The DHT-dependent cell functions depend on the availability of weak androgens, their conversion to more potent androgens via the action of 5α-reductase, low enzymatic activity of androgen-inactivating enzymes, and functionally active AR present in high numbers. The predisposed scalp exhibits high levels of DHT and increased expression of the AR. Conversion of testosterone to DHT within the dermal papilla plays a central role, while androgen-regulated factors deriving from dermal papilla cells are believed to influence growth of other components of the hair follicle.

Finally, the limited success rate of treatment of androgenetic alopecia with modulators of androgen metabolism, such as oral finasteride, and of hair growth promoters, such as topical minoxidil solution, means that further pathogenic pathways must be taken into account.[7] Among these, the role of oxidative stress, and of follicular microinflammation and fibrosis have gained more recent attention.

Naito et al.[8] analyzed the effect of the lipid peroxides on hair follicles and observed that the topical application of linolein hydroperoxides, one of the lipid peroxides, leads to the early onset of the catagen phase in murine hair cycles. Furthermore, they found that lipid peroxides induced apoptosis of hair follicle cells. They also induced apoptosis in human epidermal keratinocytes by upregulating apoptosis-related genes. These results indicate that lipid peroxides, which can cause free radicals, induce the apoptosis of hair follicle cells, and this is followed by early onset of the catagen phase. Ultimately, Bahta et al.[9] cultured dermal hair papilla cells (DPCs) from balding and nonbalding scalp and demonstrated that balding DPCs grow slower in vitro than nonbalding DPCs. Loss of proliferative capacity of balding DPCs was associated with changes in cell morphology, expression of senescence-associated beta-galactosidase, decreased expression of proliferating cell nuclear antigen and Bmi-1, upregulation of p16(INK4a)/pRb, and nuclear expression of markers of oxidative stress and DNA damage, including heat shock protein-27, super oxide dismutase catalase, ataxia-telangiectasia-mutated (ATM) kinase, and ATM- and Rad3-related protein. The finding of premature senescence of balding DPC in vitro, in association with expression of markers of oxidative stress and DNA damage, suggests that balding DPCs are particularly sensitive to environmental stress, such as cigarette smoking or ultraviolet radiation (UVR).

Eventually, a population-based cross-sectional survey among Asian men 40 years or older showed statistically significant positive associations between moderate or severe androgenetic alopecia and smoking status, current cigarette smoking of 20 cigarettes or more per day, and smoking intensity.[10] The odds ratio of early onset history for androgenetic alopecia grades increased in a dose–response pattern. Risk for moderate or severe androgenetic alopecia increased for family history of first-degree and second-degree relatives, as well as for paternal relatives.

Even though the consequences of yet another environmental stress, namely, sustained UVR on unprotected skin, are well appreciated, mainly photocarcinogenesis and solar elastosis, the effects of UVR on the evolution of androgenetic alopecia have only recently found attention.[11] However, some clinical and morphological observations suggest that UVR has some negative effect on hair growth. Histopathologically, elastosis is regularly found in scalp biopsies, especially in alopecic conditions, but so far has largely been ignored. To date, no controlled study has been performed on the degree of scalp elastosis in relation to the pace of development, duration, or grade of androgenetic alopecia, though it would seem to be a good marker for exposure to UVR penetrating the skin.

The implication of microscopic follicular inflammation in the pathogenesis of androgenetic alopecia has emerged from several independent studies[12–14]; an early study referred to an inflammatory infiltrate of activated T cells and macrophages in the upper third of the hair follicles, associated with an enlargement of the follicular dermal sheath composed of collagen bundles (perifollicular fibrosis), in regions of actively progressing alopecia. Horizontal section studies of scalp biopsies indicated that the perifollicular fibrosis is generally mild, consisting of loose, concentric layers of collagen that must be distinguished from cicatricial alopecia. The term *microinflammation* has been proposed,[13] because the process involves a slow, subtle, and indolent course, in contrast to the inflammatory and destructive process in the classical inflammatory scarring alopecias. The significance of these findings has remained controversial. However, morphometric studies in patients with male androgenetic alopecia treated with minoxidil showed that 55% of those with microinflammation had regrowth in response to treatment, in comparison to 77% in those patients without inflammation and fibrosis.[14] Surprisingly, so far, the inflammatory component has not been included in treatment protocols for male androgenetic alopecia.

EVIDENCE-BASED MEDICINE-GUIDED TREATMENT OF MALE ANDROGENETIC ALOPECIA

Although testing medical interventions for efficacy has existed since the time of Avicenna's (980–1037) "The Canon of Medicine" in the eleventh century, it was only in the twentieth century with the works of Alvan R. Feinstein (1925–2001) and Archie Cochrane (1909–1988) that this effort evolved to impact almost all fields of health care and policy.[15,16] Evidence-based medicine (EBM) aims for the ideal that healthcare professionals should make conscientious, explicit, and judicious use of the best available evidence gained from the scientific method in clinical decision making. It seeks to assess the strength of the evidence of risks and benefits of diagnostic tests and treatments, using techniques from science, engineering, and statistics, such as the systematic review of medical literature, meta-analysis, risk-benefit analysis, and randomized controlled trials.

As EBM guidelines on hair loss are rare, a European consensus group recently developed guidelines for treatment of androgenetic alopecia. It conducted a systematic literature review of Medline, Embase, and Cochrane databases upto August 2008.[17] There were 1370 publications found; 51 were added by hand search. Eight-five publications fulfilled the following inclusion criteria for the guideline: prospective study with a number of patients ≥20 (no minimal patient number required in twin studies), age ≥12 years, with confirmed diagnosis of androgenetic alopecia (diagnosis either clinically or by further diagnostic evaluations, e.g., trichogram, TrichoScan, or biopsy). Objective outcome measures of efficacy described for drug therapy were mean change from baseline hair count in target area or measurement of hair growth/loss in target area by global photography.

The guideline revealed excellent evidence levels (randomized, double-blind, comparative clinical studies of high quality, e.g., sample size calculation, flowchart of patient inclusion, intent-to-treat [ITT] analysis, sufficient size, or meta-analysis, which includes at least one randomized double-blind, comparative clinical study of high quality) for the therapeutic use of topical minoxidil solution and for oral finasteride, low evidence levels (little to missing systematic evidence) for hormonal or surgical treatments, and insufficient, respectively, lacking, evidence for a broad panel of miscellaneous treatments available claiming effectiveness. Table 6.3 summarizes the EBM-guided recommendations for treatment of male androgenetic alopecia, and Table 6.4 lists miscellaneous treatments with insufficient or lacking evidence for efficacy.

Finasteride is a competitive inhibitor of type 2 5α-reductase and inhibits the conversion of testosterone to DHT. The rationale for the use of finasteride to treat AGA in men is based on the absence of androgenetic alopecia in men with congenital deficiency of type 2 5α-reductase, and the presence of increased 5α-reductase activity and DHT levels in balding scalp.[18]

Minoxidil promotes hair growth through increasing the duration of anagen. It causes hair follicles at rest to grow, and enlarges suboptimal follicles. Minoxidil was developed for treatment of hypertension, and this feature of the drug's action is best understood; its mechanism of

Table 6.3 Treatment Recommendations for Male Androgenetic Alopecia

Topical minoxidil solution

- Topical minoxidil 2%–5% solution 1 mL twice daily is recommended to improve or to prevent progression of androgenetic alopecia in male patients older than 18 years with mild to moderate androgenetic alopecia (Hamilton-Norwoo IIv-V).
- Use of 5% solution is suggested for greater efficacy.
- There is not enough data to recommend the 5% minoxidil foam instead of the 5% solution.
- The response to treatment should be assessed at 6 months. If successful, treatment needs to be continued to maintain efficacy.

Oral finasteride

- Oral finasteride 1 mg a day is recommended to improve or to prevent progression of androgenetic alopecia in male patients older than 18 years with mild to moderate androgenetic alopecia (Norwood–Hamilton IIv–V).
- The response to treatment should be assessed at 6 months, although in some men it may not become evident until 12 months. If successful, treatment needs to be continued to maintain efficacy.
- There is insufficient evidence to support the use of topical finasteride.
- For greater efficacy, the combination of oral finaseride 1 mg/1 × /d and topical minoxidil 2%–5% solution, 2 × /d can be considered.

Hormonal treatments

- The use of oral estrogens or androgen-receptor-antagonists is inappropriate to improve or prevent progression of androgenetic alopecia in male patients.
- There is insufficient evidence to support the use of topical alfatradiol to improve or prevent progression of androgenetic alopecia in male patients.
- It is suggested that topical fluridil or topical fulvestrant should not be used in male patients with androgenetic alopecia.

Surgical treatments

- Surgery, especially follicular unit transplantation (FUT), can be considered in male patients with sufficient donor hair.
- It is suggested that FUT to be combined with finasteride 1 mg daily to achieve a better clinical outcome.

Source: Adapted from Blumeyer A, Tosti A, Messenger A et al. *J Dtsch Dermatol.* 2011;Ges;9 Suppl 6:S1–S57.

action on hair growth is poorly understood. Minoxidil is a potassium-channel opener and vasodilator, and it has been reported to stimulate the production of vascular endothelial growth factor (VEGF) in cultured dermal papilla cells.[19] There is evidence that this effect is mediated by adenosine and sulfonylurea receptors, which are well-known target receptors for adenosine-triphosphate-sensitive potassium channel openers.[20]

Table 6.4 Miscellaneous Treatments with Insufficient or Lacking Evidence for Efficacy and Proposed Mechanisms of Action in Treatment of Androgenetic Alopecia

Promotion of hair regrowth

- Amino acids
- Iron supplements in absence of efficiency
- Vitamins (biotin, niacin derivates)
- Proanthocyanidines
- Millet seed (silic acid, amino acids, vitamins, minerals)
- Marine extract and silicea component
- Chinese herbals
- Ginkgo biloba
- Aloe vera
- Ginseng
- Bergamot
- Hibiscus
- Sorphora
- Caffeine
- Melatonin
- Retinoids
- Ciclosporine
- Electromagnetic/electrostatic field
- Low-level laser

Improved perifollicular vascularization

- Prostaglandins (viprostol, latanoprost)
- Aminexil
- Glyceroloxyesters and silicium
- Minerals
- Niacin derivatives
- Mesotherapy

DHT-inhibitory activity

- Saw palmetto
- ß-sitosterol
- Polysorbate 60
- Green tea
- *Cimicifuga racemosa*

Anti-inflammatory activity

- Ketoconazol
- Zinc pyrithione
- Corticosteroids

Improved hair nutrition

- Vitamins (biotin, niacin derivates)
- Trace elements (zinc, copper)

Others

- Botulinum toxin

Source: Adapted from Blumeyer A, Tosti A, Messenger A et al. *J Dtsch Dermatol.* 2011;Ges;9 Suppl 6:S1–S57.

Autologous hair transplantation represents the only treatment that can produce substantial improvement in patients with advanced hair loss and can give satisfactory results, as long as the patient has a realistic expectation regarding the treatment results.[21] Hair line design, evaluation of the donor and recipient areas, as well as discussion of graft numbers, are basic parts of the hair transplant consultation. There are two donor hair harvesting techniques that are performed under local anesthesia: in one technique, a strip of scalp skin is taken from the occipital area, which then is divided into mini- or micrografts, each containing 1–4 hairs. The grafts are then planted into tiny slits in the desired recipient area. The other technique is follicular unit extraction (FUE): multiple follicles are harvested with small 1-mm punches and planted in the target area, avoiding the occipital linear scar of the strip technique. However, FUE is more labor intensive and therefore usually more expensive. A natural looking result can be achieved with both procedures. One or two sessions usually provide good coverage of a balding recipient area. Final results are usually seen 6–8 months after the surgery.

BEYOND EVIDENCE-BASED MEDICINE

Although EBM has become the gold standard for clinical practice, there are a number of limitations of its use (summarized in Table 6.5).

In EBM, the expert opinion is considered to be the least valid form of evidence. Nevertheless, knowledge gained from clinical research does not directly answer the primary clinical question of what is best for the patient at hand, and suggests that EBM should not discount the value of clinical experience. Good medical practice means integrating individual clinical expertise with the best available external clinical evidence from EBM.

For successful management of male androgenetic alopecia, one must remain open-minded for the possibility of a multitude of cause-relationships underlying hair loss, and accordingly for the potential of combination treatments.[22] It is important to manage male androgenetic alopecia strategically, with the variety of current therapeutic options depending on the individual's needs. Ultimately, combination treatments with topical minoxidil, oral finasteride, nutritional supplements, surgery, low-level laser therapy, and appropriate scalp care may act synergistically. The scientific rationale for such an approach is given, but—again—there is a need for clinical studies to establish an increase in efficacy of combination regimens and adjuvant treatments.

Table 6.5 Limitations of EBM

- EBM guidelines do not remove the problem of extrapolation to different populations or longer time frames
- Even if several top-quality studies are available, questions always remain about how far, and to which populations, their results may be generalized
- Certain groups have been historically underresearched, such as racial minorities and people with comorbid diseases, and thus the literature is sparse in areas that do not allow for generalizing
- EBM applies to groups of people, but this does not preclude clinicians from using their personal experience in deciding how to treat an individual subject

Finally, the influence of the prescribing physician should be kept in mind, because inspiring confidence versus skepticism and fear clearly impacts the outcome of treatment.[22] Treatment success relies on patient compliance that, on its part, relies on comprehension of treatment benefit, confidence, and motivation. A positive physician–patient relationship and regular follow-up visits (at 3, 6, 12, and 24 months; Figure 6.1a–e), including standardized photographic assessments, are the most important factors in determining the degree of patient compliance. The overall goal is to gain short-term compliance as a prerequisite to long-term adherence to treatment. Recommendations for improvement of patient compliance are summarized in Table 6.6.

More recently, the post-finasteride syndrome has been claimed to occur in men who have taken oral finasteride to treat either hair loss or benign prostatic hyperplasia. Reported symptoms include persistent loss of libido, erectile dysfunction, reduction in penis size, penile curvature or reduced sensation, gynecomastia, muscle atrophy, cognitive impairment, severely dry skin, and depression. The condition allegedly may have a life-altering impact on sufferers and their families, such as job loss and the break-up of romantic relationships or marriages, while also being linked to suicides.[23] As yet, the condition is not recognized by the scientific community, although individuals who suffer from the syndrome do present with distinctive and relatively homogenous symptoms. Even though the incidence of persistent sexual, mental, and physical side effects which continue despite quitting finasteride is unknown, it is likely that over 1000 men worldwide are experiencing the effects. This estimate is based on the number of registered users on the Internet forum www.propeciahelp.com. The Post-Finasteride Syndrome Foundation (www.pfsfoundation.org) is a nonprofit organization dedicated to helping fund research on the characterization, underlying biologic mechanisms, and treatments of the post-finasteride syndrome, while improving public awareness of the condition.

There are no predictive factors for the risk of development of post-finasteride syndrome, and there are no known treatments for the disorder. Preliminary recommendations for the prescription of oral finasteride in the treatment of male androgenetic alopecia are summarized in Table 6.7.

HAIR CARE

A majority of current treatments associated with thinning hair, such as androgenetic alopecia and aging hair,

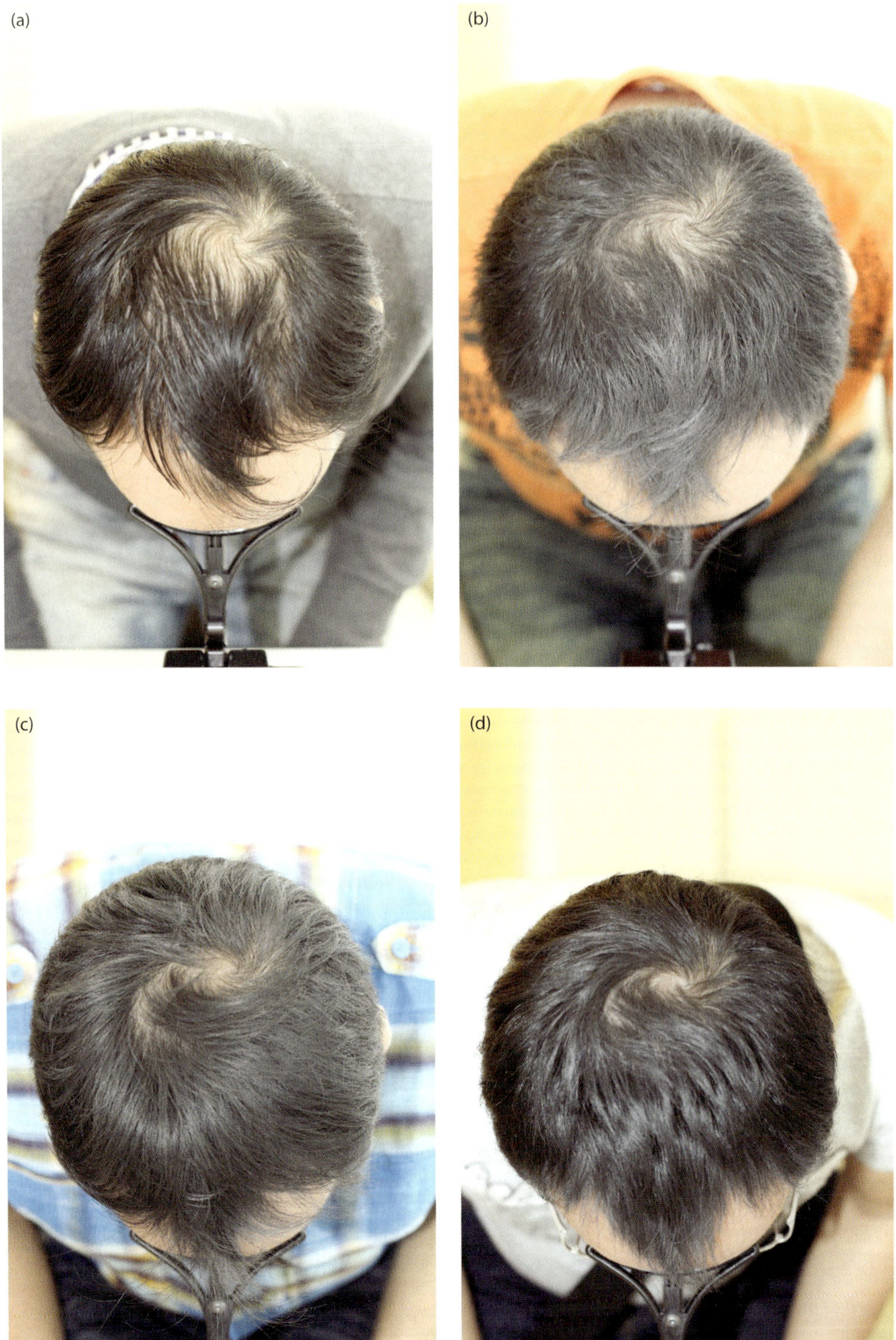

Figure 6.1 (a–e) Photographic documentation of successful combination treatment in a 45-year-old male with 1-mg oral finasteride and topical 5% minoxidil solution bid, (a) before, (b) after 3 months, (c) 6 months, (d) 12 months, and (e) 24 months. *(Continued)*

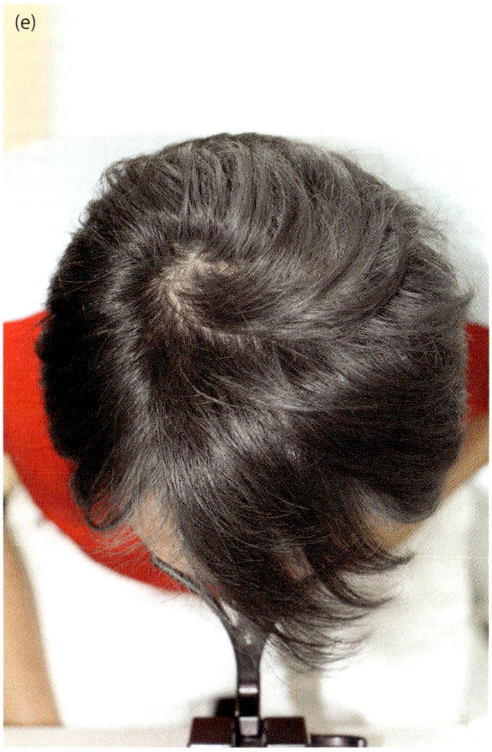

Figure 6.1 (Continued) (a–e) **Photographic documentation of successful combination treatment in a 45-year-old male with 1-mg oral finasteride and topical 5% minoxidil solution bid, (a) before, (b) after 3 months, (c) 6 months, (d) 12 months, and (e) 24 months.**

are focused on improving scalp hair density, and on preventing further damage of the hair fiber. The efficacy of hair growth-promoting agents in shampoo form is questionable, given their dilution with water and short contact time, unless they can be absorbed in effective quantities. Nevertheless, since hair fiber diameter has been recognized to represent another key contributor to hair thinning, a novel leave-on technology has been developed that combines caffeine, niacinamide, panthenol, dimethicone, and an acrylate polymer (CNPDA) to affect the diameter and behavior of individual scalp hair fibers as an approach to improve decreasing fiber diameter. Utilizing a laser scan micrometer for assessment of fiber diameter measures, and tensile break stress and torsion pendulum testing for assessment of behavioral properties, it was found that CNPDA significantly increased the diameter of individual terminal scalp hair fibers by 2–5 μm, which yields an increase in the cross-sectional area of approximately 10. Beyond the increase in hair fiber diameter, the CNPDA-thickened fibers demonstrated enhanced mechanical properties characteristic of thicker fibers, such as increased suppleness/

Table 6.6 Recommendations for Improvement of Patient Compliance

- Only recommend treatments that are effective in circumstances when they are required
- Prescribe the minimum number of different medications (e.g., combining active ingredients into a single compound)
- Simplify dosage regimen by selecting different treatment or using a preparation that needs fewer doses during the day
- Select treatments with lower levels of side effects or fewer concerns for long-term risks
- Discuss possible side effects, and whether it is important to continue medication regardless of those effects
- Advise on minimizing or coping with side effects
- Provide regular follow-up for reassurance on drug safety and treatment benefits
- Develop trust so patients do not fear embarrassment or anger if unable to take a particular drug, allowing the doctor to propose a more acceptable alternative

Source: With kind permission from Springer Science+Business Media: *Male Alopecia. Guide to Successful Management*, Cham, 2014, Switzerland: Springer International Publishing, Trüeb RM, Lee W-S.

Table 6.7 Recommendations for Prescription of Oral Finasteride in Treatment of Male Androgenetic Alopecia

- Note that efficacy and safety of oral finasteride for treatment of male androgenetic alopecia in men aged 18 through 40 with mild to moderate androgenetic alopecia (Hamilton–Norwood IIv–V) have been demonstrated.[a]
- Refrain from prescribing oral finasteride to a patient with a personal history of depression, sexual dysfunction, or fertility problems.
- When fertility is an issue, consider performing a sperm count before and during treatment with oral finasteride.
- In any case of adverse effects, immediately stop oral finasteride treatment.
- In all men 45 and over, perform PSA before starting therapy with oral finasteride, after starting therapy, and thereafter on a twice-yearly basis. The level should drop by ca. 50% upon initiation of therapy. In case of increase >0.4 ng/mL per year, refer to a urologist to check prostate condition.
- Note that for men who choose regular prostate-cancer screening, the use of oral finasteride meaningfully reduces the risk of prostate cancer.[b]

Source: With kind permission from Springer Science+Business Media: *Male Alopecia. Guide to Successful Management*, Cham, 2014, Switzerland: Springer International Publishing, Trüeb RM, Lee W-S.

[a] See also Finasteride Male Pattern Hair Loss Study Group. *Eur J Dermatol.* 2002;12:38–49.

[b] See also LeFevre A. *N Engl J Med.* 2013;369:670–671.

pliability and better ability to withstand force without breaking.[24]

In summary, although cosmetic treatments will not reverse the process of androgenetic alopecia, new technologies help to mitigate the effects of androgenetic alopecia-related thinning of hair.

CONCLUDING REMARKS

Mainstream scientists are currently working on gene polymorphisms diagnostics for prediction of risk, prevention, diagnosis, and targeted treatment development for male androgenetic alopecia, on stem cell technologies, and on bioengineering of the hair follicle. Meanwhile, healthcare providers are becoming increasingly aware of a more holistic approach toward successful treatment of hair loss in men, to include awareness, lifestyle, environmental factors, nutrition, EBM-guided pharmacotherapy and medical devices, surgery, and hair care.

REFERENCES

1. Trüeb RM, de Viragh PA, and Swiss Trichology Study Group. Status of scalp hair and therapy of alopecia in men in Switzerland. *Praxis (Bern 1994)*. 2001;90:241–248.
2. Trüeb RM. The difficult hair loss patient: A particular challenge. *Int J Trichoology*. 2013;5:110–111.
3. Descartes R. *Rules for the Direction of the Mind*. Indianapolis, Indiana: Bobbs-Merrill Co.; 2000.
4. Norwood OT. Male-pattern baldness. Classification and incidence. *South Med J*. 1975;68:1359–1370.
5. Paus R, Cotsarelis G. The biology of hair follicles. *N Engl J Med*. 1999;341:491–497.
6. Kaufman KD. Androgen metabolism as it affects hair growth in androgenetic alopecia. *Dermatol Clin*. 1996;14:697–711.
7. Trüeb RM. Molecular mechanisms of androgenetic alopecia. *Exp Gerontol*. 2002;37:981–990.
8. Naito A, Midorikawa T, Yoshino T, Ohdera M. Lipid peroxides induce early onset of catagen phase in murine hair cycles. *Int J Mol Med*. 2008;22:725–729.
9. Bahta AW, Farjo N, Farjo B, Philpott MP. Premature senescence of balding dermal papilla cells *in vitro* is associated with p16(INK4a) expression. *J Invest Dermatol*. 2008;128:1088–1094.
10. Su L-S, Chen T H-H. Association of androgenetic alopecia with smoking and its prevalence among Asian men. *Arch Dermatol*. 2007;143:1401–1406.
11. Trüeb RM. Is androgenetic alopecia a photoaggravated dermatosis? *Dermatology*. 2003;207:343–348.
12. Jaworsky C, Kligman AM, Murphy GF. Characterisation of inflammatory infiltrates in male pattern alopecia: Implication for pathogenesis. *Br J Dermatol*. 1992;127:239–246.
13. Mahé YF, Michelet JF, Billoni N et al. Androgenetic alopecia and microinflammation. *Int J Dermatol*. 2000;39:576–584.
14. Whiting DA. Diagnostic and predictive value of horizontal sections of scalp biopsy specimens in male pattern androgenetic alopecia. *J Am Acad Dermatol*. 1993;28:755–763.
15. Feinstein AR. *Clinical Judgement*. Philadelphia, PA: Williams & Wilkins; 1967.
16. Cochrane AL. *Effectiveness and Efficiency: Random Reflections on Health Services*. London: Nuffield Provincial Hospitals Trust; 1972.
17. Blumeyer A, Tosti A, Messenger A et al. Evidence-based (S3) guideline for the treatment of androgenetic alopecia in women and in men. *J Dtsch Dermatol*. 2011;Ges;9 Suppl 6:S1–S57.
18. Kaufman KD, Olsen EA, Whiting D et al. Finasteride in the treatment of men with androgenetic alopecia. Finasteride male pattern hair losss study group. *J Am Acad Dermatol*. 1998;39:578–589.
19. Lachgar S, Charveron M, Gall Y, Bonafe JL. Minoxidil upregulates the expression of vascular endothelial growth factor in human hair dermal papilla cells. *Br J Dermatol*. 1998;138:407–411.
20. Li M, Marubayashi A, Nakaya Y, Fukui K, Arase S. Minoxidil-induced hair growth is mediated by adenosine in cultured dermal papilla cells: Possible involvement of sulfonylurea receptor 2B as a target of minoxidil. *J Invest Dermatol*. 2001;117:1594–1600.
21. Bunagan MJ, Banka N, Shapiro J. Hair transplantation update: Procedural techniques, innovations, and applications. *Dermatol Clin*. 2013;31:141–153.
22. Trüeb RM, Lee W-S. *Male Alopecia. Guide to Successful Treatment*. Cham, Switzerland: Springer International Publishing; 2014.
23. Irwig MS. Persistent sexual side effects of finasteride: Could they be permanent? *J Sex Med*. 2012;9:2927–2932.
24. Davis MG, Thomas JH, van de Velde S et al. A novel cosmetic approach to treat thinning hair. *Br J Dermatol*. 2011;165 Suppl 3:24–30.

7 Management of female androgenetic alopecia

Bianca Maria Piraccini and Aurora Alessandrini

Female androgenetic alopecia (AGA) is the most common form of alopecia in women, occurring in up to 50% of women in the course of their life.[1] It appears in most cases after the age of 60, but onset in young adult females is not rare.[2] Rapid appearance of patterned thinning in a premenopausal woman should always suggest a possible hormonal disease. Progression is also slower than in males, with generally a more diffuse involvement of the scalp. Patients usually complain of progressive hair thinning, and/or loss of hair volume, or about a continuous or intermittent hair shedding.

In women three different patterns[3] can be observed: (1) diffuse thinning of the crown region with maintenance of the frontal hairline (Ludwig type) (Figure 7.1); (2) thinning and widening of the central part of the scalp with breach in the frontal hairline (Christmas tree pattern) (Figure 7.2); (3) more rare, thinning associated with bitemporal recession (Hamilton type) (Figure 7.3), usually observed in postmenopausal women and in women with hyperandrogenism.

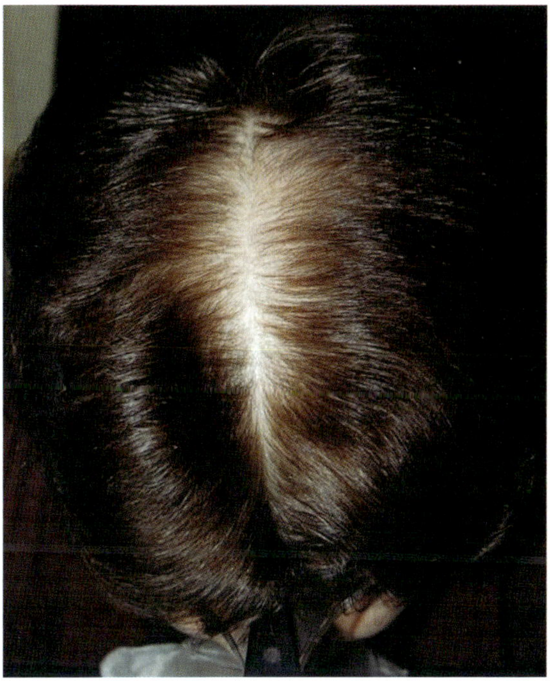

Figure 7.1 **Ludwig-type androgenetic alopecia: widening of the medial hairline.**

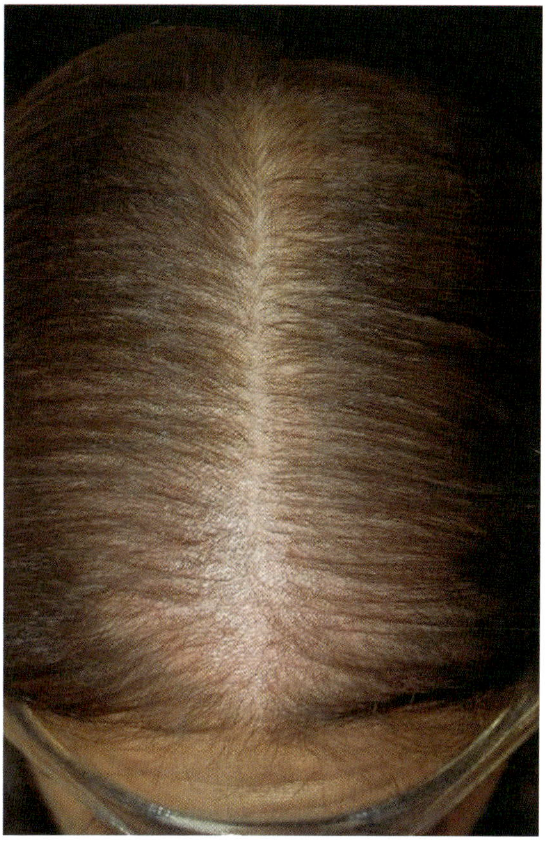

Figure 7.2 **Christmas tree pattern: widening of the central line from the back to the frontal area.**

Involvement of the parietal and occipital scalp with diffuse alopecia can be seen as well.

The hairs of the affected regions are both decreased in number, and reduced in diameter, length, and pigmentation; they are less evident and therefore no more able to cover the scalp adequately. Complete miniaturization only affects a percentage of the hair, which assumes the appearance defined as *vellus*, while the majority of hair acquires border-line characters, keeping the pigment and reaching partially intermediate thickness, between vellus hairs and normal ones.

Hair thinning has an important impact on a woman's quality of life, and a treatment should always be advised.[4]

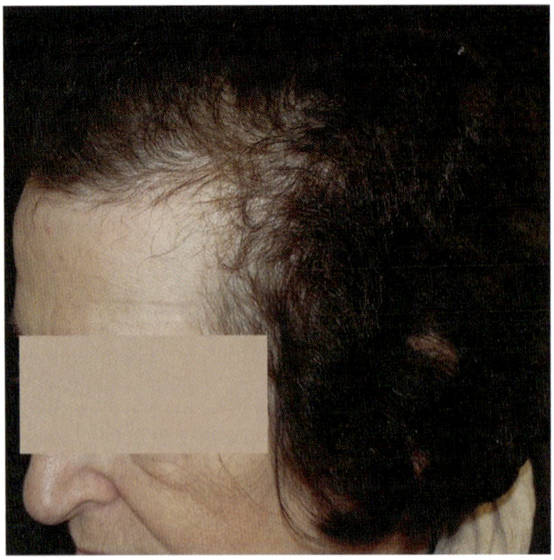

Figure 7.3 **Androgenetic alopecia in a female with a male pattern: receding frontotemporal hairline.**

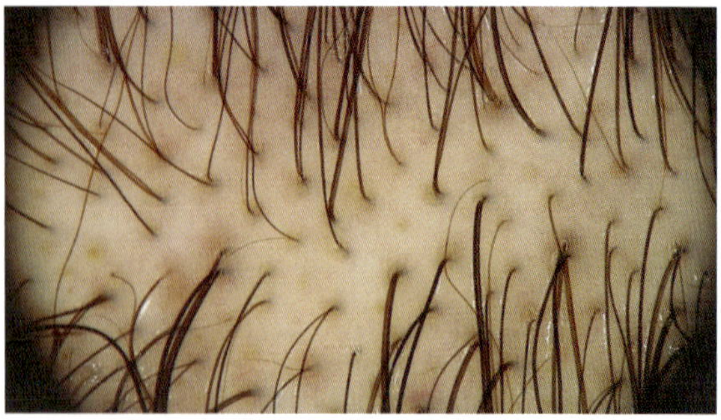

Figure 7.4 **Scalp videodermoscopy of female androgenetic alopecia: hair diameter variability, yellow dots, and perifollicular halos.**

FIRST STEP FOR CORRECT MANAGEMENT OF FEMALE ANDROGENETIC ALOPECIA (AGA): ESTABLISH THE DIAGNOSIS

Diagnosis of AGA is simple in most cases. The patient complains of a slowly progressive hair thinning, which is not generally associated with increased hair shedding. Patients usually report a change in consistency and thickness of the hair, which appears thinner. The history of acute hair shedding is indicative of an associated acute telogen effluvium. Telogen effluvium may in fact be associated with AGA, and in some cases it may induce the onset of the condition or its worsening. It is therefore important to understand if the patient complains of thinning alone or of an associated hair shedding. Causes of this acute telogen effluvium may include drugs, crush diets, systemic disease, and childbirth.

Clinical examination should start with evaluation of the density of hair in the different areas of the scalp. Comparing the density of hair in the crown region with that of the occipital region can be very helpful to differentiate mild forms of AGA from diffuse hair loss. The pull test may be negative or may reveal an increased telogen shedding. The presence of telogen hairs, shorter than 3 cm, representing the telogen phase of miniaturized follicles, is diagnostic for AGA. Variation in the hair shaft diameter is typical of AGA and is an important feature for early diagnosis of the disease. This can be better visualized using scalp dermoscopy[5] (Figure 7.4). The dermoscopic features of AGA are variation of the hair shaft diameter, empty follicles phenomenon, peripilar depressions, pigmentation, and inflammation of the scalp. (1) Variation of the diameter of the hair is diagnostic of AGA. A variation in diameter affecting >20% of hair in androgen regions is seen. Under the effect of androgens, hair follicles undergo a progressive miniaturization and produce a hair shaft that is gradually thinner and less pigmented. Follicular miniaturization initially involves the adjacent follicles in a different extent: in the initial forms of androgenetic alopecia, using scalp dermoscopy, we can see in the same area hair of normal diameter, hair slightly thinner, and very thin and short hair (diameter <0.3 mm). A diagnosis of early forms, which are not recognized by clinical examination alone, is then possible. In the most severe forms of AGA, the miniaturization affects follicles diffusely, and the hair shafts are uniformly thin. (2) The empty follicle phenomenon is another pathogenetic factor of AGA. Empty follicles appear as yellow spots (yellow dots) on the scalp. The yellow color is due to the fact that the follicular ostium, more or less dilated, contains sebum produced by sebaceous glands associated with the follicle. They can be seen especially in the frontal area. (3) Peripilar depressions, also called *peripilar halos*, appear as dark halos extended approximately 1 mm around the follicular ostium from which the hair emerges. They are specific and characteristic of androgenetic alopecia and occur more often in patients with mild forms of androgenetic alopecia, with a high density of hair.

A scalp biopsy is very useful in doubtful cases: in longitudinal sections the detection of the miniaturized follicles is diagnostic. Important findings are a decrease of terminal hairs, anagen hairs, and an increase of vellus-like hairs, telogen hairs, and fibrous streamers. A mild to moderately dense perifollicular lymphohistiocytic inflammatory infiltrate may be seen around the infundibulum.

SECOND STEP FOR CORRECT MANAGEMENT OF FEMALE AGA: DEFINE SEVERITY OF DISEASE

According to the classification proposed by Ludwig, female AGA can be divided into three grades of severity.[6] The first grade is characterized by a slight thinning of hair located in the central-parietal region. In the second grade, we observe an accentuation of thinning hair in the vertex and central-parietal regions. In the third grade, there is a more pronounced thinning of the hair in the central and parietal regions, up to a stage of severe alopecia, in which the frontal and occipital areas are still preserved, with hair thinning also involving the regions in front of the ears and at the sides of the head. This grade of severity scarcely benefits from medical cure, as whatever the improvement the patient achieves, the alopecia remains evident. Hair transplantation is a possible solution in these cases.[7]

THIRD STEP FOR CORRECT MANAGEMENT OF FEMALE AGA: VERIFY PRESENCE OF HYPERANDROGENISM

In premenopausal women, AGA may be a cutaneous sign of hyperandrogenism, together with acnes, hirsutism, irregular menses, and signs of virilization (Figure 7.5). In patients with severe AGA, it is important to rule out disorders associated with excessive production of androgens, such as polycystic ovary syndrome (PCOS), found in about 30% of women with AGA. Other more rare conditions characterized by excessive androgen production are congenital adrenal hyperplasia and ovarian cancers. Laboratory investigations are necessary only in those patients with signs of hyperandrogenism, like acnes and/or hirsutism, in which several examinations are mandatory (FSH, LH, Testosterone, free testosterone, DHEA, DHEA-S, androstenedione, 17OH- progesterone, prolactin, SHBG, cortisol, ACTH test, thyroid function, ovary scan).

DECIDE BEST TREATMENT FOR PATIENT

If used correctly, available medical treatments for AGA arrest the progression of the disease and reverse

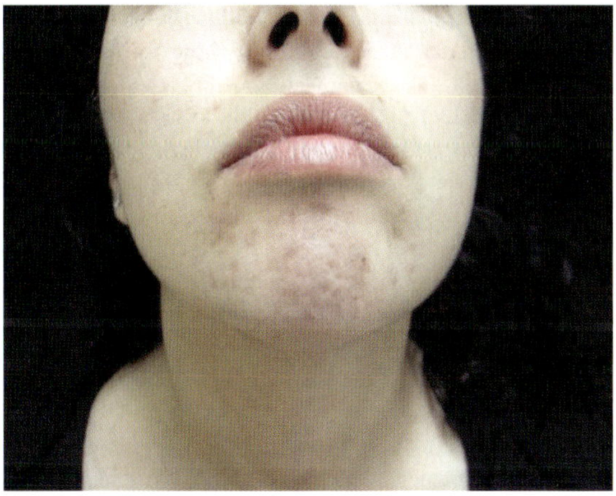

Figure 7.5 **Signs of hyperandrogenism in a young women with androgenetic alopecia: acnes and hirsutism.**

miniaturization in most cases.[8] As advanced stages are unlikely to benefit from medical treatment, hair replacement surgery should be discussed in these cases.

Topical minoxidil

Minoxidil, 2,6-diamino-4-piperidinopyrimidine 1-oxide, exerts its effects via its active metabolite minoxidil sulfate, which is produced in some tissues, including the hair follicle. The drug mechanism of action on the follicles is still unclear, but is not androgen-dependent: the drug probably increases the anagen phase duration and promotes the increase of hair diameter. This results in progressive reversion of miniaturization. Topical minoxidil at 2% or 5% concentrations should be applied twice a day on the affected areas. A recent study in women showed that once a day application of minoxidil 5% is not inferior, and is as effective for stimulating hair growth as twice a day application of minoxidil 2%, and is associated with several aesthetic and practical advantages.[9] Another recent study[10] confirms the data of the literature and the evidence coming from years of clinical experience, that twice a day topical application of 5% minoxidil solution is effective in the treatment of male and female androgenetic alopecia, with evident efficacy already visible after 6 months. Minoxidil is the drug of choice in normoandrogenic premenopausal women, and is also useful in postmenopausal women.[11]

Side effects of topical minoxidil include scalp irritation, allergic contact dermatitis, and reversible hypertrichosis, located on the face and due to local contamination, or on distal regions, like arms, suggesting drug absorption. Irritant or allergic contact dermatitis due to minoxidil solution presents as scalp itching: in these patients, it is useful to perform patch testing with minoxidil alone and with propylene glycol at 30%. Minoxidil 5% in a foam vehicle is a good alternative option for patients with contact allergy to propylene glycol.

According to the package insert, minoxidil is contraindicated during pregnancy and breastfeeding, because only a few studies have defined the safety profile of minoxidil when taken during pregnancy. The drug is capable of crossing biologic barriers, accumulating in the lipids, so that brain and fetal concentrations may be higher than those found in serum.

Treatments should be continued for at least 6 months before assessing efficacy. Dermoscopy allows better visualization of the initial hair thickening. Regular drug use is mandatory for maintaining results. Minoxidil interruption often produces an acute telogen effluvium that starts 3–4 months after discontinuation of the drug. Drug withdrawal leads to loss of all beneficial effects after 6 months.

Systemic antiandrogens

They include androgen receptor antagonists, such as cyproterone acetate, flutamide, and spironolactone, and 5-alpha reductase inhibitors, such as finasteride and dutasteride. They are commonly used in women with signs of hyperandrogenism, because they compete with androgens for androgen receptors or reduce serum concentrations of dihydrotestosterone (DHT).

Cyproterone acetate acts by interfering with the binding of 5-alpha DHT to the androgen receptor and by inhibiting the secretion of FSH and LH, as the result of its progestinic action. A dose of 100 mg a day, administered in the first 10 days of the menstrual cycle,[12] and at the dose of 50 mg a day in postmenopausal women,[13] can be useful in women with biochemical hyperandrogenism. Contemporary administration of estrogen (ethynyl estradiol or oral contraceptives) is mandatory, due to the potential of these drugs to feminize a male fetus. Side effects include loss of libido, mood swings, fatigue, mastodynia, hypertension, and weight gain. It is contraindicated in patients with liver disease.

Spironolactone is an aldosterone antagonist and also an inhibitor of androgen synthesis. A dose of 200 mg a day is effective in inducing hair growth in women with loss of hair.[14] In the event that spironolactone is used, recall that it is pregnancy category D: patients should ideally be on birth control. The drug can increase serum potassium levels.

Finasteride is a selective inhibitor of type 2 5-alpha reductase, which catalyzes the conversion of testosterone in DHT. By this inhibition, serum and scalp levels of DHT become lower, while scalp levels of testosterone increase. In females, oral finasteride should only be prescribed in postmenopausal women or in women willing to use oral contraceptives. The drug is contraindicated in women who may become pregnant (or are pregnant), because it can cause feminization of a male fetus. A recent study has shown that oral finasteride, 5 mg a day, may be an effective and safe treatment for normoandrogenic women with AGA.[15]

Dutasteride acts by blocking both isoenzymes of 5-alpha reductase (type I and II). In men, dutasteride seems to be three times more potent then finasteride in the inhibition of type II alpha reductase and more than 100 times more potent in the inhibition of type I isoenzyme, decreasing serum DHT levels of 90% versus 70%.[16] Studies with this drug in women are lacking, and a single case report has been published.[17]

PROGNOSIS

Family history is of great importance for prognosis. AGA is a progressive disease that, if left untreated, tends to worsen with time. Progression of the disease can be slow or very fast, especially in patients with a strong family history or with hormonal disturbances. Rapid progression of AGA is also observed after any pathological condition that induces telogen effluvium.

REFERENCES

1. Gan DC, Sinclair RD. Prevalence of male and female pattern hair loss in Maryborough. *J Investig Dermatol Symp Proc.* 2005;10:184–189.
2. Messenger AG. Hair through the female life cycle. *Br J Dermatol.* 2011;165:2–6.
3. Blume-Peytavi U, Blumeyer A, Tosti A et al. European consensus group. S1 guideline for diagnostic evaluation in androgenetic alopecia in men, women and adolescents. *Br J Dermatol.* 2011;164:5–15.
4. Zhuang XS, Zheng YY, Xu JJ et al. Quality of life in women with female pattern hair loss and the impact of topical minoxidil treatment on quality of life in these patients. *Exp Ther Med.* 2013;6:542–546.
5. Ross EK, Vincenzi C, Tosti A. Videodermoscopy in the evaluation of hair and scalp disorders. *J Am Acad Dermatol.* 2006;55:799–806.
6. Ludwig E. Classification of the types of androgenetic alopecia (common baldness) occurring in the female sex. *Br J Dermatol.* 1977;97:247–254.
7. Unger RH. Female hair restoration. *Facial Plast Surg Clin North Am.* 2013;21:407–417.
8. van Zuuren EJ, Fedorowicz Z, Carter B et al. Interventions for female pattern hair loss. *Cochrane Database Syst Rev.* 2012;5:CD007628.
9. Blume-Peytavi U, Hillmann K, Dietz E et al. A randomized, single-blind trial of 5% minoxidil foam once daily versus 2% minoxidil solution twice daily in the treatment of androgenetic alopecia in women. *J Am Acad Dermatol.* 2011;65:1126–1134.
10. Piraccini B, Starace M, Alessandrini A et al. Efficacy and tolerability of 5% minoxidil solution (Carexidil®) in male and female androgenetic alopecia: A 6-month open multicentric study. *G Ital Dermatol Venereol.* 2011;146(6 suppl 1):1–8.
11. Camacho-Martínez FM. Hair loss in women. *Semin Cutan Med Surg.* 2009;28:19–32.
12. Dinh QQ, Sinclair R. Female pattern hair loss: Current treatment concepts. *Clin Interv Aging.* 2007;2:189–199.
13. Price VH. Androgenetic alopecia in women. *J Investig Dermatol Symp Proc.* 2003:8;24–27.
14. Sinclair R, Wewerinke M, Jolley D. Treatment of female pattern hair loss with oral antiandrogens. *Br J Dermatol.* 2005;152:466–473.
15. Oliveira-Soares R, E Silva JM, Correia MP, André MC. Finasteride 5 mg/day treatment of patterned hair loss in normo-androgenetic postmenopausal women. *Int J Trichology.* 2013;5:22–25.
16. Olsen EA, Hordinsky M, Whiting D et al. The importance of dual 5α-reductase inhibition in the treatment of male pattern hair loss: Results of a randomized placebo-controlled study of dutasteride versus finasteride. *J Am Acad Dermatol.* 2006;55:1014–1023.
17. Olszewska M, Rudnicka L. Effective treatment of female androgenic alopecia with dutasteride. *J Drugs Dermatol.* 2005;4:637–640.

8 Management of diffuse alopecia

Pierre Bouhanna

The term *diffuse alopecia* refers to hair loss affecting the entire scalp, with acute or chronic evolution, whose etiologic diagnosis requires thorough investigation.

Telogen effluvium is the most common hair-loss condition that presents to the dermatologist, and it is seen in all races and ethnic groups.

PATHOPHYSIOLOGY

Telogen effluvium, or excessive loss of normal hair, reflects a disturbance of the hair cycle (Figure 8.1).[1,2] At the onset of telogen effluvium, the patient presents with a perceived loss greater than 25% of scalp hair density. The shedding results in a diffuse loss with a more prominent central, frontal, and subauricular scalp loss. The hair cycle begins with the anagen growth phase of the hair follicle. The time of this phase of growth is highly variable from one individual to another, according to age, sex, and anatomical region. The anagen phase ends with the catagen phase of acute irreversible follicular involution. The hair cycle ends with the telogen or resting phase, characterized by the presence of a normal mature hair.

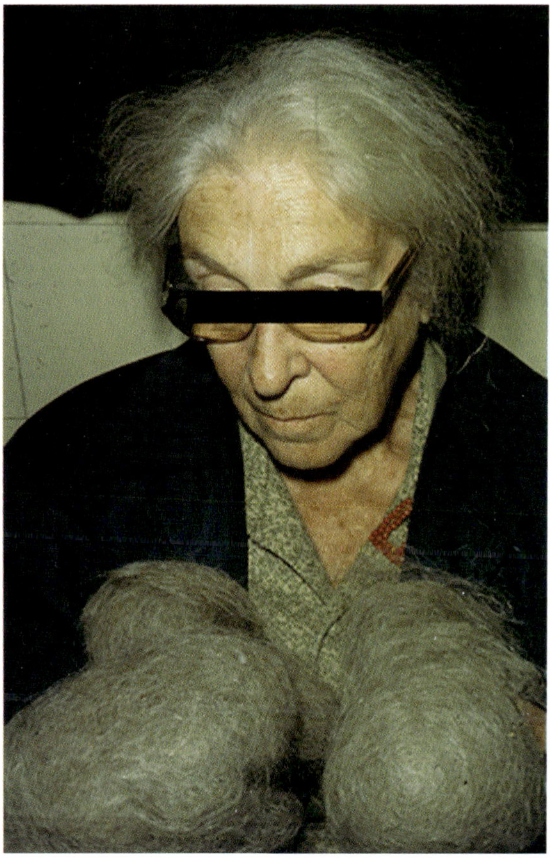

Figure 8.1 **Diffuse alopecia in a woman showing her hair loss through the hairs collected during a 2 week time period.**

The mechanisms involved in the determination of diffuse alopecia are variable and could correspond to at least five functional types of effluvium:

Type I: Premature ending of the anagen phase. This common form of telogen effluvium starts quickly, in 3–5 weeks, and is caused by some drugs, high fever, or psychological stress.

Type II: The anagen phase is unusually long; this phenomenon underlies telogen effluvium in the postpartum period.

Type III: The short anagen phase syndrome is characterized by a distinct but prolonged effluvium. Hair loss becomes clinically apparent only after a decrease of at least 50% of the duration of the anagen phase.

Type IV: Follicles in the telogen phase eliminate mature hair prematurely. This premature removal could be triggered by an extrinsic factor, such as a drug. (It seems that this phenomenon is triggered by local application of minoxidil.)

Type V: Extension of the telogen phase. This phenomenon allows the elimination of winter coats in some animals. It is triggered by the increased exposure to light and can be observed in a modified form in humans.

When a trigger is identified and removed or treated, the patient experiences diminished shedding and later regrowth of hair (Table 8.1). On occasion, the telogen effluvium will unmask an underlying androgenetic alopecia, autoimmune disease, or other disorder.

CLINICAL DIAGNOSIS

Clinical examination

The diagnosis of telogen effluvium is based on the clinical presentation and the confirmation of excess telogen hair loss. The specific time of onset is important to establish it. Telogen effluvium can start 2 weeks after a trigger but peaks between 6 and 8 weeks and then tapers off in about 6–8 weeks if the trigger is removed or treated.

Table 8.1 Telogen Effluvium Triggers

Scalp inflammation	Endocrine disorders
Seborrheic dermatitis	Hormonal changes
Nutritional deficiencies	Poor health/illness
Iron storage anemia, low zinc	Drugs
Physiological stress	Surgery
Metabolic stress	Heredity

The examination should begin with a detailed examination, specifying in particular the consumption of drugs.

The onset and the history of hair loss should be determined; abrupt onset of telogen effluvium is generally associated with a specific factor. However, a more gradual onset may reflect short anagen phase syndrome and should rule out other conditions such as alopecia areata, androgenic alopecia, and diffuse scarring alopecia.

The hair and scalp surface should be inspected. Normally, the hair diameter is uniform, and less than 10% of hair is of reduced diameter.

Additional tests

The pull-test is to do a gentle traction between the thumb and forefinger on a lock of 50–60 hairs. Normally, the number of mature hairs does not exceed five hairs (see Chapter 2) (Table 8.2).[3,4]

A trichoscopy may be helpful for a better diagnosis of the etiology.

A trichogram can detail hair loss and indicate its intensity. It confirms the telogen effluvium (cf Chapter 2).

A digital phototrichogram can be essential to assess changes in hair density. If there are numerous dystrophic anagen hairs, the diagnosis is an anagen effluvium.

Scalp biopsy is indicated when the diameter of the hair is reduced (possible androgenetic alopecia) or when there is doubt about the presence of an inflammatory alopecia (alopecia areata, for example).

Table 8.2 Telogen Effluvium Diagnostic Techniques

Clinical inspection
Visual
Wood light
Dermoscopy
Demonstration of telogen effluvium
Hair collection
Hair pull-test
Trichoscopy
Digital phototrichogram
Trichogram
Scalp biopsy

Table 8.3 Telogen Effluvium: Laboratory Evaluation

Basic
Complete blood count
Comprehensive metabolic panel
Ferritin >70
TSH, T4, antimicrosomal ab
Zinc
Extended
Androgen excess screen
Others dependent on personal and family history

Histological findings of telogen effluvium

Telogen effluvium of inflammatory origin is mainly due to infectious causes (e.g., syphilis, ringworm) and also due to certain drugs. The causes of noninflammatory telogen effluvium have the same histological characteristics: an increase in the number of follicles in the telogen phase. A 4 mm punch sample can provide evidence of this. Combined vertical and transverse sections of the biopsy contain 25–50 follicles. The proportion of follicles in the telogen phase normally does not exceed 12%–15%—if greater than 25%, a diagnosis of diffuse alopecia is favored (see Chapter 2).

Laboratory evaluation

- Ferritin–TSH–zinc
- Complete blood count
- Comprehensive metabolic panel (Table 8.3)

ETIOLOGIC DIAGNOSIS

Acute diffuse alopecia

The target factor for the telogen effluvium precedes the loss by 2–4 months. The sudden baldness predominant on the temples is reversible in 4–6 months (Table 8.4).[4–8]

The main causes are

- An important psychological stress (a serious accident, death, divorce, etc.), which in the most severe

Table 8.4 Drug Causes

Allopurinol	Beta blockers
Androgens	Ergots
Antibiotics	
Anticholesterol-statins	Dopa
Anticoagulants	Immunomodulators
Anticonvulsants	Retinoids, vitamin A
Antifungals	Psychotropics
Antihistamines H2	Minoxidil
Anti-inflammatory	Heavy metals
Antithyroid	Thallium, arsenic

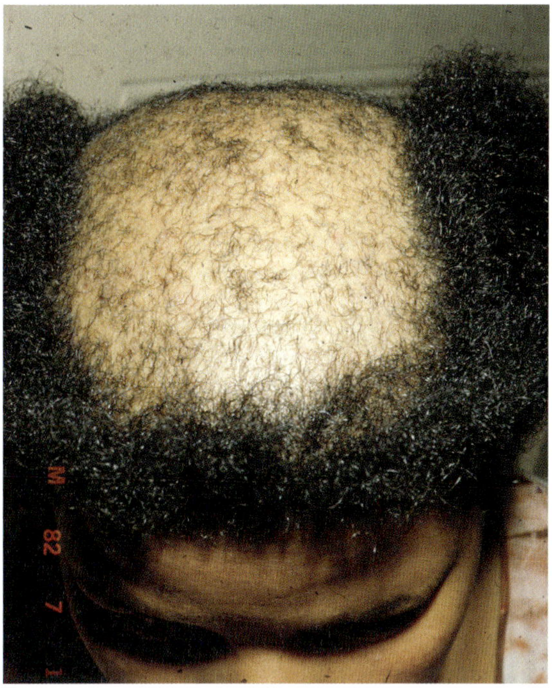

Figure 8.2 **Alopecia of the vertex, appearing suddenly in a woman after a major emotional shock (the kidnapping of her child).**

cases leads to effluvium capillorum of Sabouraud (Figure 8.2).

- Dietary history with particular attention to the "healthy diet"[9] (Figure 8.3).
- Acute hemorrhage, shock, or acute iron deficiency.[10]
- Childbirth (Figure 8.4), miscarriage, or termination of breastfeeding (progression to the hair being restored to the previous state is not certain).
- Recent medical illness with hyperthermia greater than 39.5°C[11] (Figure 8.5).
- Recent surgery under general anesthesia.
- Recent hair transplant surgery.

Toxic drug abuse (Table 8.4) is also a cause.

With *drug alopecia*,[12,13] the mode of action of the drugs that can be involved is variable:

- Inhibition of mitosis of the germinal centers.
- Disturbances of keratinization.
- Acceleration of the hair cycle with early catagen or early telogen.

Antimitotic drugs have varying potential to cause hair loss, so prevention is possible (Figure 8.6a and b). Before attributing alopecia to a drug, it should be verified that the time of onset fits with the drug administration.

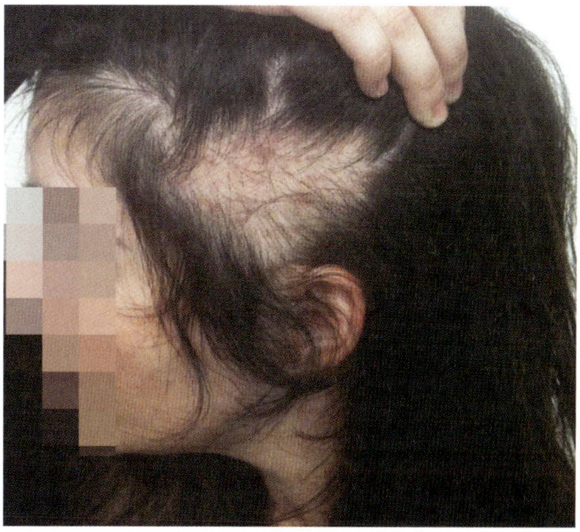

Figure 8.3 **Alopecia after "healthy diet."**

Prevention of *chemotherapy-induced alopecia* can be attempted by use of a cooling helmet or pneumatic tourniquet.

Food alopecia may be related to the ingestion of various kinds of plants containing cytostatic ingredients or antimetabolites (such as cashews).

Alopecia by occupational poisoning may occur with drugs such as thallium (used in rat poison), borax (detergents), chloroprene (rubber), or arsenic.

Radiotherapy is responsible for a reversible or permanent alopecia depending on the dose.

Chronic diffuse alopecia

Chronic diffuse alopecia can derive from persistence of acute alopecia, or have a general endocrine or metabolic cause.[14] Androgenetic alopecia in both male and female is discussed in Chapters 6 and 7 (Figures 8.7 and 8.8).

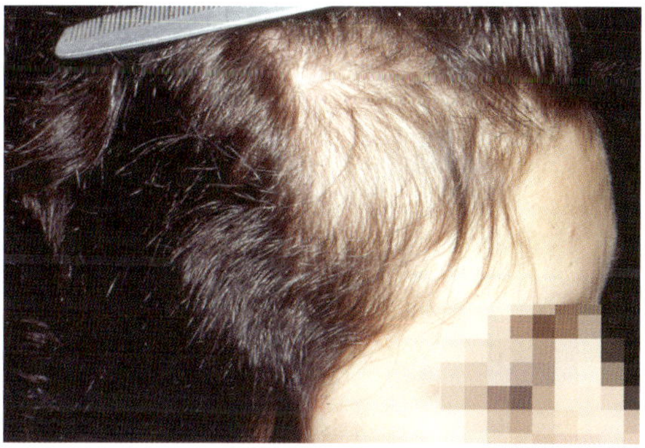

Figure 8.4 **Alopecia postpartum, appearing in the 2 months following childbirth.**

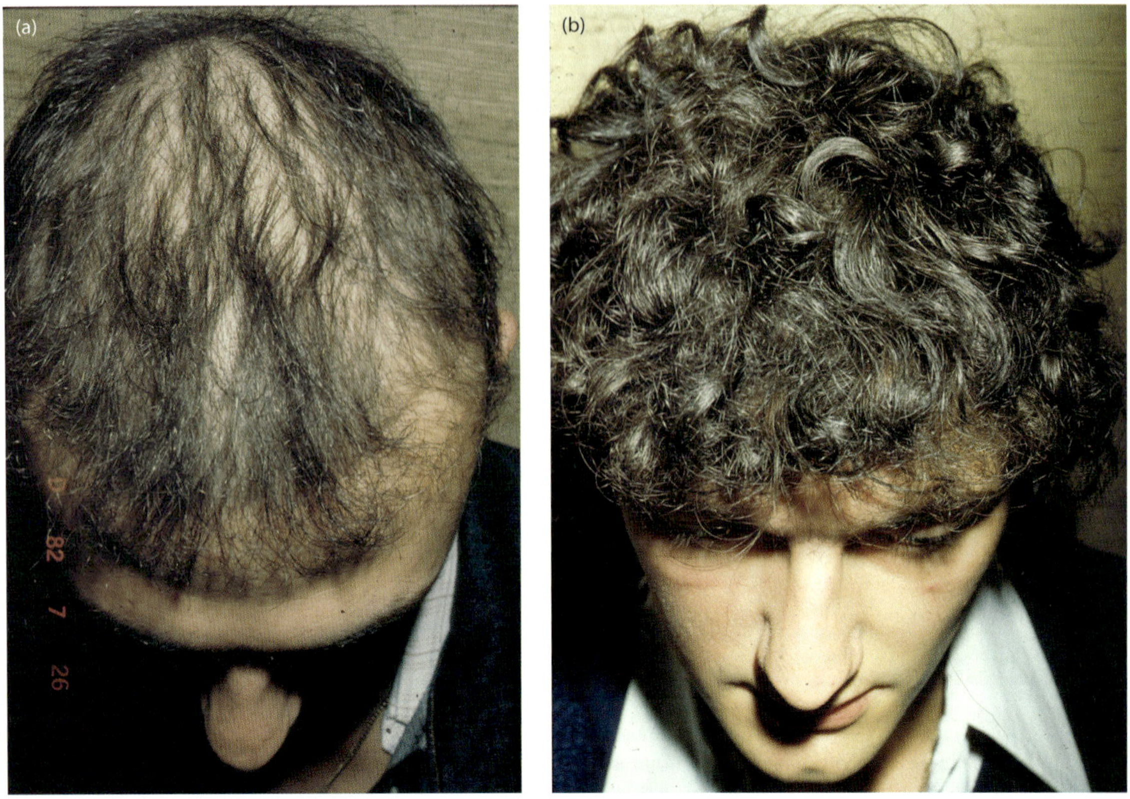

Figure 8.5 **(a) Acute diffuse alopecia in a young adult patient with acute febrile pneumonia. (b) Same patient with complete regrowth after healing of pneumonia.**

Endocrine causes

- Hyperthyroidism: Hair is thin and brittle, appearing silky.
- Hypothyroidism (Figure 8.9): Diffuse alopecia with sometimes eyebrow loss, axillary and pubic hair loss, and nail brittleness.
- Hypoparathyroidism: Hair is fine, and the nails opaque, lined, and brittle.
- Hypopituitarism: The skin is pale and associated with fine and dry hair.
- Hyperadrenocorticism: There is associated hirsutism in women.
- Uncontrolled diabetes.
- Cushing syndrome.
- Acromegaly.
- Hyperprolactinemia.

Metabolism and nutrition causes

These cause the hair to become thin, brittle, and dull:

- Iron deficiency is best studied by the dosage of ferritin rather than by determining serum iron. Blood levels less than 30 mg ferritin/mL can cause a chronic telogen effluvium (Figure 8.10).
- Folate deficiency or vitamin B_{12}.
- Vitamin D deficiency.
- Zinc deficiency,[15] acrodermatitis enteropathica.
- Nutritional deficiencies, dieting, malabsorption syndromes, parenteral nutrition.
- Spasmophilia, kidney failure, liver failure.

More rarely

- Systemic lupus erythematosus or other collagenosis syndrome.
- Secondary syphilis causes "patchy" alopecia that differs from other alopecias. It has many bald patches scattered from 1 to 3 cm in diameter, like a "clumsy scissors" cut on the temporoparietal regions (Figure 8.11).

Do not confuse

- External or traumatic causes (frequent brushings, hairstyles that involve the hair being pulled backwards (Figure 8.12), or chemicals (dyes and repeated "perm" stylings).
- Psychological causes (emotional stress, bereavement) can take over from organic causes (Figure 8.2).
- Diffuse alopecia without obvious cause can arise in 5%–40% of cases depending on the series studied.[16,17]

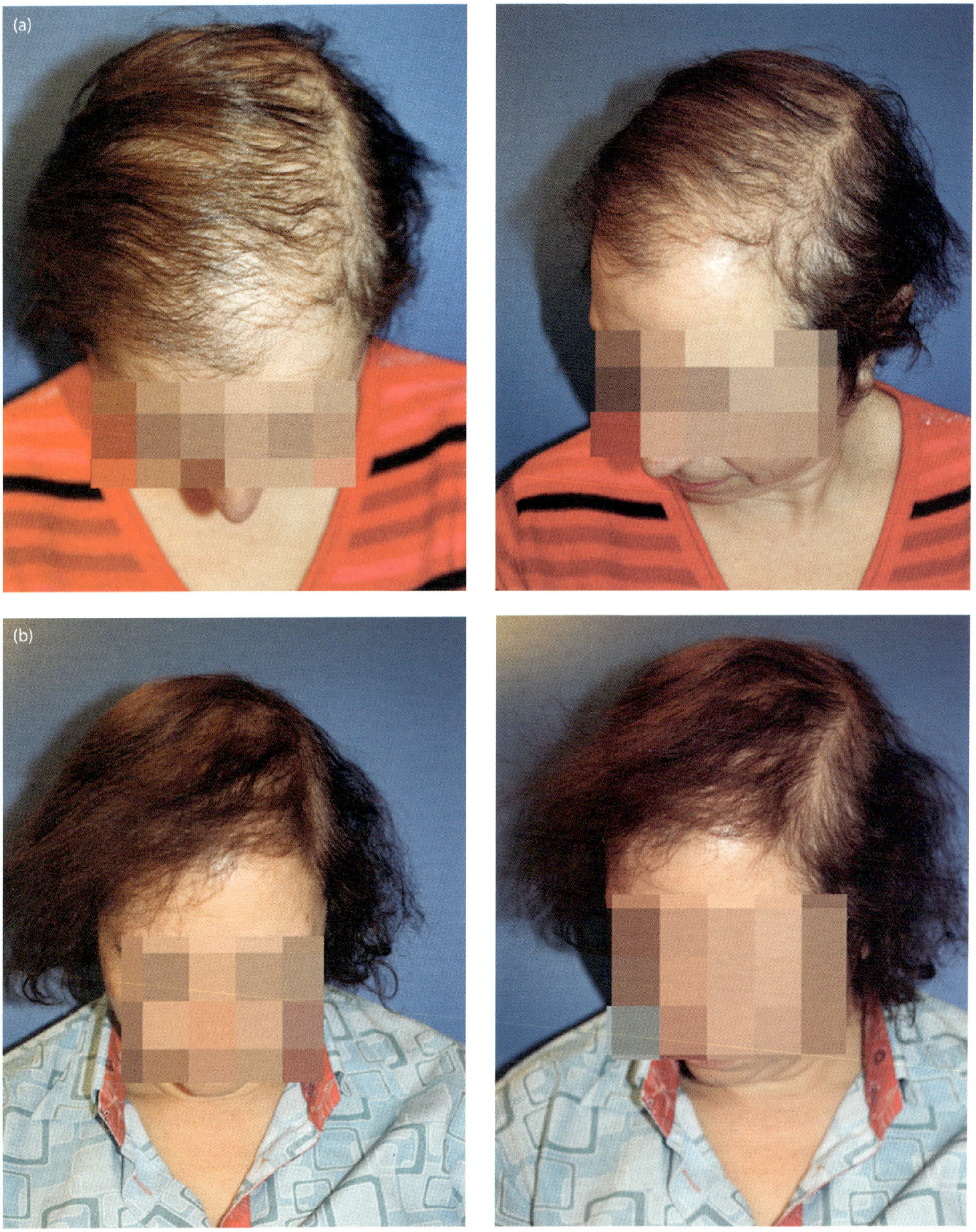

Figure 8.6 (a) Diffuse alopecia after chemotherapy for breast cancer. (b) Some regrowtth after 6 months of minoxidil 2% treatment.

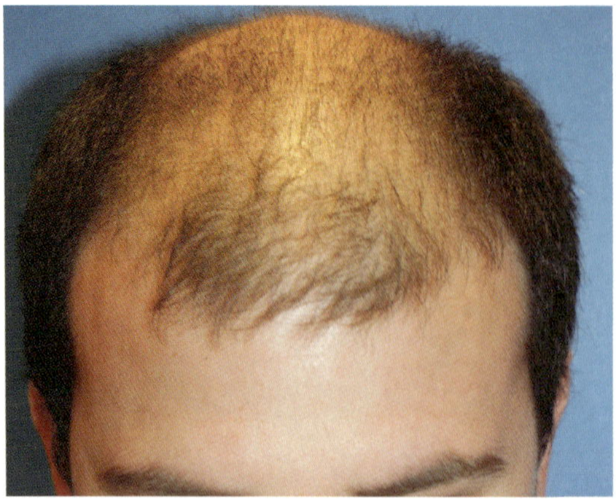

Figure 8.7 Male androgenetic alopecia (note the miniaturization of hair on the balding area).

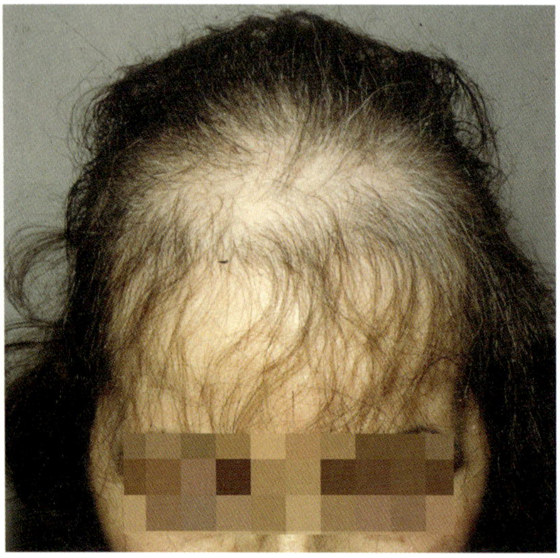

Figure 8.8 Female androgenetic alopecia (note the hair miniaturization and the persistence of a frontal hairline).

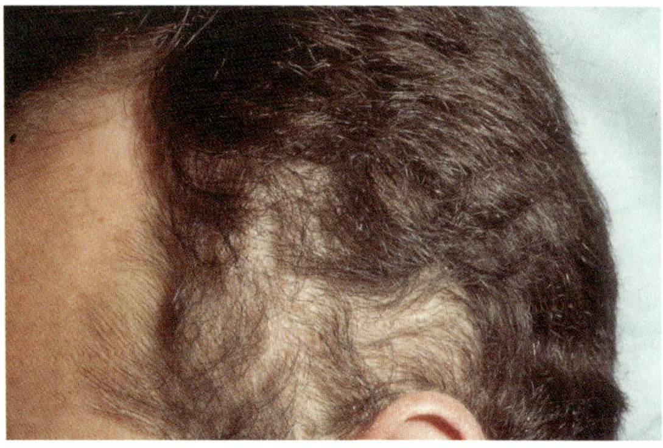

Figure 8.9 Diffuse alopecia in a man with hypothyroidism.

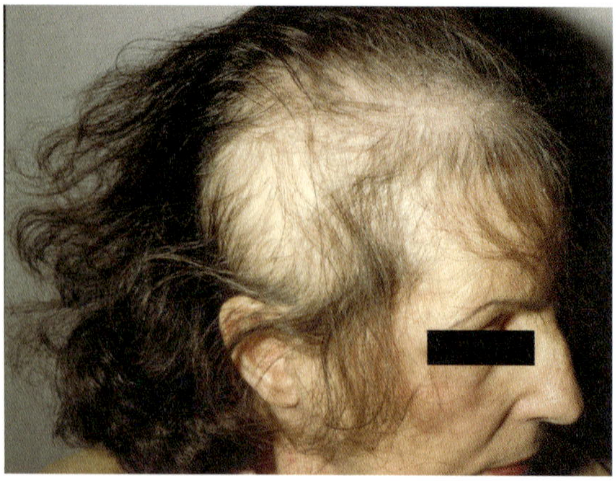

Figure 8.10 Diffuse alopecia in a woman with a blood iron deficiency.

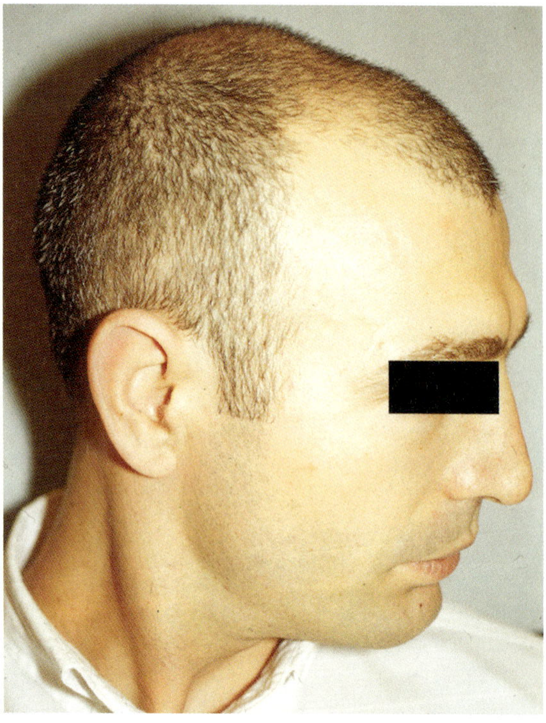

Figure 8.11 Alopecia with syphilis in a typical "clumsy scissors" appearance in a patient with androgenetic alopecia.

PROGNOSIS AND TREATMENT

Prognosis

The prognosis of telogen effluvium varies by functional type. In most patients, it is a phenomenon of limited duration which corrects spontaneously, especially during shorter anagen phase (caused by drugs or acute physiological events) or during seasonal extensions of the telogen phase.

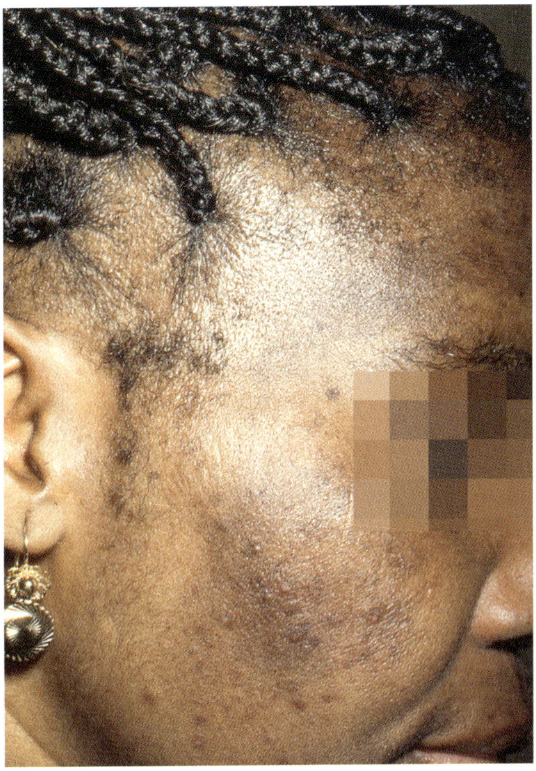

Figure 8.12 **Alopecia secondary to traction styling (the hair pulled back in excessive braiding).**

Treatment

The treatment is based on psychological support and education of the patient, to whom the follicular cycle and the mechanism of telogen effluvium should be explained.

Minoxidil in topical applications can extend the cycle in the short anagen phase syndrome:

- Treatment of the cause is to be implemented whenever possible.
- Dietary supplements are based on
  - Iron, L-lysine, biotin, pantothenic acid, vitamin B_6, vitamin D, copper, zinc, soy
  - Sulphur amino acids (cystine) or vitamin B (biotin, bepanthen) administered orally or intramuscularly
  - Vegetal gelatin
  - Iron as fumarate or protoxalate if there is iron deficiency.
- Additional local treatments in the form of lotions or shampoos can be added to specific etiologic treatment.

The use of cosmetic approaches to camouflage diffuse alopecia include a variety of methods, such as hairstyling, styling agents, coloring, camouflage prostheses such as wigs and hairpieces, and scalp coloring products such as tints, powders, lotions, and sprays (Chapter 18).

CONCLUSION

The treatment of telogen effluvium is guided by the clinical evaluation and the identification of triggering events. The physician's primary focus is to remove and to treat or inhibit the trigger(s) of the telogen effluvium.

The expected results of any therapy should be diminished telogen effluvium after 2 months and evidence of regrowth at 4–6 months.

REFERENCES

1. Camacho F, Montagna W. *Trichologie-maladies du follicule pilosébacé*. Madrid, Spain: Grupo Aula Médica SA; 1997.
2. Bouhanna P. Alopécies diffuses. In: Bouhanna P, Reygagne P, ed. *Pathologie du cheveu et du cuir chevelu*. Paris, France: Masson; 1999:76–82.
3. Ferrando J. *Alopecias: Guia de diagnostico y tratamiento*. Barcelona, Spain: Pulso; 2000.
4. Bouhanna P. Conduite à tenir devant une alopécie diffuse: Enquête, étiologies et traitements. In: Bouhanna P, ed. *Les alopécies—de la clinique au traitement. Collection Guide Pratique de Dermatologie*. Paris, France: Med'Com; 2004.
5. Fiedler VC, Gray AC. Diffuse alopecia: Telogen hair loss. In: Olsen EA, ed. *Disorders of Hair Growth: Diagnosis and Treatment*. New York, NY: McGraw-Hill; 2003:303–320.
6. Headington JT. Telogen effluvium. New concepts and review. *Arch Dermatol*. 1992;130(2):256–263.
7. Olsen EA. *Disorders of Hair Growth—Diagnosis and Treatment*. New York, NY: McGraw-Hill; 1997.
8. Rook A, Dawber R. *Diseases of the Hair and Scalp*. Oxford: Blackwell Scientific Publications; 1982.
9. Skolochenco M. Crash dieting associated with telogen effluvium. *Geriatrics*. 2000;55(7):16.
10. Trost LB, Bergfeld WF, Calogeras E. The diagnosis and treatment of iron deficiency and its potential relationship to hair loss. *JAAD*. 2006;54:824–844.
11. Almagro M, del Pozoi, Garcia-Silva J et al. Telogen effluvium as a clinical presentation of human immunodeficiency virus infection. *Am J Med*. 2002;112(6):508–509.
12. Tosti A, Misciali C, Piraccini BM, Peluso AM, Bardazzi F. Drug induced hair loss and hair growth. Incidence, management and avoidance. *Drug Saf*. 1994;10(4):310–317.
13. Reygagne P. Alopécies toxiques et médicamenteuses. In: Bouhanna P, Reygagne P, ed. Pathologie du cheveu et du cuir chevelu. Paris, France: Masson; 1999:83–100.
14. Whiting DA. Update chronic telogen effluvium. *Exp Dermatol*. 1999;135(9):1123–1124.
15. Arnaud J Beani FC, Favier AE, Embliard R. Zinc status in patients with telogen effluvium. *Acta Derm Venereol*. 1995;75:248–249.
16. Trueb RM. Idiopathic chronic telogen effluvium in the woman (review). *Hautarzt*. 2000;51(12):899–905.
17. Guarrera RA, Baldari M, Vecchio F. Distinguishing androgenetic alopecia from chronic telogen effluvium when associated in the same patient; a simple noninvasive method. *Arch Dermatol*. 2005;141(10):1243–1245.

9 Management of noncicatricial circumscribed alopecia

Ralph M. Trüeb

COGNITION LIES IN THE EYE OF THE BEHOLDER

The skin and hair are gratifying for diagnosis. One has but to look, and recognize, since everything to be named is in full view. Looking would seem to be the simplest of diagnostic skills, and yet its simplicity lures one into neglect. To reach the level of artistry, looking must be a skillful, active undertaking. The skill comes in making sense out of what is seen, and it comes in the quest for the underlying cause, once the disorder has been named. In many instances, a specific diagnosis is made in a fraction of a second if it is a simple matter of pattern recognition. The informed look is the one most practiced by dermatologists; it comes from knowledge, experience, and visual memory. Where the diagnosis does not come from a glance, the diagnostic tests come in (i.e., the dermatological techniques of examination, and the laboratory evaluation).

By definition, alopecia is the acquired condition of recognizable hair loss. The term derives from Greek with reference to the loss of hair in patches in foxes afflicted with sarcoptic mange. Traditionally, the alopecias have been classified into generalized or circumscribed alopecia, congenital or acquired alopecia, and alopecia with or without evidence of scarring.

When examining the scalp, the distribution of hair loss, the presence and characteristics of associated anomalies, and the presence of scarring should be noted.

In the case of congenital absence or lack of hair, the correct terms are *atrichia* and *hypotrichosis*, respectively.

Aquired hair loss in patches signifies either alopecia areata, traumatic alopecia, trichotillomania, or scarring alopecia.

Finally, increased fragility of the hair shaft may lead to pseudoalopecia from breakage of hair, particularly in regions with higher friction, such as the occiput.

Congenital triangular alopecia (of Sabouraud), also known as temporal alopecia or temporal triangular alopecia, is a congenital disorder that usually appears in childhood as a focal patch of fine vellus hairs with a usually triangular configuration in the temporal region of the scalp (Figure 9.1). The condition basically represents the most common of a variety of congenital circumscribed hypotrichoses of the scalp, and may appear either uni- or bilaterally. The suggested frequency for this condition in the general population has been estimated around 0.11%. The majority of cases are detected in childhood between the ages of 2 and 9 years.[1]

The condition presents usually as an isolated finding; rare cases have been associated with *Setleis syndrome* that is characterized by scar-like, circular depressions on the temples (Figure 9.2), which may resemble forceps marks and (much as with aplasia cutis congenita) give rise to litigations with respect to alleged obstetrical injury.[2]

A patchy type of hair loss, particularly over the cranial sutures, and associated with cutaneous atrophy of the scalp, is a typical finding of the *Hallermann–Streiff syndrome* (oculomandibular dyscephaly). Patients have a typical bird-like face, due to a sharply curved, thick, pointed nose, and mandibular hypoplasia. Associated anomalies, believed to derive from a developmental defect of the branchial arch, are brachycephaly, dental, and ocular abnormalities.[3]

Hair restoration surgery using follicular unit transplantation is usually successful for treatment of congenital triangular alopecia.[4]

Alopecia areata is a common hair loss condition characterized by an acute onset of nonscarring hair loss in usually sharply defined areas. Any hair-bearing area can be affected, but the most noticeable are the scalp, the beard area, and the eyebrows. The characteristic patch of alopecia areata is usually round or oval and is completely bald and smooth (Figure 9.3a). Some patients lose hair in only a small patch, while others may have more extensive or less frequently diffuse involvement. Some patients show a reticular pattern of alopecia resulting from confluence of multiple small patches of alopecia (Figure 9.3b). Ophiasis is a form of alopecia areata characterized by the loss of hair in the shape of a wave at the circumference of the head (Figure 9.3c). The name derives, again, from the Greek word for snake, because of the apparent similarity to a snake shape and the pattern of hair loss. Occasionally, alopecia areata may progress to complete baldness, which is referred to as alopecia totalis, and when the entire body suffers from complete hair loss, it is referred to as alopecia universalis.

Alopecia areata is considered to be of autoimmune origin with an organ-specific, T cell-mediated assault on the hair follicle at the level of the bulb. The hair bulb is an immune protected site with deficient major histocompatibility complex (MHC) expression. There is circumstantial evidence suggesting that alopecia areata results from

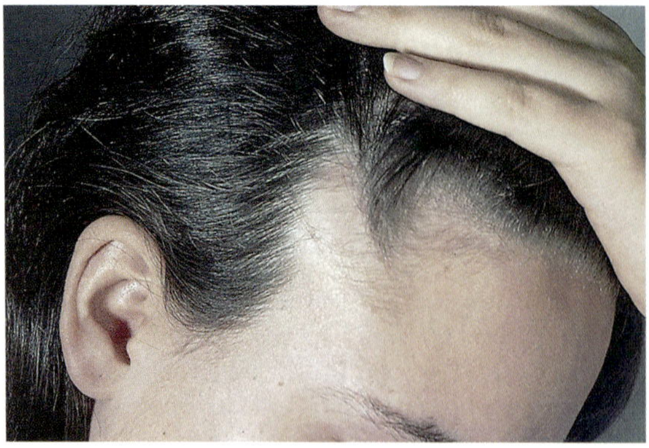

Figure 9.1 **Congenital triangular alopecia. (Reproduced from Trüeb RM. *Haare Praxis der Trichologie*. Steinkopff, Darmstadt 2003. With permission.)**

loss of immune privilege with presentation of autoantigens. A peribulbar lymphocytic infiltrate induces hair follicle keratinocytes to undergo apoptosis resulting in inhibition of cell division in the hair matrix.

The progress of alopecia areata in an individual patient is unpredictable, though a large surface area, a long disease duration, and associated nail abnormalities (nail pitting, and trachyonychia, rarely onychomadesis) have been associated with a poor prognosis.

With respect to treatment of alopecia areata, a recent meta-analysis of published trials states that only a few treatments have been well evaluated in randomized trials.[5] The authors found no randomized controlled trials on the use of diphenylcyclopropenone (DCP), intralesional corticosteroids, or dithranol, although commonly used in clinical practice. Although topical steroids and minoxidil are widely prescribed and appear to be safe, there is no convincing evidence that they are beneficial in the long term. Most trials have been reported poorly and are so small that any important clinical benefits are inconclusive. Of 17 trials including 6–85 participants with a total of 540 participants assessing a range of interventions that included topical and oral corticosteroids, topical ciclosporin, photodynamic therapy, and topical minoxidil, none showed significant treatment benefit in terms of hair growth when compared with placebo. The authors came to the conclusion that considering the possibility of spontaneous remission, especially for those in the early stages of the disease, the options of not being treated therapeutically or, depending on individual preference, of wearing a wig may be alternative ways of dealing with this condition.

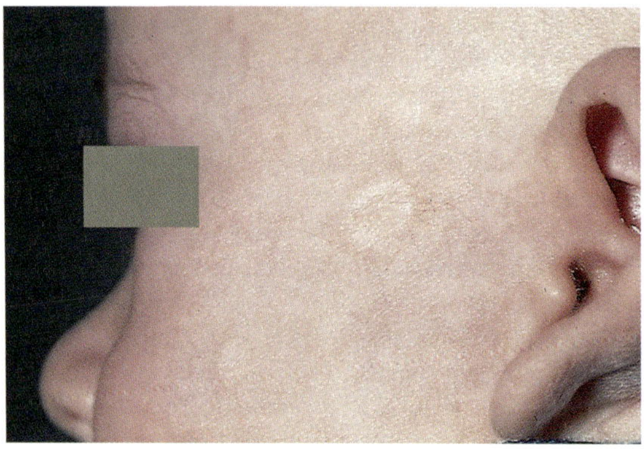

Figure 9.2 **Setleis syndrome. (Reproduced from Trüeb RM. *Haare Praxis der Trichologie*. Steinkopff, Darmstadt 2003. With permission.)**

The spontaneous remission rates for patchy alopecia areata are one-third within 6 months, half within one year, and two-thirds within 5 years; thereafter, complete remissions are rare. Recurrence rates within 5 years are 80%, and within 20 years are 100%. Total remission rates for alopecia totalis or universalis with a disease duration of 5 years or more are 1% in children and less than 10% in adults.

Nonetheless, depending on patient age, surface area, and disease duration, a treatment algorithm can be designed: Single patches of alopecia areata are best treated with intralesional triamcinolone acetonide 10 mg/mL by jet injector or insulin syringe on a monthly basis, for an average of three to a maximum of six consecutive treatments (in children 5 mg/mL, for eyebrows 2.5–5 mg/mL, and for beard 5 mg/mL by insulin syringe).

With pulse corticosteroid therapy (500 mg IV methylprednisolone on 3 consecutive days, in three cycles 4 weeks apart) within 6 months of disease onset remission rates are 88% for multilocular alopecia areata with a surface area <50%, 59.4% with a surface area >50%, and 21.4% in alopecia totalis. After 6 months of disease onset the remission rate is 15.8%.[6]

With 0.05% topical clobetasol ointment under occlusion (Saran wrap) on 6 consecutive nights per week over 6 months, regrowth of hair is achieved in alopecia totalis or universalis in 17.8%. Despite positive clinical results obtained using clobetasol ointment with occlusive dressing, this approach has a low patient compliance, especially in patients with residual hair.[7]

More recently, 0.05% clobetasol foam applied twice daily on 5 consecutive days per week proved to also be an effective, safe, and well-tolerated treatment with good cosmetic acceptance and patient compliance.[8]

In a retrospective study of 68 patients with severe alopecia areata (>40% scalp hair loss) treated for at least 5 months with topical diphenylcyclopropenone (DCP), Pericin and Trüeb[9] found an overall response rate of 70.6%, with 30.9% complete remission and 39.7% partial remission. Among the investigated prognostic factors for the outcome of DCP therapy, only the extent of alopecia areata at the time of initiation of treatment was found to be of significance. Total remission rates were as follows:

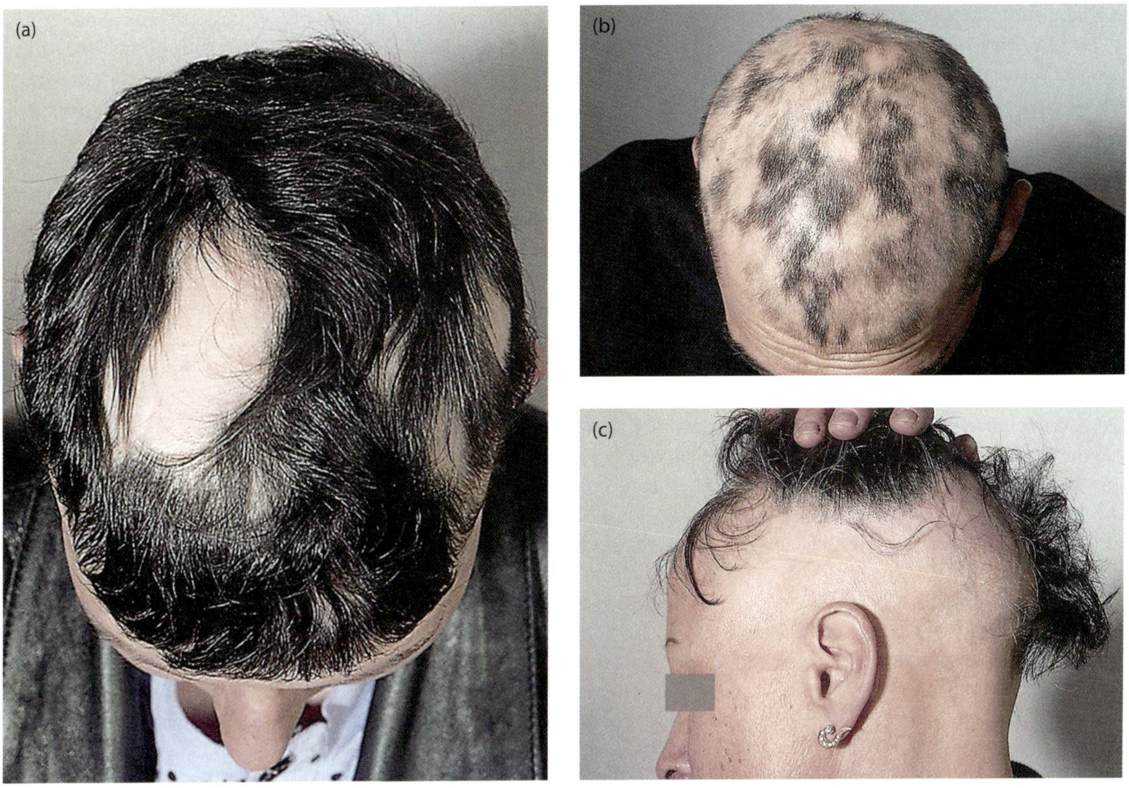

Figure 9.3 **Alopecia areata: (a) typical bald patch of alopecia areata, (b) reticular pattern, and (c) ophiasis pattern. (Reproduced from Trüeb RM. *Haare Praxis der Trichologie*. Steinkopff, Darmstadt 2003. With permission.)**

for multilocular alopecia areata were 43.8%, for subtotal alopecia areata and ophiasis 33.3%, and for alopecia totalis or universalis 21.4%, irrespective of disease duration.

Joly[10] proposed the use of methotrexate (MTX) alone or in combination with low doses of oral corticosteroids in the treatment of alopecia areata totalis and universalis, with an overall success rate of 64%. Best results are achieved with subcutaneous MTX in the maximal dosage of 30 mg weekly in combination with 20 mg oral prednisone daily, with regrowth of hair beginning within 2 to 4 months of therapy. Drug toxicities are to be carefully weighed against treatment benefit.

Ultimately, the options available for adapting to the disease rather than treating in an effort to cure are to be taken into consideration in selected long-standing widespread cases or recurrent small spot disease.

New drug treatment opportunities, based on the results of genome-wide association studies that implicate T cell and natural killer cell activation pathways, are paving the way to new approaches in future clinical trials for alopecia areata. Currently, there are ongoing studies with the CTLA4-Ig fusion protein abatacept (blocks costimulation of T cells), anti-IL15Rβ monoclonal antibodies (blocks activation of $CD8^+$ T cells), and the Janus Kinase (JAK) 3 inhibitor tofacitinib and JAK 1/3 inhibitor ruxolitinib (block signal transduction at the IL-15 receptor).[11]

Platelet-rich plasma (PRP) is blood plasma that has been enriched with platelets. As a concentrated source of autologous platelets, PRP contains and releases through degranulation several growth factors and cytokines. These include PDGF, TGFb, FGF, IGF-1 and IGF-2, VEGF, EGF, IL-8, and KGF. PRP has gained popularity among a limited number of dermatologists with a primary commercial interest, though the use and clinical validation of the method for diverse dermatologic conditions is still in the early stages. Results of basic science and preclinical trials have yet to be confirmed in large-scale controlled clinical trials. A Cochrane review on PRP has been performed in chronic wounds.[12] Even if the conclusion of the respective review was positive, this would have not been surprising, because blood platelets have a physiologic role in wound healing. In contrast, it is more difficult to comprehend the role of platelet-derived growth factors and cytokines for hair growth and treatment of hair growth disorders. For this reason, a stringent evaluation of existing data in favor of PRP for treatment of hair-related disorders is indispensable. There exists a single, double-blind, placebo- and active-controlled, half-head study to evaluate the effects of PRP on alopecia areata published in 2013.[13] However, in an era in which a more comprehensive understanding of the immunologic basis of alopecia areata has opened the venue to more targeted treatments of alopecia areata, in the opinion of the more stringent scientific community, the proposal of PRP, with its poorly defined mode of action, rather represents an intellectual step backward.

TRAUMATIC ALOPECIA

Traction alopecia is defined as hair loss resulting from either prolonged or repetitive pulling force to the hair. Clinically, traction alopecia most often affects the frontal and temporal scalp areas. However, it has been extensively reported in the literature to occur on many different regions of the scalp, depending on an individual's hair grooming practices, which may or may not be related to the ethnic or cultural background. The condition was originally described in female subjects in Greenland who developed hair loss along the hairline from wearing tight ponytails. In 1958, Slepyan[14] reported alopecia in American girls wearing ponytails, and stated that the patches of baldness need not be limited to the margins of the scalp, since alopecia may occur along any line of traction. Traction alopecia is also seen occasionally in long-haired people who use barrettes to keep the hair out of their faces. The more recent literature has focused on traction alopecia from African hair-braiding styles. It has been pointed out that in African females the likelihood of developing traction alopecia increases when traction is applied to chemically processed hair. The risk of developing traction alopecia also increases in the presence of androgenetic alopecia, and with age. With androgenetic alopecia, the hair seems to be less resistant to traction, while with age, traction alopecia is likely to result from a longer history of the aforementioned hair practices.[15] Finally, the risk of developing traction alopecia is substantial in hair weaves, that are worn to conceal hair loss, usually resulting from androgenetic alopecia. Hair weaving involves creating a braid around the head below the existing hairline, to which a hairpiece is attached. Since the hair of the braid is still growing, it requires frequent maintenance, which involves the hairpiece being removed, the natural hair braided again, and the piece tightly reattached. The tight braiding and snug hairpiece cause tension in the hair that is already at risk.

Traction alopecia generally does not present any diagnostic difficulties, provided the possibility is considered. Diagnostic challenges may be encountered if the clinical suspicion is not high or if no history of traction is obtained. The earliest clinical manifestation of continuous traction on hair is perifollicular erythema. Occasionally, keratin cylinders may surround the hairs just above the scalp surface. Not infrequently patients complain of localized dandruff with itching. Eventually the erythema around the follicles will evolve into folliculitis and minute folliculopustules may become evident. In general, patients who develop any symptoms, including pain, pimples, stinging, or crusts with hairdressing are at increased risk of developing traction alopecia. The process gradually leads to loss of hair, which becomes irreversible after sustained traction. By the time the alopecia is evident, the scalp usually no longer shows inflammatory changes. Although the hair loss has become permanent, the skin does not have the quality common to the usual types of cicatricial alopecia, remaining soft and pliable. On close inspection there is a decrease in the density of follicular orifices. In traction alopecia of the marginal hair line, Mirmirani et al. made the observation that the presence of retained hairs along the frontal and/or temporal rim, which they termed the fringe sign (Figure 9.4), may be a useful clinical marker seen in 85% of women with the condition.[16]

Treatment of traction alopecia depends on whether or not long-standing traction has resulted in permanent loss of hair. Accordingly, management of traction alopecia is divided into prevention, treatment of early disease, and treatment of long-standing disease. Prevention is key in girls, and involves educating parents on the importance of loosening the hairstyle. Brushing the affected area with the misbelief of stimulating hair growth should be avoided as well. In adults with early traction alopecia, the hairstyle should also be loosened. Moreover, chemicals or heat are to be avoided. Intralesional triamcinolone and oral tetracycline antibiotics may be beneficial in suppressing perifollicular inflammation, while added topical minoxidil may promote hair growth in some patients. Ultimately, with long-standing disease, surgical procedures, such as hair transplants in the form of micrografting, minigrafting, and follicular unit transplantation, may be considered.

Postoperative pressure alopecia represents yet another peculiar form of traumatic alopecia frequently mistaken

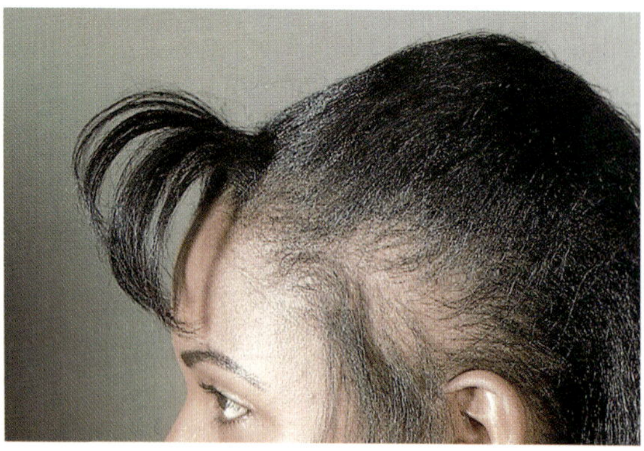

Figure 9.4 **Fringe sign in traction alopecia. (With kind permission from Springer Science+Business Media: Female Alopecia. *Guide to Successful Management*, 2013, Berlin, Germany, Springer, Trüeb RM.)**

for alopecia areata, localized to the occipital scalp (Figure 9.5). Patients typically complain of occipital pain and tenderness within 24 hours of surgery. Signs observed within the first week after surgery may be focal swelling, edema, crusting, and ulceration. The hair loss sets in between 2 and 3 weeks after surgery and is complete within 28 days. The condition was originally reported after open cardiac surgery, and is now increasingly observed following lengthy plastic surgical procedures. It occurs after prolonged pressure on the scalp during general anesthesia with intubation, with the head fixed in one position, and is understood to be due to pressure-induced ischemia. Risk factors for hair loss and scarring include length of the anesthesia, prolonged endotracheal intubation, prolonged head immobilization, intraoperative use of the Trendelenburg position, and additional factors potentially aggravating ischemia of the scalp, such as severe hypotension, massive blood loss, and use of vasoconstrictors.[17]

The most important aspect of prevention of this complication of surgery is knowledge of its existence and pathophysiology. A prospective study that incorporated head repositioning every 30 minutes in cardiac surgical patients significantly reduced the incidence of alopecia from a prospectively determined value of 14% to 1%.[18] Fortunately, the condition is self-limiting in most cases with spontaneous regrowth of hair occurring within 3 months. In cases of necrosis, ulceration, and scarring, the alopecia is permanent.

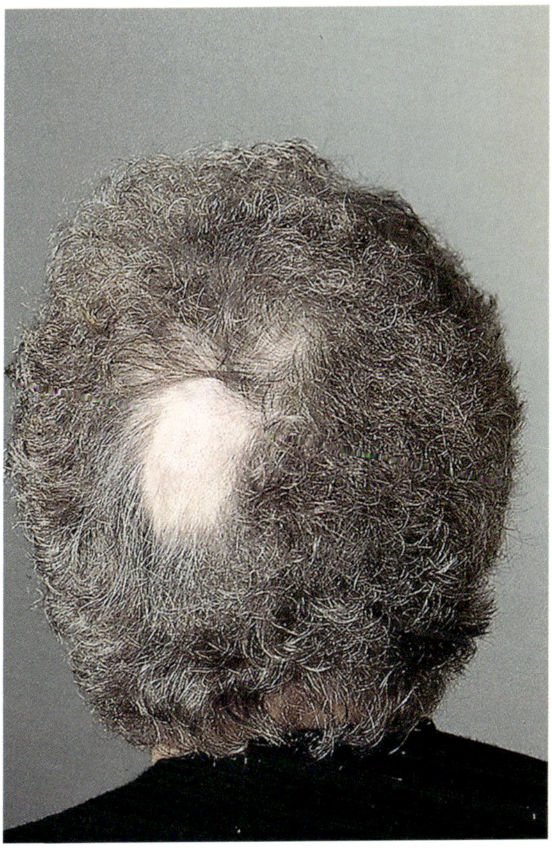

Figure 9.5 Postoperative pressure alopecia. (Reproduced from Trüeb RM. *Haare Praxis der Trichologie*. Steinkopff, Darmstadt 2003. With permission.)

Temporary radiation-induced epilation following neuroradiologically guided embolization procedures represents yet another condition frequently mistaken for alopecia areata. Since the anagen hair follicle is highly susceptible to x-ray exposure, loss of hairs results from acute damage to the actively dividing matrix cells of anagen follicles (dystrophic anagen effluvium). Hair loss occurs within the area exposed to x-rays, and most patients notice hair loss 2 to 3 weeks following radiation exposure (Figure 9.6). Hair loss occurs on hair-bearing skin with doses above 300 to 400 cGy and is permanent only with a single dose above 1200 cGy, and if the dose is fractionated, not until the dose exceeds 4500 cGy. Krasovec and Trüeb[19] originally reported temporary radiation-induced epilation following a neuroradiologically guided embolization procedure in the dermatologic literature. Endovascular procedures have become a widely used treatment of cerebral vascular malformation. Transient radiation-induced alopecia following neuroradiologically guided therapeutic embolization of cerebral vascular malformation is probably underreported, since it seems not to be uncommon. It has been misinterpreted to be due to arterial occlusion; moreover, excluding the differential diagnosis of alopecia areata may be difficult, since the bald patch is devoid of inflammatory signs, and hair loss is characterized by dystrophic hair. The patient history, chronology of events, and localization and geometry of the bald patch usually allow correct diagnosis.

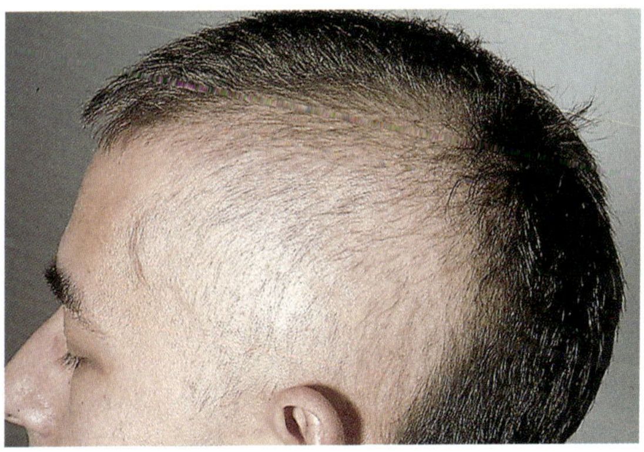

Figure 9.6 Temporary radiation-induced alopecia. (Reproduced from Trüeb RM. *Haare Praxis der Trichologie*. Steinkopff, Darmstadt 2003. With permission.)

Because the hair loss is temporary, complete hair regrowth occurs spontaneously 2 to 4 months after x-ray exposure, and patient education is paramount to prevent needless anxiety.

TRICHOTILLOMANIA AND RELATED DISORDERS

Trichotillomania involves the repetitive, uncontrollable pulling of one's hair, resulting in noticeable hair loss. It represents a disorder of impulse control. The disorder usually begins between early childhood and adolescence. It occurs six to seven times more frequently in children than in adults, before the age of 6 males predominate, thereafter females. Most commonly, scalp hair is pulled, resulting in ill-defined areas of incomplete hair loss. In the affected areas, there are different lengths of hair, short, longer, and normal. When the hair is pulled in the centroparietal area of the scalp, sparing the lateral margins and the nape of the neck, a tonsural pattern may result, that has been termed tonsure trichotillomania (Figure 9.7).[20]

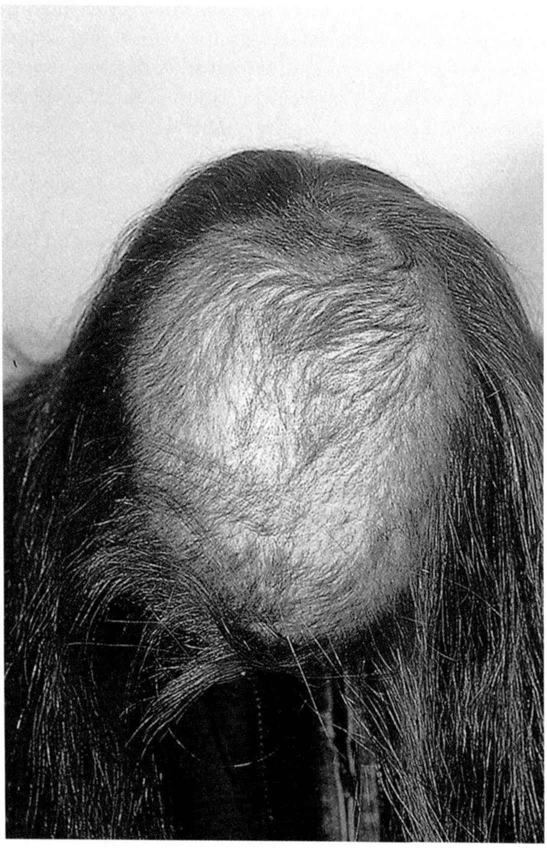

Figure 9.7 **Tonsure trichotillomania. (Reproduced from Trüeb RM. *Haare Praxis der Trichologie*. Steinkopff, Darmstadt 2003. With permission.)**

In younger children, trichotillomania results from a mild form of frustration in a climate of psychosocial stress, and soon becomes a habitual practice. From puberty onward, trichotillomania is related to more severe pathologic psychodynamics, and prognosis is more guarded, particularly tonsure trichotillomania in the female adolescent.

The younger the patient, the smaller the percentage of cases referred to a psychiatrist; the rest are treated by the dermatologist who applies his or her own psychiatric knowledge (liaison psychiatry). A proper follow-up is required to establish whether improvement has actually occurred. When the symptom is present in adolescents or adults, competent help from a psychiatrist should be sought. The primary treatment approach for trichotillomania is habit reversal combined with stress management and behavioral contracting. Parents can help by recognizing the problem in its early stages and getting involved in its treatment. Treatment may involve self-monitoring of hair-pulling episodes as well as the feelings and situations that are most likely to lead to hair pulling. Youngsters are then systematically introduced to new behaviors; for example, squeezing a ball or tightening their fist whenever they feel the urge to pull at their hair. Relaxation training and other stress-reduction techniques may also be used, including reward charts that help track and monitor a child's progress with the added incentive of earning small rewards for continued progress. In addition, cognitive therapy is found to be effective.

Children with trichophagy should be screened for iron deficiency as part of their evaluation, since the association of pica—an unusual craving for nonfood items—and iron deficiency has been reported. The compulsive oral behavior characteristically resolved with the oral administration of therapeutic doses of iron. It must be kept in mind though, that iron deficiency may either be a cause of trichophagy or result from gastrointestinal bleeding in the case of trichobezoar.

In a dermatologic setting, a pharmacologic approach may be most feasible for patients who refuse to be referred elsewhere. Basically, the same pharmacologic agents are used for the treatment of trichotillomania as for obsessive–compulsive disorder: the older tricyclic antidepressants imipramine and clomipramine, and the newer selective serotonin reuptake inhibitors (SSRIs) fluoxetine, fluvoxamine, sertraline, and paroxetine. Physicians using SSRIs for treatment of patients with obsessive–compulsive disorders or trichotillomania are cautioned that the duration of treatment is critical in determining adequate treatment. Improvement continues to occur when the drugs are taken beyond 8- or 12-week trials. A patient showing a partial response after 4–6 weeks would be expected to continue to improve during the following weeks. Cessation of pharmacotherapy results in a relapse in the majority of patients. Despite success with SSRIs, patients with obsessive–compulsive disorders tend to respond to medication with only partial symptom reduction, suggesting that obsessive–compulsive disorders may be a neurobiological heterogeneous disorder that may require alternative treatment options in the individual patient. For example, successful treatment of five adult trichotillomania patients with a combination of the SSRI escitalopram with the anticonvulsant topiramate was originally reported. Subsequently, Lochner et al.[21] performed an open-label pilot study to investigate the efficacy and safety of topiramate in 14 adults with trichotillomania. They found that topiramate may be useful in the treatment of trichotillomania, and suggested that future studies should investigate the efficacy of topiramate in an appropriately powered randomized placebo-controlled trial.

An interesting new therapy is based on the glutamate modulator *N*-acetylcysteine.[22] It is hypothesized that *N*-acetylcysteine, an amino acid, restores the extracellular glutamate concentration in the nucleus accumbens and, therefore, offers promise in the reduction of compulsive behavior. In a 12-week, double-blind, placebo-controlled study performed in 50 individuals with trichotillomania (45 women and 5 men with a mean age [SD] of 34.3 [±12.1]), Grant et al. orignially found that *N*-acetylcysteine (dosing range, 1200–2400 mg/d) demonstrated statistically significant reductions in trichotillomania symptoms. No adverse events occurred in the *N*-acetylcysteine group, and *N*-acetylcysteine was well tolerated.

To examine the efficacy of *N*-acetylcysteine for the treatment of trichotillomania in children, Bloch et al.[23] again performed a double-blind, placebo-controlled (add-on) study with a total of 39 children and adolescents aged 8 to 17 years with trichotillomania randomly assigned to receive the active agent or matching placebo for 12 weeks. No significant difference between *N*-acetylcysteine and placebo was found on outcome measures. It is noteworthy that on several measures of hair-pulling, subjects significantly improved with time regardless of treatment assignment: in the *N*-acetylcysteine group, 25% of subjects were judged as treatment responders, compared to 21% in the placebo group.

Trichotillomania in connection with alopecia areata may pose a special diagnostic challenge. It may result from scratching at the site of alopecia areata that is symptomatic with pruritus, initiating a habit-forming behavior. Alternatively, patients with a mental predisposition may artificially prolong the disfigurement as the hair on the bald patches of alopecia areata regrows, with the aim to maintain gratification of dependency needs, which were being met during alopecia areata.[24]

Traumatic alopecia due to child abuse (battered child) is, though uncommon, yet another important differential diagnosis to take into consideration in a child with unexplained hair loss and other signs of physical trauma.[25]

Trichoteiromania is the term originally coined by Freyschmidt-Paul et al.[26] for breakage of hair by forcefully rubbing an area of the scalp. The typical clinical presentation is that of a bald patch with broken hairs (Figure 9.8). In contrast to trichotillomania, traumatic changes to the hair shaft are more conspicuous, with splitting at the ends of the hairs, giving the impression of white tips. The underlying mental disorder varies among the patients, though an underlying cutaneous sensory disorder, not explained through any specific dermatological disorder, is a common denominator in all cases. Although trichotillomania is considered to be an obsessive–compulsive disorder, the underlying mental disorder in trichoteiromania represents a more heterogeneous group, including anxiety, depression, or somatoform disorder.[27]

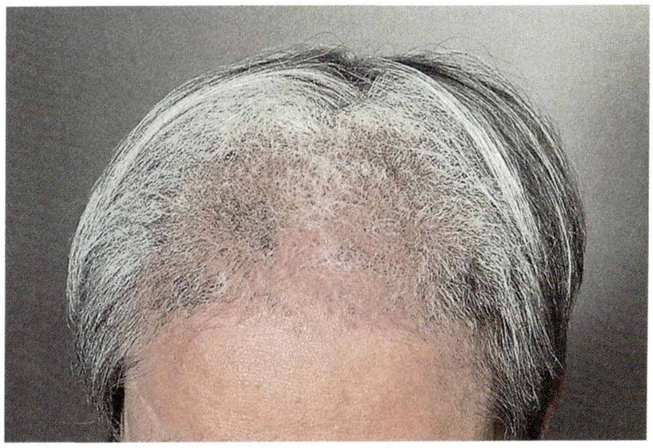

Figure 9.8 **Trichoteiromania. (Reproduced from Trüeb RM. *Haare Praxis der Trichologie*. Steinkopff, Darmstadt 2003. With permission.)**

Cooperation with the psychiatrist is indicated, as much as the management and prognosis of trichoteiromania will depend on recognition of the underlying mental disorder and its specific psychotherapeutic and pharmacological treatment.

Trichotemnomania is an area of cut-off hair as just one of varied manifestations of factitious disorder. Factitious disorder with physical symptoms is a condition in which the patient creates lesions on the skin to satisfy a psychological need of which he or she is not consciously aware, usually a need to be taken care of by assuming the sick role. Patients with factitious disorder create the lesions for psychological reasons, and not for monetary or other discrete objectives as in the case of malingering. Patients knowingly fake symptoms but will deny any part in the process. They desire the sick role and may move from physician to physician in order to receive care. They are usually loners with an early childhood background of trauma and deprivation. The majority of patients suffer from borderline personality disorder. The condition for which dermatologists are consulted often has already occasioned many visits to other physicians. The patient typically presents a bundle of normal investigative findings and a shopping bag filled with oral and topical medications. Though the possibilities are limitless, consistent is a "hollow" history—a term that refers to the patient's vagueness and inability to give details of how the lesions evolved.

With respect to treatment, the essential and probably most difficult step is to secure an enduring and stable patient–physician relationship. For achieving this goal most clinicians advocate a nonconfrontational strategy, reframing the factitious manifestation as a "cry for help." An interesting approach is that of "contract conference." In this approach the psychiatrist emphasizes the need for the patient to express himself or herself in the common language of difficult relationships, feelings, and problems in living instead of the (factitious) language of illness. After that the patient and clinician can focus their efforts on resolving those real problems. Once a stable relationship is installed, the management of the disorder must be oriented to avoid unnecessary hospitalizations and medical procedures. Another important issue in the management of this condition is recognition and adequate treatment of frequently associated disorders, such as personality disorders, depression, drug and/or alcohol abuse and dependency, etc. Occlusive dressings are used as a diagnostic tool rather than an effective therapeutic intervention, because success is only of temporary nature. Some case reports focus on the use of pharmacological agents. A good response has been reported to the antipsychotic drug pimozide; other clinicians, because of the resemblance to the obsessive–compulsive disorder, advocate the use of clomipramine, or the SSRIs fluoxetine and fluvoxamine maleate. In the vast majority of patients, the condition remains chronic.

LOOSE ANAGEN HAIR

Loose anagen hair, characterized by easily pluckable anagen hairs, is a disorder predominantly observed in children. The diagnosis is based on the following criteria: on pull-test, painless extraction of >10 anagen hairs (devoid of hair root sheaths), and in the trichogram >80% of plucked hairs are anagen hairs devoid of sheaths.[28] Clinically, the hair may show uneven ends. Additionally, there may be variations in hair texture, and the hair is often dry and lustreless (Figure 9.9). Loose anagen hair has originally been reported in girls but may be under diagnosed in males simply because of hairstyle differences between boys and girls. The condition often recedes with age but can be seen in adulthood, either as a continuation of the disorder that has lingered since childhood, or as late-onset loose anagen hair.

There is no specific treatment for loose anagen hair, except for careful grooming of the hair to avoid extracting the loose anagen hairs. Oral biotin may be beneficial for the strength and texture of the hair.

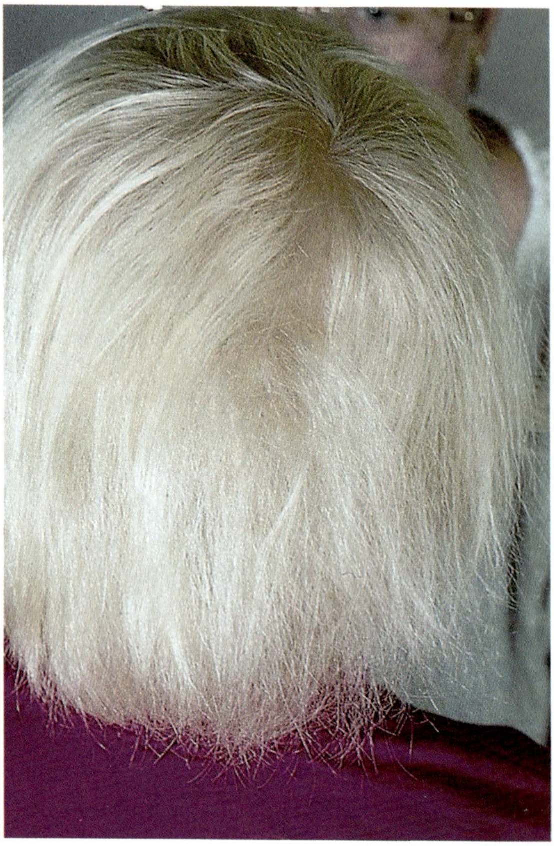

Figure 9.9 **Loose anagen hair. (Reproduced from Trüeb RM. *Haare Praxis der Trichologie*. Steinkopff, Darmstadt 2003. With permission.)**

ALOPECIA PARVIMACULATA

Alopecia parvimaculata (of Dreuw) represents yet another peculiar form of circumscribed alopecia in the pediatric population, in which hair is lost in very small, irregularly shaped patches (Figure 9.10). The etiology has remained obscure, but in its original description may have been related to small epidemic outbreaks of parasitic infection.[29] In 90% regrowth of hair occurs spontaneously, in 10% alopecia is permanent and is understood to represent a pediatric variant of the pseudopeladic state of Degos (i.e., the nonspecific end stage of a variety of scarring alopecias).

PSEUDOALOPECIA FROM HAIR BREAKAGE

Finally, circumscribed patches of hair loss can result from hair breakage (pseudoalopecia) that is either due to an inherent weakness of the hair shaft, or results from excessive trauma to the hair shaft. The patches of hair loss are usually in areas of higher friction. Already 15 minutes of hair scratching will cause hair to break.

A simple hair-feathering test is used to determine abnormal hair fragility with hair shaft breakage. The distal 2–3 cm of the hairs are grasped between the thumb and index finger. After rubbing the distal hair ends between the thumb and index finger, a brisk pull is made

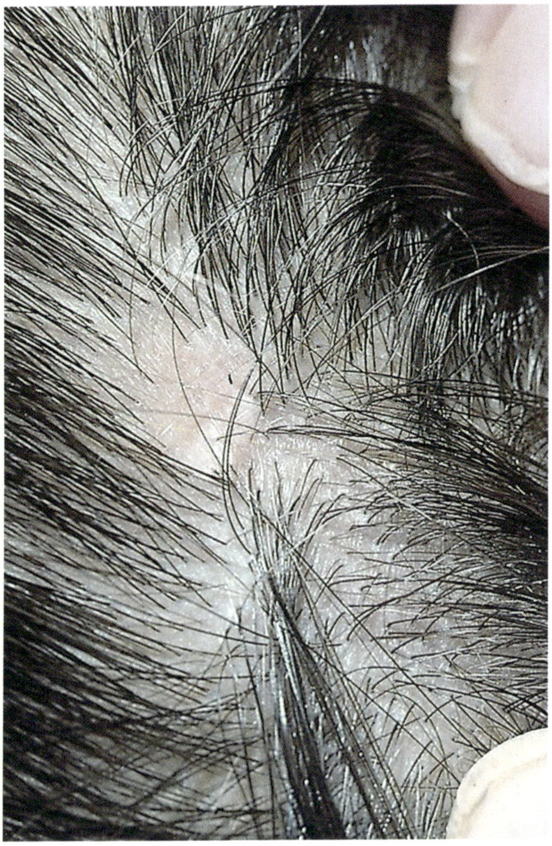

Figure 9.10 Alopecia parvimaculata. (Reproduced from Trüeb RM. *Haare Praxis der Trichologie*. Steinkopff, Darmstadt 2003. With permission.)

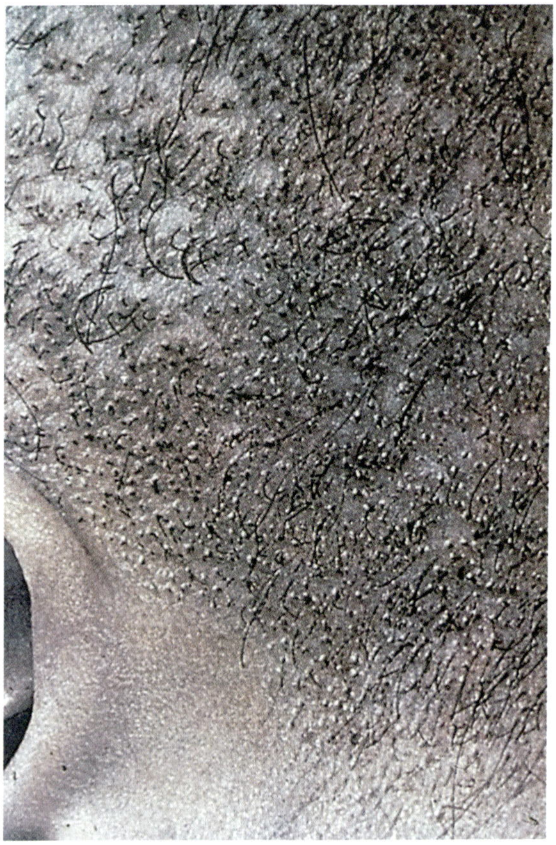

Figure 9.11 Monilethrix. (Reproduced from Trüeb RM. *Haare Praxis der Trichologie*. Steinkopff, Darmstadt 2003. With permission.)

on the ends of the hairs. The thumb and index finger are then checked for short broken hair fragments. In case of increased hair fragility in the hair-feathering test, a light microscopic study of the hair shaft usually reveals the hair shaft defect underlying abnormal breakage.

Hair shaft abnormalities result from genetic conditions and/or exogenous factors affecting the integrity of the hair shaft.[30] Definitive diagnosis is based on microscopic examination of the hair shaft, though dermoscopy represents an effective tool for quick diagnosis of hair shaft disorders on the patient. Hair shaft abnormalities with increased fragility and hair breakage that can be visualized by dermoscopy include the following:[31]

Monilethrix is characterized by a beaded appearance of the hair due to periodic thinning of the shaft. The uncommon hereditary condition results in hair fragility and patchy dystrophic alopecia. The alopecia is more severe in the occipital region that is more exposed to friction. Typically, the occipital scalp also presents follicular keratosis (Figure 9.11).

Pili torti is characterized by hair that is flattened and twisted through 180° on its axis at varying intervals; the hair can additionally be grooved and has then also been termed *pili torti et canaliculi* or twisting dystrophy. The hair shaft anomaly can be seen as an isolated hereditary trait, in a number of genetic syndromes, including Menkes kinky hair syndrome, Björnstad syndrome (with sensorineural deafness), and the ectodermal dysplasias. Twisting dystrophy in a progressive patch of alopecia in the vertex region is a typical finding in Marie Unna's hereditary hypotrichosis (Figure 9.12).[32]

Trichorrhexis invaginata or bamboo hair is the marker for Netherton syndrome, a rare autosomal recessive condition with bamboo hair, ichthyosis, and atopic dermatitis. The hair shaft shows multiple nodes along its length. The nodes consist of a proximal cup-shaped portion and a distal ball-shaped portion, resembling the joint of bamboo. Hair breakage corresponds to the nodes. Eyebrows are affected as well as scalp hair. Simple examination of eyebrow hairs may increase the likelihood of early

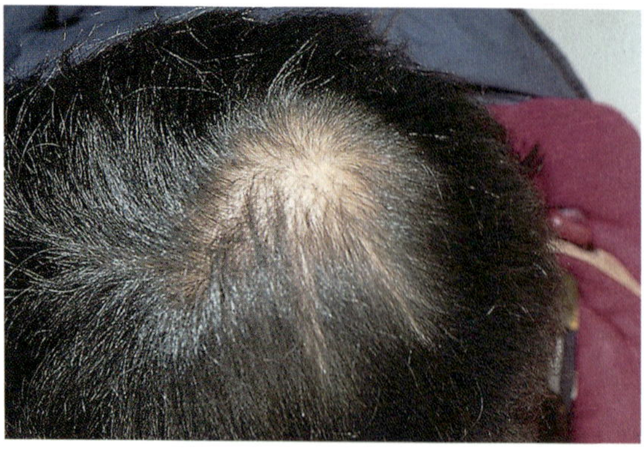

Figure 9.12 **Marie Unna's hereditary hypotrichosis. (Reproduced from Trüeb RM. *Haare Praxis der Trichologie*. Steinkopff, Darmstadt 2003. With permission.)**

diagnosis of Netherton syndrome in the newborn with congenital erythrodermic ichthyosis.

Trichorrhexis nodosa refers to white knots with transverse fractures along the hair shaft. Dermoscopy reveals brush-like hair fracturing. In general, trichorrhexis nodosa is an unspecific finding related to excess stress of hair in relation to its fragility. It can be observed in hair shaft abnormalities with increased fragility, or more frequently as a consequence of hair weathering.

Pili annulati are defined by characteristic alternating light and dark banding in the hair shaft, due to air-filled spaces between the macrofibrillar units of the hair cortex. A priori, not a hair shaft anomaly with increased fragility, the significance of pili annulati lies in that affected hair is more susceptible to weathering, particularly in combination with androgenetic alopecia. With onset of hair thinning due to androgenetic alopecia, progressive reduction of hair shaft diameter may cause increased fragility and trichorrhexis nodosa-like hair shaft fracturing.[33]

For treatment, trauma must be minimized, and hair care products and conditioning agents that improve the structural integrity of damaged hair fibers and increase tensile strength are available.

REFERENCES

1. Yamazaki M, Irisawa R, Tsuboi R. Temporal triangular alopecia and a review of 52 past cases. *J Dermatol*. 2010;37:360–362.
2. Dunn PM. Litigation over congenital scalp defects. *Lancet*. 1992;339:440.
3. Mirshekari A, Safar F. Hallermann-Streiff syndrome: A case review. *Clin Exp Dermatol*. 2004;29:477–479.
4. Wu WY, Otberg N, Kang H, Zanet L, Shapiro J. Successful treatment of temporal triangular alopecia by hair restoration surgery using follicular unit transplantation. *Dermatol Surg*. 2009;35:1307–1310.
5. Delamere FM, Sladden MM, Dobbins HM, Leonardi-Bee J. Interventions for alopecia areata. *Cochrane Database Syst Rev*. 2008;16(2):CD004413.
6. Nakajima T, Inui S, Itami S. Pulse corticosteroid therapy for alopecia areata: Study of 139 patients. *Dermatology*. 2007;215:320–324.
7. Tosti A, Piraccini BM, Pazzaglia M, Vincenzi C. Clobetasol propionate 0.05% under occlusion in the treatment of alopecia totalis/universalis. *J Am Acad Dermatol*. 2003;49:96–98.
8. Tosti A, Iorizzo M, Botta GL, Milani M. Efficacy and safety of a new clobetasol propionate 0.05% foam in alopecia areata: A randomized, double-blind placebo-controlled trial. *J Eur Acad Dermatol Venereol*. 2006;20:1243–1247.
9. Pericin M, Trüeb RM. Topical immunotherapy of severe alopecia areata with diphenylcyclopropenone: Evaluation of 68 cases. *Dermatology*. 1998;196:418–421.
10. Joly P. The use of methotrexate alone or in combination with low doses of oral corticosteroids in the treatment of alopecia totalis or universalis. *J Am Acad Dermatol*. 2006:55:632–636.
11. Petukhova L, Duvic M, Hordinsky M et al. Genome-wide association study in alopecia areata implicates both innate and adaptive immunity. *Nature*. 2010;466:113–117.
12. Martinez-Zapata MJ, Martí-Carvajal AJ, Solà I et al. Autologous platelet-rich plasma for treating chronic wounds. *Cochrane Database Syst Rev*. 2012;17(10):CD006899.
13. Trink A1, Sorbellini E, Bezzola P et al. A randomized, double-blind, placebo- and active-controlled, half-head study to evaluate the effects of platelet-rich plasma on alopecia areata. *Br J Dermatol*. 2013;169:690–694.
14. Slepyan AH. Traction alopecia. *Arch Derm*. 1958;78:395–398.
15. Khumalo NP, Jessop S, Gumedze F, Ehrlich R. Determinants of marginal traction alopecia in African girls and women. *J Am Acad Dermatol*. 2008;59:432–438.
16. Samrao A, Price VH, Zedek D, Mirmirani P. The "Fringe Sign"—A useful clinical finding in traction alopecia of the marginal hair line. *Dermatol Online J*. 2011;17:1.
17. Abel R, Lewis G. Postoperative (pressure) alopecia. *Arch Dermatol Syphilol*. 1960;81:34–42.
18. Lawson N, Mills N, Oscher J. Occipital alopecia following cardiopulmonary bypass. *J Thorac Cardiovasc Surg*. 1976;71:342–347.
19. Krasovec M, Trüeb RM. Temporary roentgen epilation after embolization of a cerebral arteriovenous malformation. *Hautarzt* 1998;49:307–309.
20. Sanderson KV. Tonsure trichotillomania. *Br J Dermatol*. 1970;82:343–350.

21. Lochner C, Seedat S, Niehaus DJ, Stein DJ. Topiramate in the treatment of trichotillomania: An open-label pilot study. *Int Clin Psychopharmacol.* 2006;21:255–259.
22. Grant JE, Odlaug BL, Kim SW. *N*-acetylcysteine, a glutamate modulator, in the treatment of trichotillomania: A double-blind, placebo-controlled study. *Arch Gen Psychiatry.* 2009;66:756–763.
23. Bloch MH, Panza KE, Grant JE, Pittenger C, Leckman JF. *N*-acetylcysteine in the treatment of pediatric trichotillomania: A randomized, double-blind, placebo-controlled add-on trial. *J Am Acad Child Adolesc Psychiatry.* 2013;52:231–240.
24. Trüeb RM, Cavegn B. Trichotillomania in connection with alopecia areata. *Cutis.* 1996;58:67–70.
25. Trüeb RM. Differential diagnosis in pediatric dermatology: Trichotillomania/battered child syndrome. *Eur J Pediatr Dermatol.* 1993;3:134–139.
26. Freyschmidt-Paul P, Hoffmann R, Happle R. Trichoteiromanie. *Eur J Dermatol.* 2001;11:369–371.
27. Reich S, Trüeb RM. Trichoteiromanie. *J Dtsch Dermatol Ges.* 2003;1:22–28.
28. Hamm H, Traupe H. Loose anagen hair of childhood: The phenomenon of easily pluckable hair. *J Am Acad Dermatol.* 1989;20:242–248.
29. Hoefer W. Sporadic occurrence of alopecia parvimaculaa. *Dermatol Wochenschr.* 1964;149:381–386.
30. Whiting DA. Structural abnormalities of the hair shaft. *J Am Acad Dermatol.* 1987;16:1–25.
31. Miteva M, Tosti A. Dermatoscopy of hair shaft disorders. *J Am Acad Dermatol.* 2013;68:473–478.
32. Roberts JL, Whiting DA, Henry D, Basler G, Woolf L. Marie Unna congenital hypotrichosis: Clinical description, histopathology, scanning electron microscopy of a previously unreported large pedigree. *J Investig Dermatol Symp Proc.* 1999;4:261–267.
33. Hofbauer GF, Tsambaos D, Spycher MA, Trüeb RM. Acquired hair fragility in pili anulati: Causal relationship with androgenetic alopecia. *Dermatology.* 2001;203:60–62.
34. Trüeb RM. *Haare Praxis der Trichologie.* Darmstadt, Germany, Steinkopff, 2003.
35. Trüeb RM. Female Alopecia. *Guide to Successful Management.* Berlin, Germany, Springer, 2013.

10 Traumatic alopecia

Pierre Bouhanna

Traumatic alopecia is a hair loss essentially caused by physical trauma. Schematically there are three possible etiologies for these alopecia[1]:

- Trichotillomania is a traction alopecia due to a compulsive disorder. Patients pull on and pluck hairs, often resulting in bizarre patterns of alopecia. In trichotillomania, the patient, with psychological disorders, will manipulate his or her hair, unconsciously or deliberately, but repeatedly, to cause more or less severe baldness.
- Cosmetic alopecia is caused by the excessively strong or aggressive care and handling of hair.
- Traumatic accident alopecia is easy to diagnosis.

We will not deal here with some hair dysplasias (see Chapter 4) that are responsible for brittle hair or occipital alopecia in newborn children, which present at areas of friction (Figure 10.1).

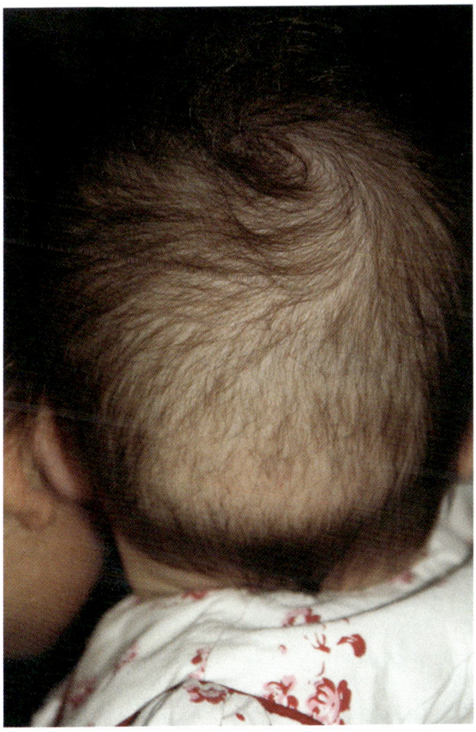

Figure 10.1 Occipital alopecia of the newborn child.

TRICHOTILLOMANIA

Psychopathological aspects

Trichotillomania is a tic of hair removal that occurs most often in boys under 6 years and in girls over 6 years (Figure 10.2).[2–4] The most severe cases occur in women between adolescence and 40 years (Figure 10.3); in these instances, the psychological disorders are major.

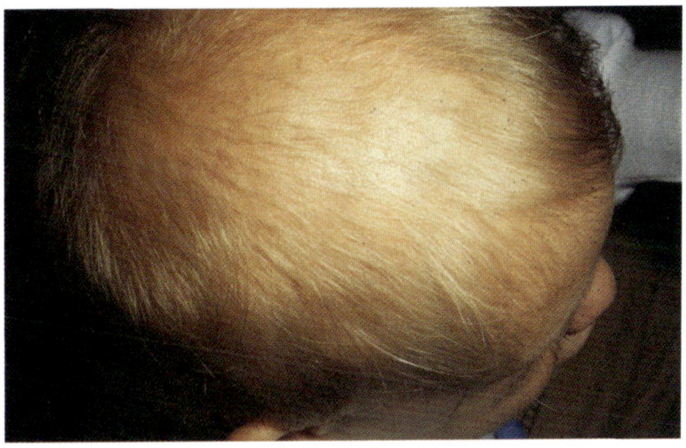

Figure 10.2 Trichotillomania in a 2-year-old child.

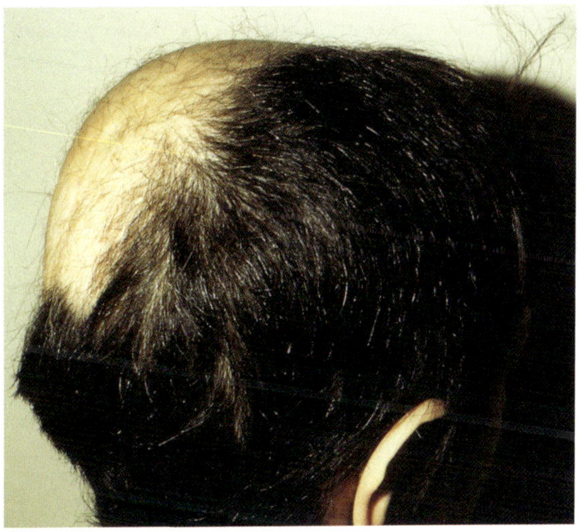

Figure 10.3 Circumscribed alopecia caused by trichotillomania located at the left half of the scalp in a young woman. (Note the angle and the rectilinear border.)

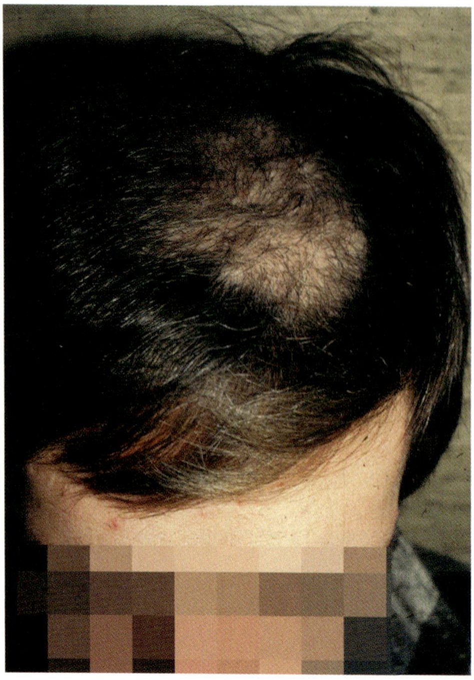

Figure 10.4 **Circumscribed alopecia caused by trichotillomania located at the vertex in a young adult. (Note the angle and the rectilinear border.)**

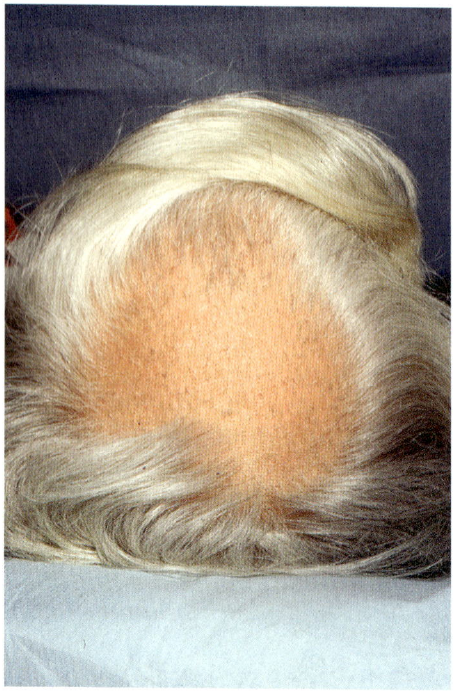

Figure 10.5 **Circumscribed alopecia caused by trichotillomania located at the vertex in an elderly woman. (Note the geometric contours.)**

Clinical aspects

Alopecia appears as an area with a clear boundary (Figure 10.4). The skin surface is normal and nonsquamous. The manipulated hairs are broken at different lengths. The parietal region is the most frequently affected.

In adults, the area of alopecia is often extensive, with short broken hairs. It can be localized to the vertex (Figure 10.5), appear unilaterally in the fronto-parietal–occipital region (Figures 10.3 and 10.6) or, exceptionally, be seen on the entire scalp.

Tics of removing eyelashes, eyebrows, or other body hair (pubic or perianal) are exceptional.

Diagnosis

Histological aspects: The most constant element is that many hair orifices are empty. In addition, telogen hairs are absent or very few. Biopsy specimens from acute lesions of trichotillomania may demonstrate perifollicular hemorrhage and fractured fibers. Later stages of trichotillomania characteristically demonstrate the presence of normal follicles surrounded by empty follicles in a noninflammatory dermis. Numerous catagen follicles (characterized by numerous apoptotic cells and a wavy surrounding vitreous membrane) and pigment casts within the upper segments of the follicle may be noted.

Trichoscopy[5,6] (Figure 10.7) is useful to confirm the evidence of pulling. The scalp presents short, coiled, fractured hairs. The broken hair shafts show longitudinal splitting (see Chapter 3).

Trichograms (1) show the almost exclusive presence of normal anagen hair (see Chapter 2).

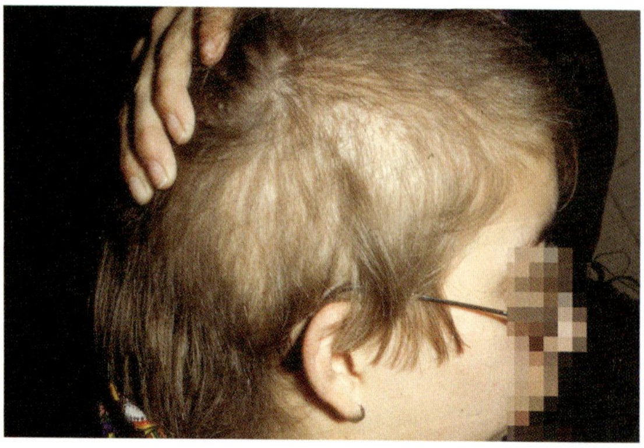

Figure 10.6 **Trichotillomania located in the parietal-occipital region in a 14-year-old boy. (Note the rectilinear or angular and geometric contours.)**

Differential diagnosis

In children, a patch caused in trichotillomania may be confused with ringworm or alopecia areata.

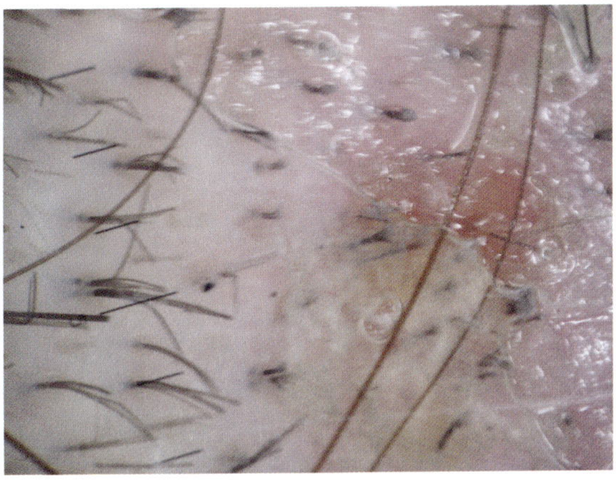

Figure 10.7 **Trichotillomania with erosion, black spots, hairs in "tulip" and hairs in "V." (Courtesy of Dr. Y. Bourezane.)**

With ringworm, the skin surface is rough. Infected hair is recognized on examination by Wood lamp and by microscopic examination.

In the case of alopecia areata, the presence of alopecia hair in "exclamation marks" is particularly evocative. Hair regrowth is fluffy and often clear or white, at first. In addition, abnormalities deriving from dystrophy of hair bulbs are visible on a trichogram.

The major forms of trichotillomania in adults should be differentiated with a careful clinical examination and a trichogram from androgenetic alopecia localized to the vertex and which can be associated (Figure 10.8).

Prognosis and treatment

In children, the tic hair removal is almost always favorably resolved after raising the issues in the presence of the parents.

In long-term cases of trichotillomania, permanent alopecia may occur.

The prognosis is more difficult in the extended forms found in the adult (Figures 10.3 and 10.5), in that they deny they are responsible for the act and often refuse psychotherapy as a solution.

COSMETIC ALOPECIA

The requirements attributed to ethnic or religious customs or the social pressure exercised by fashion cause a variety of hair damage.[7,8] Their diversity is directly proportional to the imaginative intensity of each individual (Figures 10.9a and b, 10.10a and b).

Pathogenesis

The pathogenesis of alopecia cosmetics may be attributed to

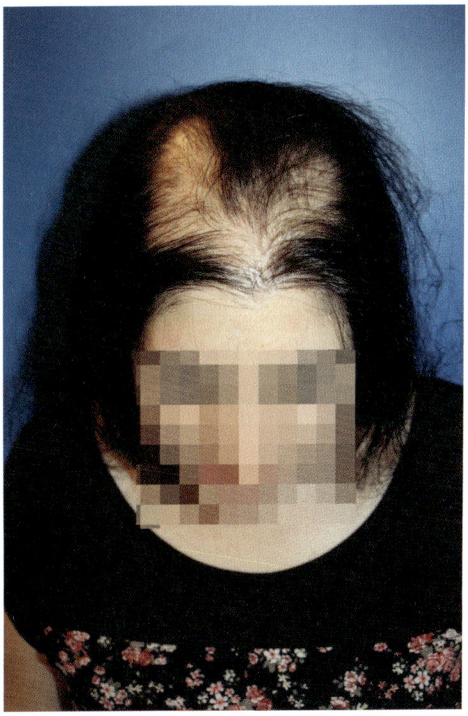

Figure 10.8 **Female androgenetic alopecia and traction alopecia. (Note the linear straight border.)**

- Breakage of hair secondary to manipulation of hair shafts, which have sometimes been weakened by chemical applications.
- Repeated traction at the shaft to stiffen it.
- Scarring alopecia induced by repeated pulling with preexisting inflammatory follicular lesions.[9]

Clinical aspects

The essential elements of frontal traction alopecia are the presence of short broken hair, folliculitis lesions, and some small scar patches located on the frontotemporal edge (Figure 10.11). This clinical form often affects women making a tightly pulled "bun," a "ponytail," or even one or two big braids (Figure 10.9a and b). Note also that parietal bald patches are often observed in nurses due to traction on the hair by clips that keep their cap in place (Figure 10.12).

The differential diagnosis is postmenopausal frontal fibrosing alopecia.

- Alopecia due to the rollers. This process, used to "curl" hair deemed too stiff, causes bald patches surrounded by broken hair and a rash if used regularly or too frequently.
- Alopecia due to wearing wigs braided to the remaining hair or attached by clips (Figure 10.13a

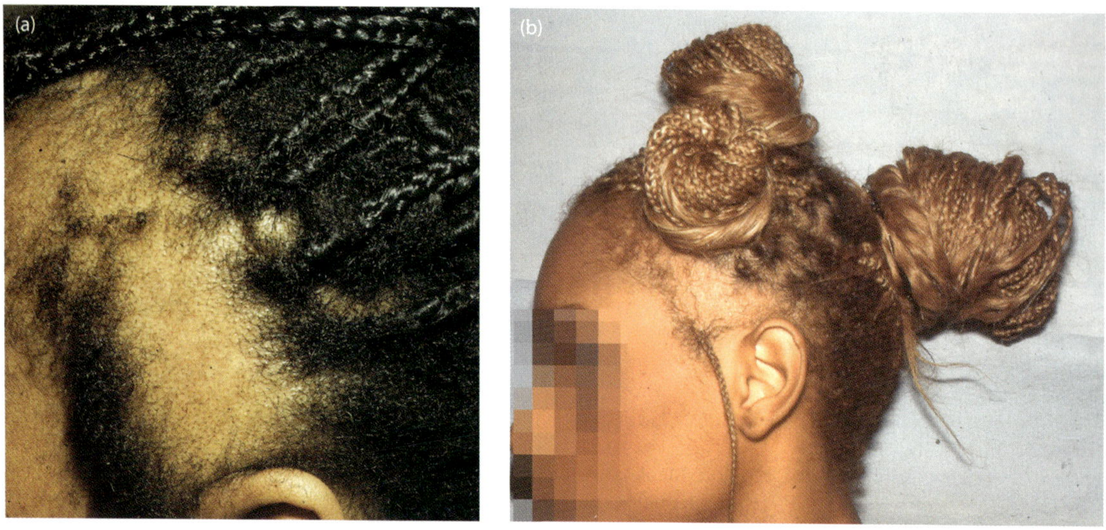

Figure 10.9 **(a,b) Alopecia from frontotemporal traction occurring in women who regularly braid their hair.**

and b). The clinical aspect of alopecia secondary to wearing a hairpiece is similar to that described above.

- Alopecia due to strong and repeated brushing. It will cause, among black patients whose hair is naturally weak (see Chapter 12), a recession of the frontotemporal line.
- Alopecia due to the use of straightening irons. Heat trauma causes a scarring alopecia gradually extending toward the vertex (Figure 10.14).
- Alopecia due to repeated friction or massage. Massage or excessive and repeated friction can cause alopecia, such as repeated rubbing of the arms of glasses (Figure 10.15).

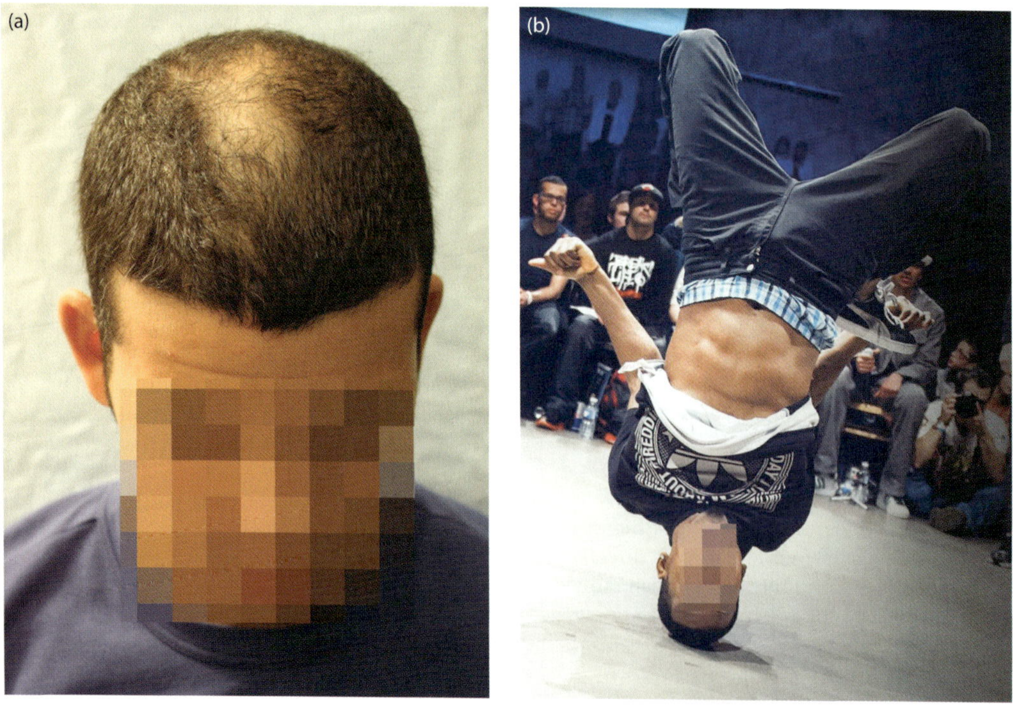

Figure 10.10 **(a) Traumatic alopecia after the break dance practice, (b) the break dance.**

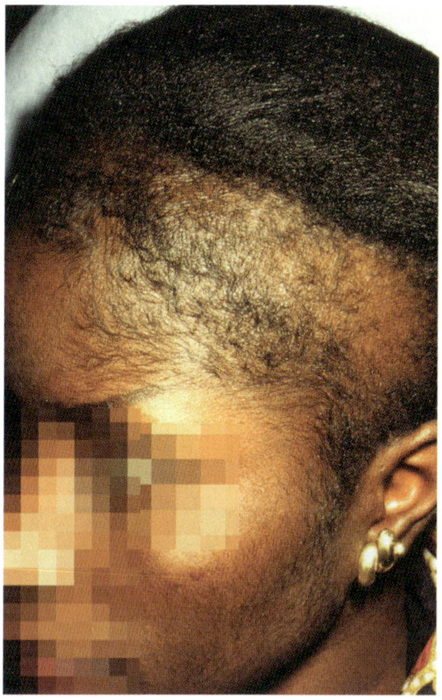

Figure 10.11 Frontotemporal alopecia after repeated hair straightening in a black patient. (Note the excess growth of vellus above the eyebrow after applying minoxidil lotion 2%.)

Differential diagnosis

The diagnosis is easily established by the results of a precise clinical examination, a trichoscopy examination, a trichogram evaluation, and eventually a biopsy.

Treatment

The treatment is obviously related to the removal of the cause and prescription of cosmetic products (such as cream

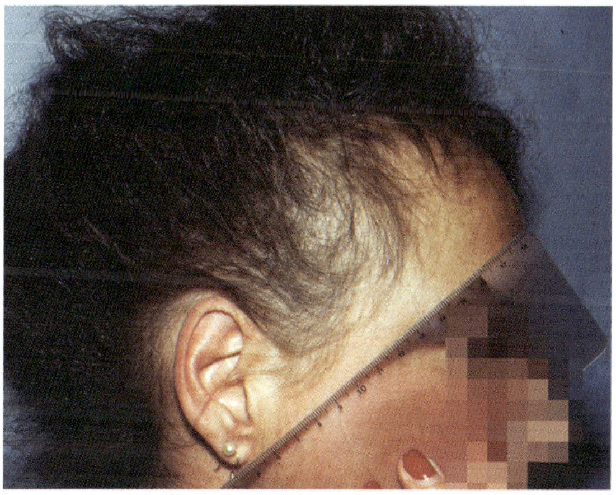

Figure 10.12 Temporoparietal alopecia in a woman after regularly wearing a cap.

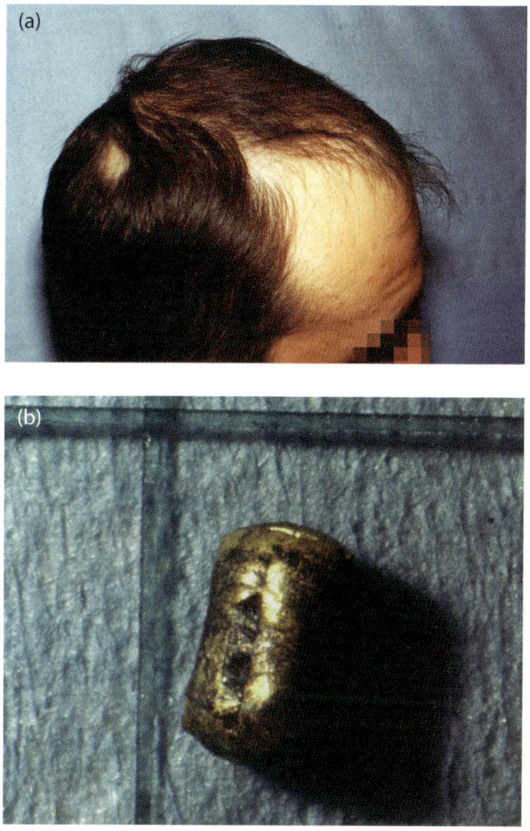

Figure 10.13 (a) Alopecia caused by traction from clips holding the hair in place. (b) Example of a small metal cylinder used to secure a prosthesis.

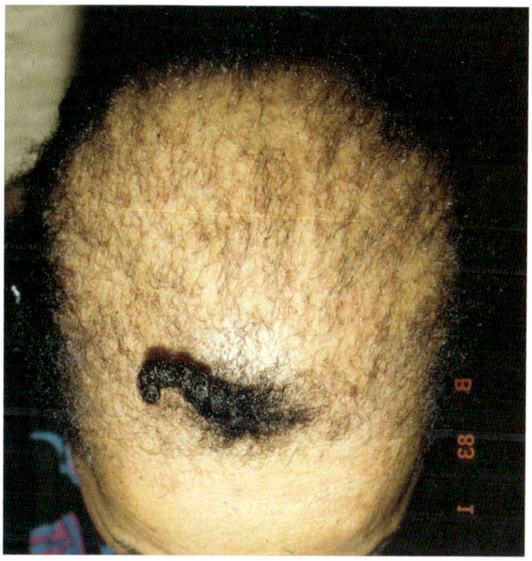

Figure 10.14 Almost complete scarring alopecia in a black woman who had been using hot hair-straightening irons for many years.

with karite) to decrease the possible underlying fragility of the hair shaft. It is not proved that the prescription of topical minoxidil encourages some regrowth because nearly all the hairs are in anagen phase, and it may increase the growth of vellus on the face of the female patient.

TRAUMATIC ACCIDENT ALOPECIA

Some traumatic accidents can cause nonscarring alopecia, for which the diagnosis of cause can be difficult; it is, most often, ischemia caused by prolonged or repeated compression of part of the scalp (Figure 10.15).[7] This can occur, for example, from compression by forceps during childbirth (Figure 10.16) or during compression by repeated and prolonged wearing of a cap or orthodontic headgear (a head cap) by a child.

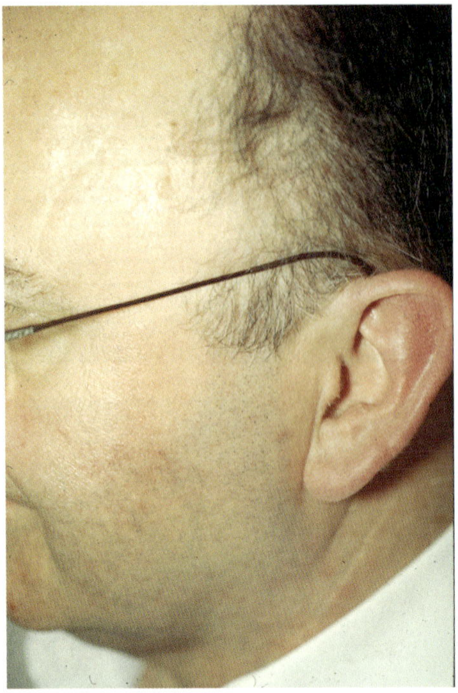

Figure 10.15 **Temporal alopecia due to repeated rubbing and compression of the glasses arms.**

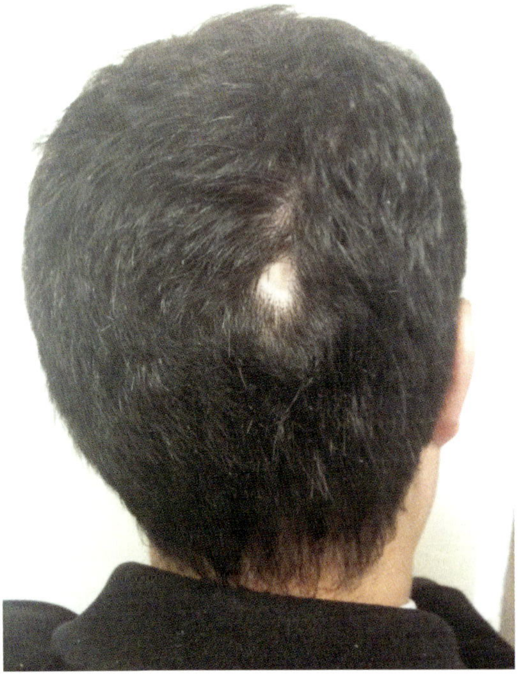

Figure 10.16 **Adult male patient with an occipital alopecia post-forceps.**

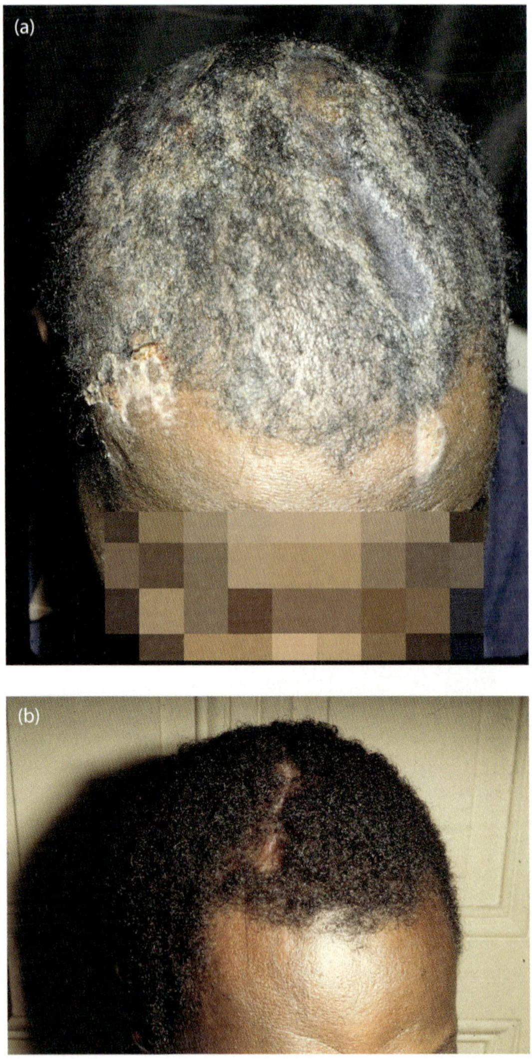

Figure 10.17 **(a) African patient after scalp burning with caustic soda. (b) Spontaneous healing without treatment.**

TRAUMATIC THERMAL, CHEMICAL, AND ISCHEMIC ALOPECIA

A variety of chemical (corrosive) and physical agents can cause permanent alopecia of the scalp. In general, any thermal, physical, or chemical injury sufficient to cause scalp necrosis can produce a permanent alopecia. In the acute stage, necrosis with crusting, an adherent eschar, or ulceration may be present (Figure 10.17a and b). Later, the scalp heals by reparative fibrosis. The result is usually an atrophic alopecic patch. Ischemic necrosis of the scalp produces a similar clinical picture. Ischemic scalp necrosis may be seen after prolonged anesthesia. The necrosis generally involves the occipital scalp and represents a pressure phenomenon. Ischemic necrosis may also occur as a result of vasoconstriction related to the infusion of pharmacologic agents such as vasopressin.

RADIATION

Radiation injury may cause transient nonscarring alopecia (epilating dose). Higher doses[9] produce permanent alopecia with scarring. Histological changes in anagen

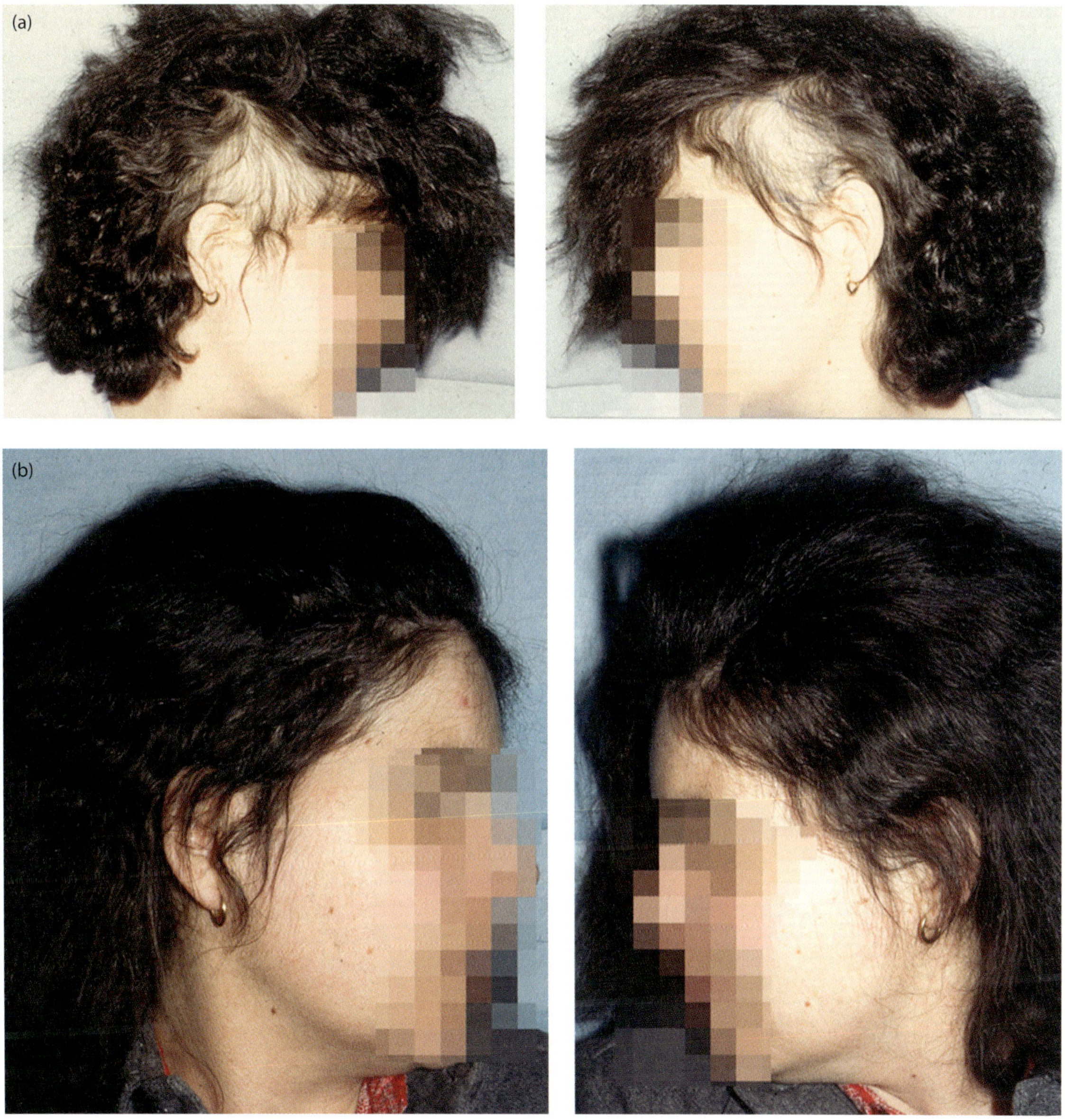

Figure 10.18 **(a) Bitemporal cicatricial alopecia after radiotherapy for brain tumor, and (b) correction after one hair transplant session.**

hair follicles can be noted as early as 4 days following radiation. Similar effects are noted with x-rays and electron beam radiation. The earliest change is thinning of the hair bulb, especially in the area of the matrix. Two or 3 weeks following irradiation, hairs with tapered shafts are apparent. The number of follicles showing radiation effects is roughly proportional to the dose of radiation. The definitive treatment is the scar excision or, better, a hair transplant restoration (Figure 10.18a and b).

CONCLUSION

Traction alopecia and trichotillomania are types of physical trauma that can lead to alopecia.

Traction alopecia is seen most commonly in black females. Trichotillomania is a traction alopecia related to a compulsive disorder. In the long term, permanent alopecia may occur.

REFERENCES

1. Rook A, Dawber R. *Diseases of the Hair and Scalp.* Oxford, UK: Blackwell Scientific Publications; 1982.
2. Camacho F, Montagna W. *Trichologie-maladies du follicule pilosébacé.* Madrid, Spain: Grupo Aula Médica SA; 1997.
3. Olsen EA. *Disorders of Hair Growth—Diagnosis and Treatment.* New York, NY: McGraw-Hill; 1997.
4. Bouhanna P. Alopécies traumatiques. In: Bouhanna P, Reygagne P, ed. *Pathologie du cheveu et du cuir chevelu.* Paris, France: Masson; 1999:145–152.
5. Tosti A, Miteva M, Torres F, Vincenzi C, Romanelli P. Hair casts are a dermoscopic clue for the diagnosis of traction alopecia. *Br J Dermatol.* 2010;163:1353–1355.
6. Tosti A. *Dermascopy of Hair and Scalp Disorders.* London: Informa Healthcare; 2007.
7. Bouhanna P. Les alopécies traumatiques, une triple orientation diagnostique. In: Bouhanna P, ed. *Les alopécies—de la clinique au traitement. Collection Guide Pratique de Dermatologie.* Paris, France: Med'Com;2004.
8. Ferrando J. *Alopecias: Guia de diagnostico y tratamiento.* Barcelona, Spain: Pulso; 2000.
9. Camacho FM, Tosti A. *Montagna tercera Edicion—Tricologia Enfermedades del foliculo pilosabaceo.* Madrid, Spain: Biblioteca Aula Medica Editions; 2014.

11 Management of acquired primary cicatricial alopecia

Salvador Villablanca and Juan Ferrando

INTRODUCTION

Human hair involves aspects of self-image, identity, ethnicity, and health, among other attributes. This is why it is no surprise that diseases that cause alopecia can cause altered self-perception and psychosocial interactions.[1]

Alopecia can be classified as cicatricial (or scarring) and noncicatricial. In turn, cicatricial alopecia (CA) is subdivided into primary cicatricial alopecia (PCA) and secondary cicatricial alopecia (SCA). The PCAs represent a rare and heterogeneous group of diseases, clinically characterized by the absence of follicular ostium and histologically by the replacement of hair follicle structures by fibrous tissue making the alopecia irreversible. From a physiopathological point of view, the scar is the end point of reparative fibrosis with permanent destruction of the preexisting tissue.[2–4] In PCA the hair follicle is the main target of the inflammatory process, as evidenced microscopically as a preferential destruction of follicular epithelium and/or adventitial dermis associated with relative preservation of interfollicular reticular dermis.[5,6]

In secondary CA, the destruction of the hair follicle is not the primary pathological event. It results from nonfollicular damage that eventually destroys the follicle. In these cases, the permanent follicular scarring develops when the involved pathological process is close to the follicular unit. Exogenous factors such as trauma (burns, radiation, and traction) and infiltrative and inflammatory endogenous processes (sarcoidosis, pemphigus vulgaris, and scleroderma) may result in secondary scarring alopecia[2,4,7] (Table 11.1).

Primary CA may become a true clinical challenge due to the limited knowledge of the natural history of the disease. Many do not have a known cause. Clinical findings often have limited useful data for the diagnosis, because of overlapping findings and lack of specific signs. This sometimes makes it difficult to distinguish between the different conditions. Also, the clinical and histological characteristics can change over time, finally resulting in most cases in hair replacement with scarring tissue.

EPIDEMIOLOGY

The epidemiology of PCA in the general population is unknown. Two retrospective studies in hair research institutions estimated prevalence between 3.2% and 7.3%.[2,3] In a recent survey performed in the United Kingdom, the estimated incidence of PCA was 6.96 per 1000 new general dermatology referrals per year, which is equivalent to about 9.6 new cases per clinician per year.[8] The ratio between PCA and SCA is estimated at 1:15, and the ratio between neutrophilic and lymphocytic PCA is 1:4.[3]

Between 30% and 40% of patients with PCA in a hair research institution are cataloged as pseudopelade (or

Table 11.1 Causes of Secondary Cicatricial Alopecia

Physical/chemical agents	• Chemical burns • Insect bites • Mechanical trauma, traction, compression or laceration • Radiation dermatitis • Thermal burns
Dermal granulomatous infiltrations (infectious origin)	• Fungic infections • Protozoa • Tuberculosis • Syphilis • Viral infections
Dermal granulomatous infiltrations (noninfectious)	• Necrobiosis lipoidica • Sarcoidosis • Amyloidosis • Actinic granuloma
Sclerosing disorders	• Lichen sclerosus et atrophicus • Morphea • Scleroderma • Sclerotic porphyria cutanea tarda
Neoplastic infiltrations	• Basal cell carcinoma • Squamous cell carcinoma • Dermatofibrosarcoma protuberans • Lymphoma • Malignant melanoma • Metastasic carcinoma • Adnexal Tumor • etc.
Inherited and congenital disorders	• Aplasia cutis, eccrine hamartoma, incontinencia pigmenti, keratosis pilaris spinulosa decalvans, neurofibromatosis, chondrodysplasia punctata, polyostotic fibrous dysplasia, cutis verticis gyrata, Darier disease, epidermal nevi, epidermolisis bullosa, hair follicle hamartoma, hypotrichosis congenita, ichthyosis (sex-linked recessive), porokeratosis of Mibelli

nonspecific cicatricial alopecia).[2] This means that one-third of cases have no specific diagnosis, becoming a true diagnostic and therapeutic "desert" for both dermatologists and patients. The diagnosis of PCA is not a purely academic exercise, because early treatment of the inflammatory component may prevent the progression of primary scarring alopecia, and the secondary fibrosis that gives the alopecia its irreversibility. Within the PCA with predominantly lymphocytic infiltrate, the most frequent condition varies depending on the different series. First and second places in frequency are always disputed between lichen planopilaris (and its variants) and cutaneous discoid lupus erythematosus, followed by pseudopelade of Brocq (PB).[2,3,9] This difference may be influenced by a discrepancy in the clinicopathological diagnostic criteria between authors, especially in regard to the classical PB (an entity in constant discussion). Among the causes of PCA with an initially neutrophilic infiltrate, we should consider folliculitis decalvans (FD) as the most common form (10% of al PCA), unlike *perifolliculitis abscedens et suffodiens capitis* (less than 5% of PCA).[10]

Table 11.2 Proposed NAHRS Working Classification of Primary Cicatricial Alopecia

Lymphocytic	Chronic cutaneous lupus erythematosus
	Lichen planopilaris
	Classic lichen planus
	Frontal fibrosing alopecia
	Graham-Little syndrome
	Classic pseudopelade (Brocq)
	Central centrifugal cicatricial alopecia
	Alopecia mucinosa,
	Keratosis follicularis spinulosa decalvans
Neutrophilic	Folliculitis decalvans
	Dissecting cellulitis/folliculitis (*perifolliculitis capitis abscedens et suffodiens*)
Mixed	Folliculitis (acne) keloidalis
	Folliculitis (acne) necrotica
	Erosive pustular dermatosis
Nonspecific	

Source: Adapted from Tan E, Martinka M, Ball N et al., *J Am Acad Dermatol.* 2004;50:25–32.

ETHIOLOGY

There is a paucity of data in the literature regarding the origin of PCA. In most of the literature, histopathology revealed the presence of inflammation affecting the upper portion of the hair, which would explain the irreversibility of the process, because at this location, stem cells are housed. This place called the protuberance or bulge is located in the infundibulum, where the hair erector muscle inserts. In some situations, the trigger of this inflammatory response is the result of an antigenic stimulation of Langerhans cells that are located in the pilosebaceous unit. Examples of a possible antigenic stimuli would be ultraviolet radiation in the case of lupus erythematosus, certain medications in the case of lichen planopilaris, and *Staphylococcus aureus* in the case of folliculitis decalvans. With the new knowledge in respect to its origin, it is known that there is a loss of immune protection of bulge stem cells,[5,11] a dysfunction in the ability of self-perpetuation of stem cells, increased autoimmune activity enhanced by pro-inflammatory cytokines, and predisposing genetic and environmental factors.[12–14] Recent data also suggest association with an altered lipid metabolism and development of the PCA, where a sebaceous gland dysfunction could play an important role in their pathogenesis. Independent of the initial event, the obliteration or permanent functional impairment of the critical elements for the reconstitution of the follicle results in permanent alopecia.[15–19]

CLASSIFICATION

Currently there are several classifications for PCA, but the most accepted is the one proposed by the North American Hair Research Society (NAHRS).[20] This classification divides the PCA into two groups according to the type of predominant inflammatory cell infiltrate (lymphocytic and neutrophilic), a concept that had been previously suggested by other authors, but was improved by this working group, adding two more subgroups: mixed and nonspecific (Table 11.2). Although there have been debates about whether this classification is satisfactory, it gives us a practical and reasonable view for basic and clinical research.

CLINICAL PATTERNS OF PRESENTATION

There is a big clinical and histopathological overlap between different entities of PCA. There are some forms of PCA whose existence per se is discussed, and among them is the pseudopelade of Brocq.

In daily practice we observe two major clinical patterns of presentations of scarring alopecia, the first correspond to patients with multiple irregular patches of scarring alopecia (Figure 11.1) on the scalp, and the second pattern correspond to patients with a central patch (Figure 11.2) surrounded by several smaller patches of scarring alopecia ("cicatricial satellitosis"). Both types of clinical presentations are final stages of cutaneous processes that previously had affected hair follicles (evidenced or not), finishing with these residual and nonspecific features that do not allow us to elucidate the etiopathogenic origin of it. We call these two classic patterns of scarring alopecia presentation a "footprints in the snow" pattern for the first and "big patch" pattern for the second. If we look at other forms of clinical presentation of scarring alopecia, there are other characteristic patterns that could be called specific patterns: marginal pattern (frontal fibrosing alopecia, and tractional alopecia),

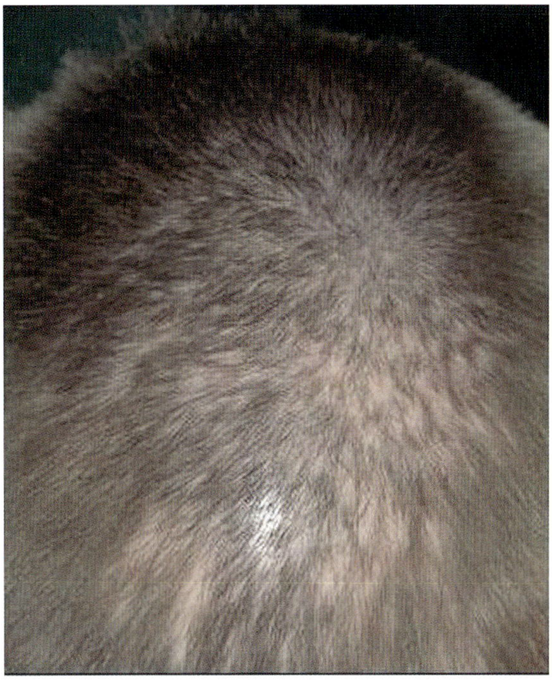

Figure 11.1 Patches of scarring alopecia as multifocal lesions ("footprints in the snow").

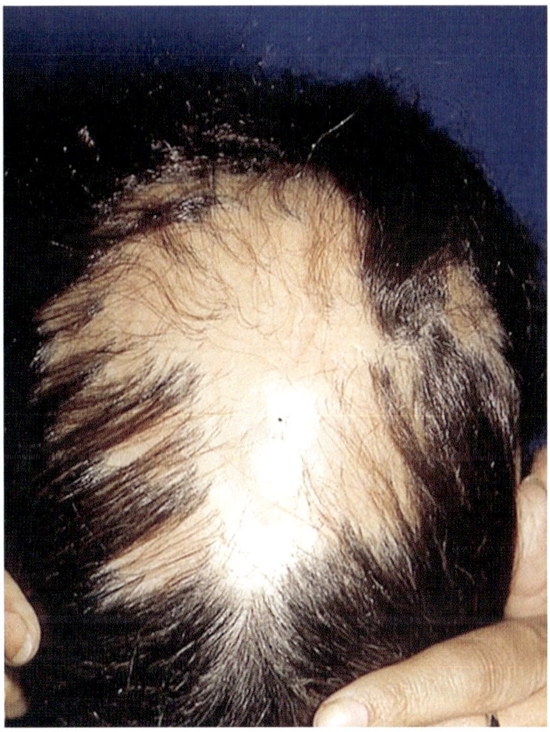

Figure 11.2 Central patch surrounded by several smaller patches of scarring alopecia at the periphery ("cicatricial satellitosis").

follicular pattern (lichen planopilaris, decalvant folliculitis, alopecia parvimaculata, acne necrotica, and tufted folliculitis), inflammatory-abscedens pattern (pustular erosive dermatosis of the scalp, perifolliculitis capitis abscedens et suffodiens), and the diffuse pattern (acute lichen planus pilaris, and the red scalp syndrome).

Primary cicatricial alopecia with an initially lymphocytic infiltrate

In early stages of primary scarring alopecia associated with lymphocytic infiltrates, the clinical features are fairly characteristic. The causes are listed in Table 11.2.

CUTANEOUS DISCOID LUPUS ERYTHEMATOSUS

Scalp involvement occurs in many cases of chronic cutaneous discoid lupus erythematosus (CDLE), but in just 10%–20% of cases as a single manifestation. It affects mainly women and usually begins between 20 and 50 years of age.[11] The lesions, which occur mainly on the sun-exposed areas of the face and ears and anywhere on the scalp, are clinically characterized by erythematous maculopapules that extend in a centrifugal way, with plugging of follicular ostia and formation of adherent scale that may be hyperkeratotic (Figure 11.3). In the evolved lesions, an atrophic component with telangiectasias is added and pigmentary changes can be seen. The early, active lesions may be sensitive and pruritic. The developed lesion exhibits a scaly crust with follicular spines attached to the under surface. The diagnosis is facilitated by the presence of lesions of CDLE in other locations, but if these lesions are not present, the differential diagnosis with follicular lichen planopilaris can be difficult, and also should include tinea capitis, psoriasis, and alopecia mucinosa. The lesion may resolve but tends

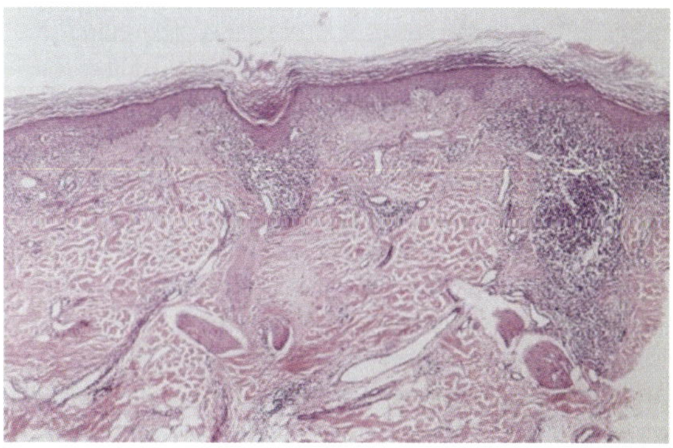

Figure 11.3 Histology of chronic discoid lupus erythematosus with involvement of the scalp. Hematoxylin and eosin stain, ×40. Atrophic epidermis with interface dermatitis changes with the presence of necrotic keratinocytes and a perivascular and periadnexal inflammatory infiltrate with lymphocyte predominance.

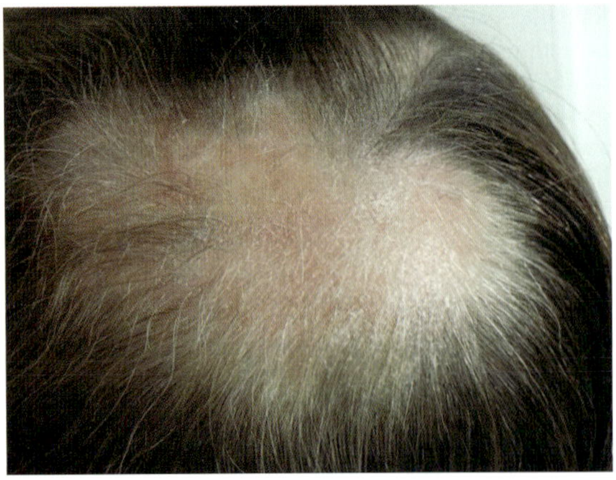

Figure 11.4 **Chronic discoid lupus erythematosus with involvement of the scalp. Erythematous patch with plugging of follicular ostia and formation of adherent scale that may be hyperkeratotic. Lesion activity is primarily in the center of the plate.**

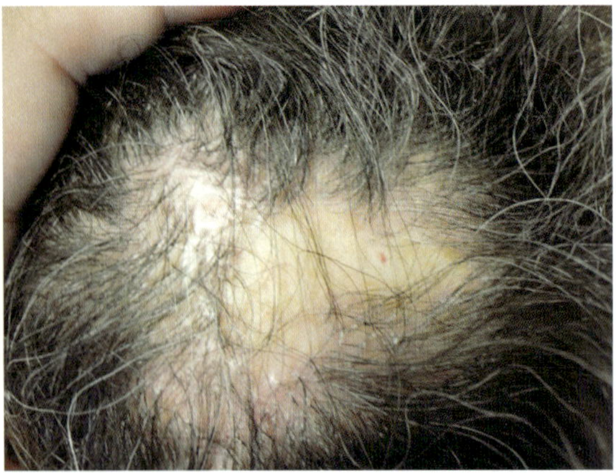

Figure 11.5 **Classical lichen planopilaris. Characterized by perifollicular erythema and hyperkeratotic follicular papules that are diffusely distributed, with isolated follicles respected in the center.**

to recur centrally, well within the previously affected atrophic patch rather than at its margin. From the histopathological point of view, cicatricial alopecia due to CDLE is characterized by perifollicular infiltrate with a lichenoid pattern.

Lupus erythematosus is characterized by the presence of vacuolar changes in the follicular epithelium and the interfollicular epidermis, with apoptotic keratinocytes, thickening of the basal membrane, the presence of dermal mucin, and periadnexal and perivascular infiltrate in the dermis (Figure 11.4). Dyskeratosis is minimal to moderate.[21–23]

LICHEN PLANOPILARIS

Lichen planopilaris is considered a variant of lichen planus and has three recognized variants: the classic follicular lichen planus, Piccardi–Lassueur–Graham-Little syndrome, and the frontal fibrosing alopecia with a marginal distribution pattern as a topographic variation.

Classical lichen planopilaris (LPP) usually appears in middle-aged women, in the form of pruritic (or painful) perifollicular erythema followed by acuminate, spinous, hyperkeratotic follicular papules that are diffusely distributed, but predominantly in the center of the scalp, which resolve leaving erythematous, atrophic polygonal-shaped patches of cicatricial alopecia areas (with intact follicles inside) with little tendency to coalesce (Figures 11.5 and 11.6).[10,21,24] The disease tends to be multifocal, with slow and progressive extension (usually with active lesions in the periphery) marked by exacerbations, which can determine an intense hair fall. Typical lesions of lichen planus are rarely observed in other skin sites or mucosa (bipolar lichen planus).[25] When the disease begins, erosions are rare, and the association with CDLE had been described. The differential diagnosis includes CDLE, alopecia areata, pseudopelade of Brocq, alopecia mucinosa, and folliculitis decalvans (although in the latter it is common to observe micropustules).

From a histopathological point of view, LPP is characterized by lichenoid infiltrate focused at the isthmus and the follicular infundibulum, with infundibular hyperkeratosis and underlying hypergranulosis, often sebaceous glands are atrophic or absent, interfollicular epidermis can be involved, and incontinentia

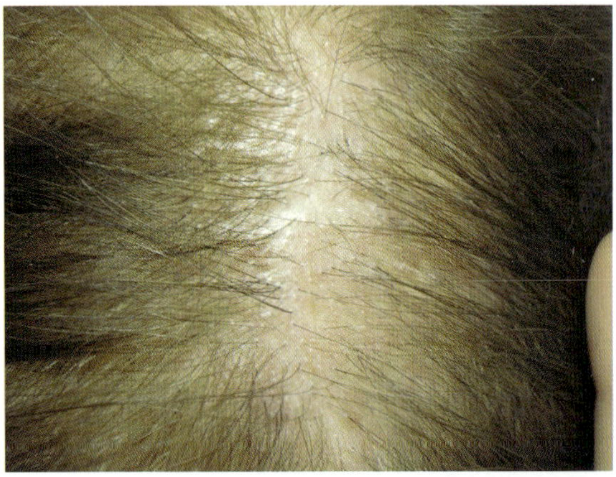

Figure 11.6 **Evolved classical lichen planopilaris. Erythematous, atrophic patches of cicatricial alopecia areas (with intact follicles inside of it) with little tendency to coalesce.**

pigmenti should be intense. Dyskeratosis is moderate to prominent. Exocytosis of cells into the epidermis is common. Perieccrine infiltrates are absent, and perivascular infiltrate may be minimal, superficial, and perifollicular. Epidermal and dermal mucin is usually absent (Figure 11.7). In evolved lesions, a destruction of the follicle with foreign body granulomas is observed, and eventually longitudinal and concentric lamellar fibrosis paths corresponding to existing follicles with minimal inflammatory infiltrate are present. In residual lesions, it is often impossible to make a specific diagnosis. In LPP diffuse dermal fibrosis is not observed, the latter being a characteristic change in CDLE.[21–23]

Piccardi–Lassueur–Graham-Little syndrome is characterized by progressive frontal scarring alopecia of the scalp associated with loss of axillary and pubic hair and rapid development of follicular keratoses on the trunk and occasionally in the lower extremities, histopathologically consistent with follicular lichen planus. It is possible that this condition is closer to a form of scarring follicular keratosis than to lichen planus or lichen planopilaris.

Frontal fibrosing alopecia (FFA), originally described by Kossard in 1994,[26] mainly affects postmenopausal women over 50 years, and is characterized by atrophic recession of the frontotemporal hairline, with remaining isolated follicles, giving it a distinctive look. The frontotemporal recession exposes pearly white looking skin that has been previously protected from the dermatoheliosis. In the recession or progression line of alopecia, perifollicular erythema and infundibular hyperkeratosis can be observed, being indistinguishable from those of classic LPP. Most patients also present with scarring alopecia in parietal areas, preauricular areas, and eyebrows, which may be accompanied by erythema (Figure 11.8). The association with androgenetic alopecia is common in postmenopausal women, and occasionally concomitant involvement of lichen planus has been described at other sites, which, together with histopathological findings,

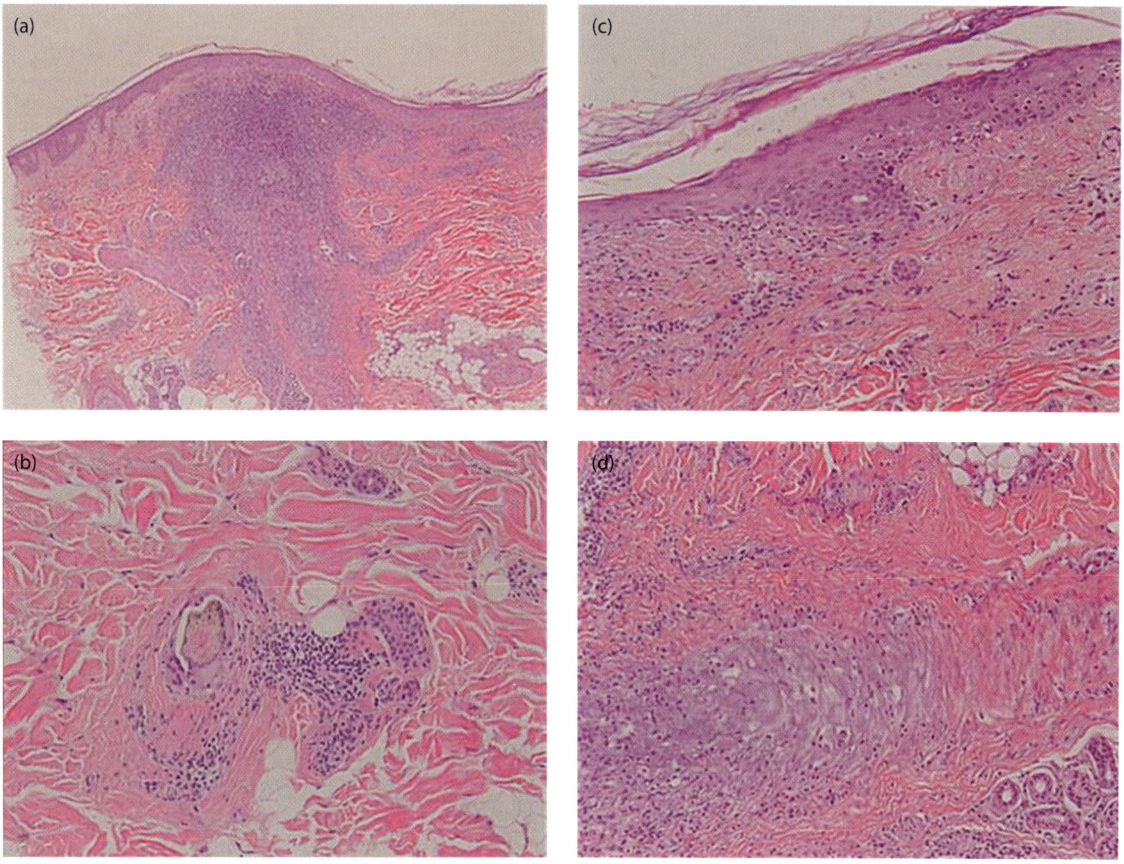

Figure 11.7 Histology of lichen planopilaris (hematoxilin and eosin stain). (a) (×40) Perifollicular lymphocytic infiltrate primarily affecting the follicular isthmus and infundibulum. (b) (×100) Vacuolar changes in the epidermis next to the follicle. (c) (×100) Lymphocytic infiltrate surrounding a follicle with incipient scarring. (d) (×100) Follicle with necrotic keratinocytes.

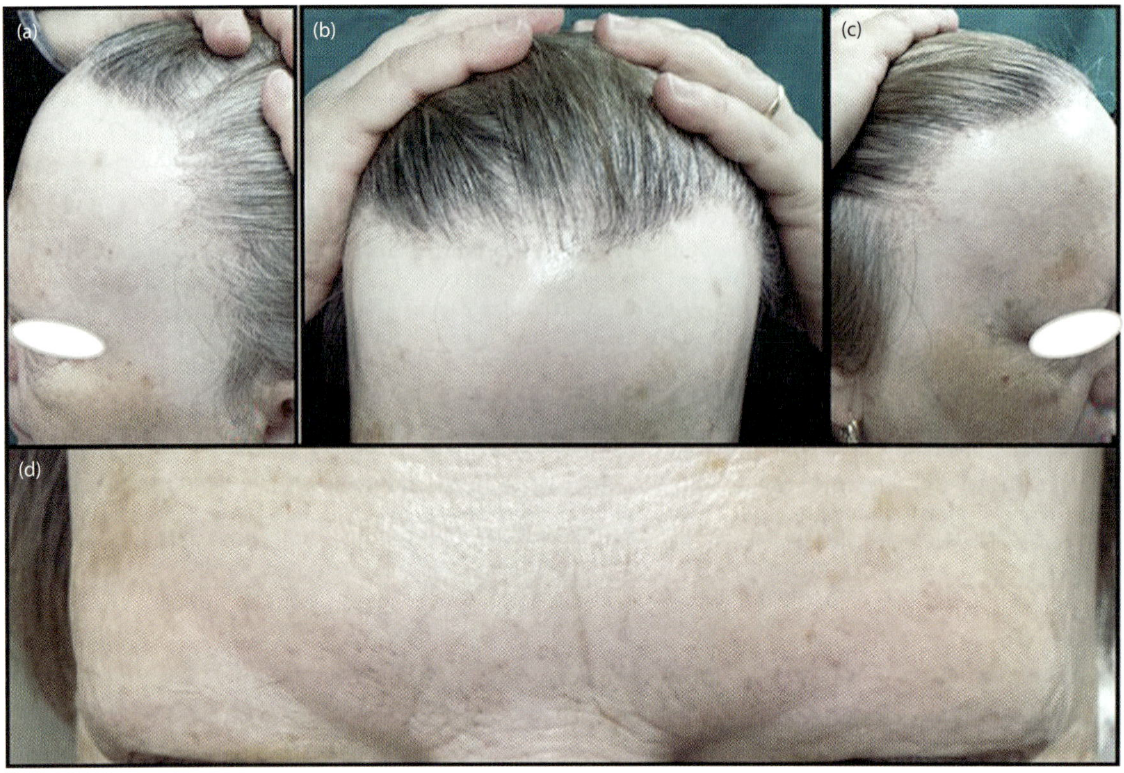

Figure 11.8 **Frontal fibrosing alopecia. Characteristic marginal pattern affecting the temporal (a and c) and frontal region (b). It is typically the partial or total involvement of the eyebrows (d).**

justifies the nosological grouping of these entities. Small papules of the face have also been described accompanying FFA, with the characteristic changes of LPP on the facial involved vellus.[27]

Fibrosing alopecia with a female androgenetic alopecia pattern distribution has been described in women about 60 years of age, proving the presence of a scarring alopecia with perifollicular erythema, loss of ostia and follicular keratosis, sometimes painful, located in the central portion of the scalp. Histologically, a lymphomononuclear infiltrate is observed in the isthmic portion of some follicles, with perifollicular lamellar fibrosis, and in a variable percentage of biopsied cases, interface dermatitis and basal vacuolar change with apoptosis of keratinocytes (Figure 11.9). Although the differential diagnosis must be made with the pseudopelade and follicular degeneration syndrome (central centrifugal scarring alopecia), this is probably either a topographic variant FFA or a hybrid form of alopecia, combining female androgenetic alopecia with a LPP.[3,10,28,29]

PSEUDOPELADE OF BROCQ

Although the concept of "pseudopelade" is used to refer to the final stage of various scarring alopecias, to avoid confusion, it has been proposed that the term be abandoned.[22,30,31] The clinical definition of the disease according to Ross et al.[10] is of a chronic form of scarring alopecia in white women that is typically presented with outbreaks of multifocal lesions (lenticular, "moth-eaten," or "footprints in the snow" pattern) predominantly of central distribution (vertex). Characteristically it presents with small size, geometrical configuration, minimal perifollicular erythema, and ivorian hypopigmentation, occasionally showing a slight depression (Figure 11.10). From the histopathological view, the Braun-Falco et al.[32] series highlights the presence of a normal epidermis with fibrous tracts in the subcutaneous tissue, the absence or decrease in number of sebaceous glands, and the absence of marked inflammation, significant follicular plugging, or widespread scarring. Although it has been described as an atrophy of the epidermis, it does not correspond to an interface dermatitis with vacuolar change. It should be considered then as a histopathological exclusion diagnosis in the context of characteristic signs. The final evolution of pseudopelade of Brocq gives clinical and histopathological features indistinguishable from other "burned" primary scarring alopecia. In summary, with this term, both forms of scarring alopecia are recognized, the small patches and the conventionally large central patch, as both are considered a final cicatricial stage of a previous inflammatory follicular process not detected at its early stage.[33,34]

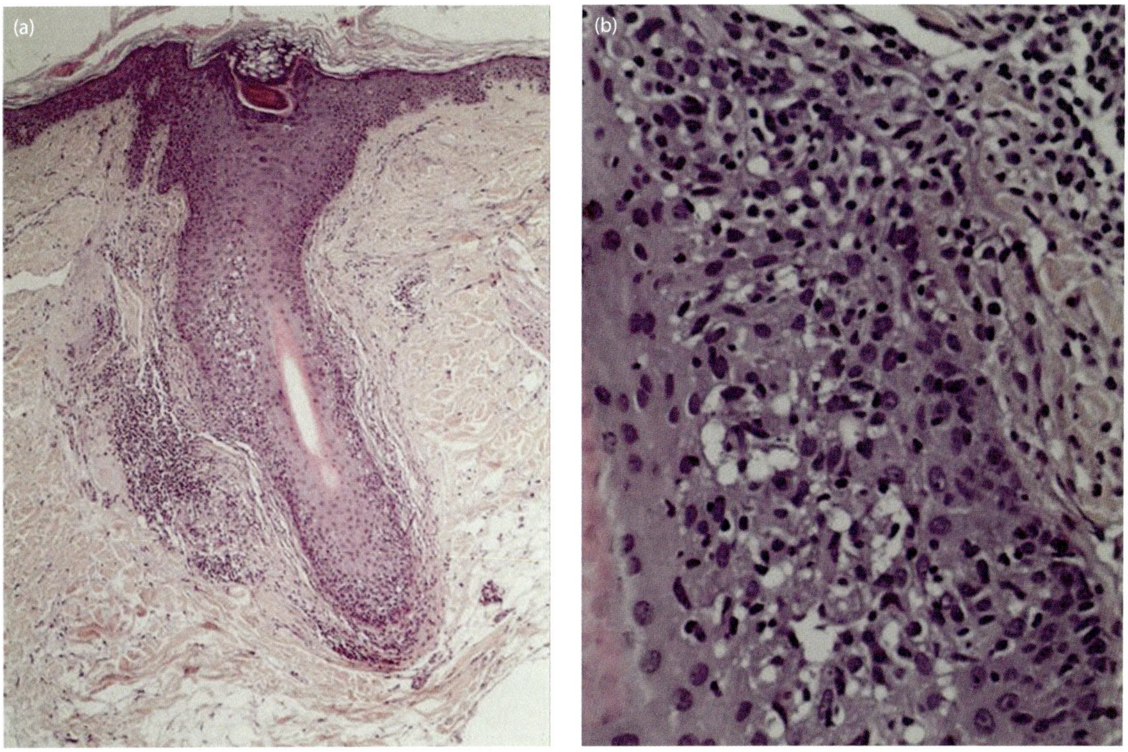

Figure 11.9 **Histology of frontal fibrosing alopecia (hematoxylin and eosin stain). (a) (×40) lymphocytic infiltrate surrounding the hair follicle. (b) (×100) Hair follicle with vacuolization of basal layer and lymphocytic infiltrate.**

CENTRAL CENTRIFUGAL CICATRICIAL ALOPECIA

The follicular degeneration syndrome was initially described in African American women who used hot combs to straighten their hair, and was then regarded as a form of traumatic alopecia. The clinical term of *central centrifugal cicatricial alopecia* (CCCA) has been set to include cases that occur in white individuals with a similar pattern of alopecia characterized by a central alopecia patch with centrifugal extension. CCCA commonly affects middle-age black women, starting as a central cicatricial alopecia over the vertex, which gradually spreads outward in a centrifugal direction (Figure 11.11).[10,35] Histopathologically it is considered characteristic of this entity of perifollicular chronic inflammation, concentric lamellar fibroplasias with eccentric epithelial atrophy (more marked in isthmus and infundibulum). Premature desquamation of the internal follicular sheath (although this is not a consistent or specific finding of this entity) and eventual destruction of the follicular epithelium, with acute and chronic perifollicular inflammation are noted, but sparse and peri-eccrine infiltrates are absent. Central centrifugal cicatricial alopecia is characterized by preservation of the elastic sheath surrounding the fibrous tracts. Dyskeratosis is absent, and pigment incontinence is minimal. Epidermal and dermal mucins are absent. The differential diagnosis includes androgenetic alopecia and trichotillomania.[35]

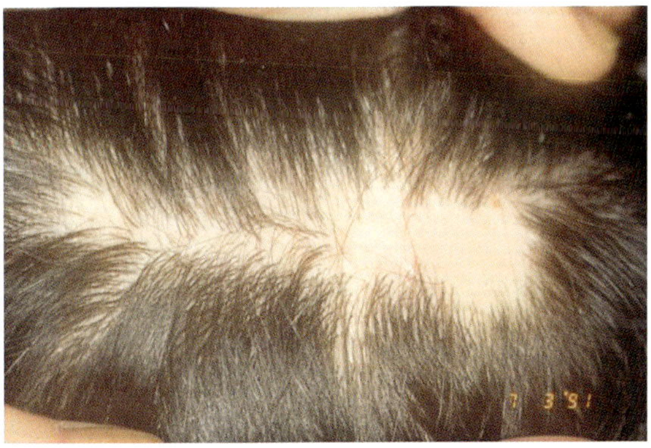

Figure 11.10 **Classic pseudopelade of Brocq. Small size patches of geometrical configuration, with minimal perifollicular erythema and ivorian hypopigmentation, occasionally showing a slight depression.**

ALOPECIA MUCINOSA

Alopecia mucinosa is usually benign and self-limiting in children and young adults, although it occasionally

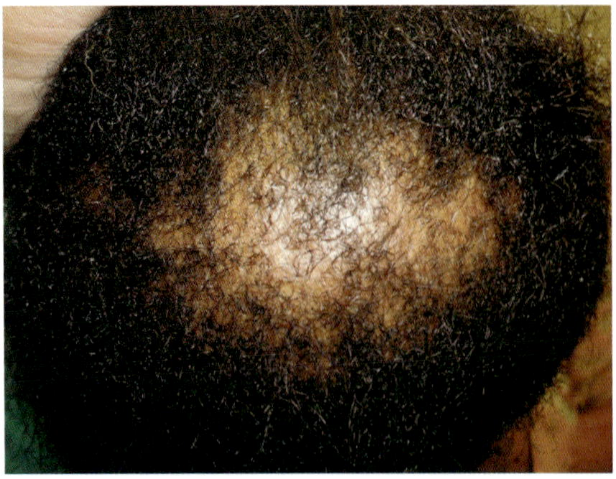

Figure 11.11 **Central centrifugal cicatricial alopecia characterized by a central cicatricial patch of alopecia over the vertex, which gradually spreads outwards in a centrifugal direction.**

results in permanent patchy alopecia. It may be associated with lymphoproliferative disorders in older patients with multiple lesions. It is characterized by scaly erythematous infiltrate plaques formed by the confluence of follicular papules, with alopecia and dilation of the ostium follicular, localized predominantly on the face, shoulders, neck, and scalp. Histopathologically, the entity is defined by the presence of follicular mucinosis, accompanying a lymphomononuclear infiltrate that in many cases (30% of cases in adults) has a clonal origin, and corresponds to a cutaneous T cell lymphoma, of relatively indolent course in many cases.[10,36]

Keratosis follicularis spinulosa decalvans

Keratosis follicularis spinulosa decalvans (KFSD) was described by Siemens in 1926. The disease is grouped with the follicular atrophic facial keratosis and the atrophoderma vermicularis under the name of *keratosis pilaris decalvans*. However, some authors postulate that they might be different stages of the same disease.

The sex-linked inheritance of KFSD has been proposed by several authors. The most severe manifestations have been observed in boys, thus confirming a sex-linked inheritance. In genetic mapping studies, the KFSD is located on chromosome Xp21.2-p22.2. Female carriers often show signs of the disease but are affected in a milder form. This type of inheritance can be explained by the inactivation escapade mechanism of X-linked genes. Some authors believe that KFSD is transmitted in autosomal dominant form with a variable expression. However, some cases may occur sporadically.[37]

They have described three stages in the development of KFSD. The onset occurs in early childhood with photophobia and follicular keratosis, then comes an active phase of progressive scarring alopecia that mainly affects the parietal and occipital region, as well as eyebrows, especially in its outer third, and eyelashes, this being a distinguishing characteristic of the disease. After puberty it may also affect axillary and pubic regions. The hair shows a dry, rough, short, and fragile aspect. This process continues until early adolescence when the progressive scarring alopecia stops and photophobia improves. During adolescence, the disease is frequently associated with hyperkeratosis of palms and soles. Other clinical features that occur in this syndrome include atopia, photophobia, and corneal abnormalities.[38]

The histological findings include intrafollicular abscesses, perifollicular and perivascular infiltrate that may contain numerous plasma cells, follicular horny plugs, and hypoplasia, or absence of sebaceous glands. The latter is a fundamental pathological substrate of the disease. The scanning electron microscope reveals a fragile constitution hair with intense severe cuticular abnormalities.

The disease has been associated with mental retardation in a few cases, sensorineural hearing loss, delayed growth, repeated bacterial infections, hyperaminoaciduria, nail changes, microcephaly, arachnodactyly, and seizures.[39]

The differential diagnosis should take into account monilethrix, trichothiodystrophy, Netherton syndrome, and ectodermal dysplasia. Although it is a rare genodermatosis, KFSD should always be considered in all cases of hyperkeratosis with congenital alopecia. The treatment of such cases should be started as early as possible (especially in the inflammatory phase) in order to delay and minimize the cicatricial phase.

Primary cicatricial alopecia with an initially neutrophilic infiltrate

The pathogenesis of the PCA with an initially neutrophilic infiltrate is unknown. It is hypothesized that *Staphylococcus aureus* may be involved because it is often isolated in pustules, but it is not clear if it is a primary or a secondary process. Other suggested causes include a possible role of bacterial superantigens or a defect in cellular immunity. Currently, the theory is that both folliculitis decalvans and dissecting folliculitis (an even acne keloidalis nuchae) may represent a different spectrum of the same disease, and depending on the difference in follicular anatomy and host immune response, one of the clinical manifestations will predominate.[40,41]

FOLLICULITIS DECALVANS

Folliculitis decalvans or Quinquaud folliculitis is a destructive and suppurative folliculitis that affects young adults of both sexes. It presents with outbreaks of multifocal, erythematous, and hyperkeratotic follicular pustules that surround multiple, slowly expanding round or oval areas of alopecia on the scalp (Figure 11.12). Sometimes it affects several neighboring follicles, which

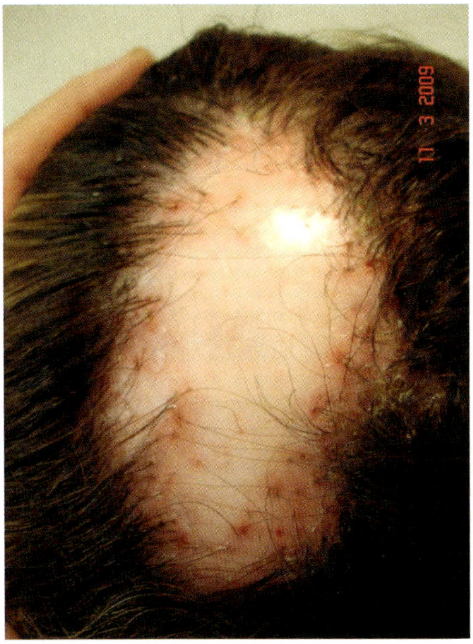

Figure 11.12 **Folliculitis decalvans. A slowly expanding oval area of alopecia on the scalp with multiple hyperkeratotic follicular pustules and crust at the periphery.**

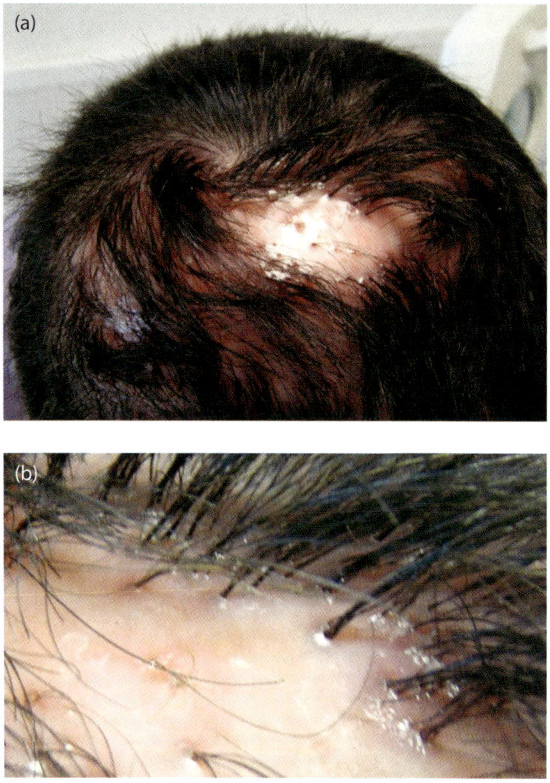

Figure 11.13 **Tufted folliculitis is a peculiar form of folliculitis decalvans where several neighboring follicles are joined in a common follicular ostium with several hairs, forming scarring alopecia patches (a) with the hairs emerging in a "bunched" way (b).**

are joined in a common follicular ostium with several hairs, forming scarring alopecia plates with these hairs emerging in a "bunched" way, which is known as tufted folliculitis (Figure 11.13). The etiological role of *Staphylococcus aureus* is under discussion, which usually appears in bacteriological cultures. Differential diagnosis must be made primarily with other bacterial folliculitis, but also fungal or viral folliculitis, CCCA, and acne necrotica. It tends to affect the vertex area and may also affect other hairy areas beyond the scalp such as the beard, pubic and axillary areas, and the inner thighs. It runs a very long course, and it is sometimes complicated by the fact that even after pustules disappear, the progressive cicatricial alopecia can continue. Histopathological examination shows intra- and perifollicular abscesses affecting the upper and middle portions of the follicle with an initial neutrophilic infiltration, with eventual follicular destruction, foreign body granuloma formation, and perifollicular dermal fibrosis (Figure 11.14). Sinus tract formation is absent, but eventually tufts of hairs may emerge through the same enlarged follicular infundibulum.[42,43]

DISSECTING FOLLICULITIS (PERIFOLLICULITIS CAPITIS ABSCEDENS ET SUFFODIENS)

Also called Hoffman disease, this is an element of the acne tetrad syndrome, along with acne conglobata, hidradenitis suppurativa, and cysta pilaris. A common etiology based on follicular obstruction with follicular rupture and secondary infection has been proposed. This most often affects young black men, and is located essentially in the vertex and occiput. Initial lesions consist on confluent pustules that form fluctuating or firm nodules, with painful suppurative follicular orifice and abscess formation, which eventually lead to scarring alopecia with sinus tracts and keloids production (Figure 11.15). Although spontaneous regression can occur, the occurrence of chronic relapses with active elements at the edges is characteristic.[44,45] The differential diagnosis is limited and must be made with Celso kerion.

Histopathologically, infundibular distention is observed with formation of intra- and perifollicular abscesses. Follicular perforation determines the production of a mixed infiltrate, composed by plasma cells and foreign body granulomas in the perifollicular dermis and superficial fat. Abscesses are lined partially by squamous epithelium that mark off the sinus tracts, that eventually lead to extensive fibrosis in the dermis and subcutaneous tissue, with possible occurrence of keloids.[10,46]

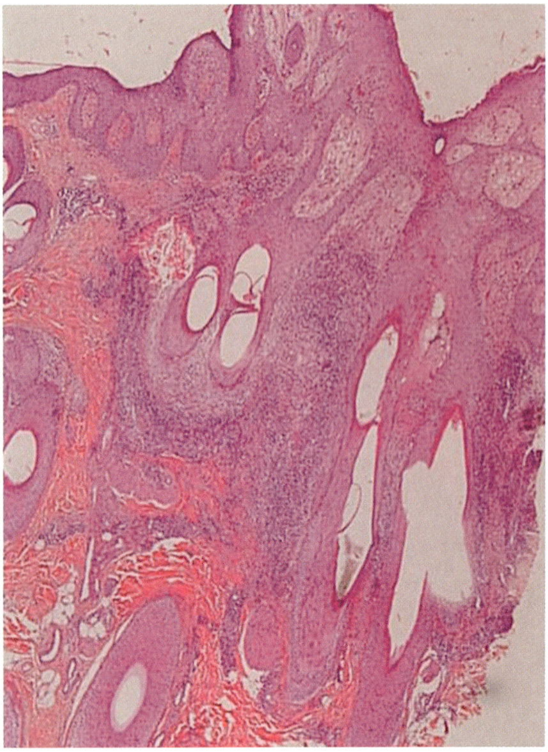

Figure 11.14 Histology of folliculitis decalvans (hematoxylin and eosin stain, ×40). Intra- and perifollicular abscesses affecting upper and middle portion of the follicle with an initial neutrophilic infiltration, with eventual follicular destruction, foreign body granulomas formation, and perifollicular dermal fibrosis.

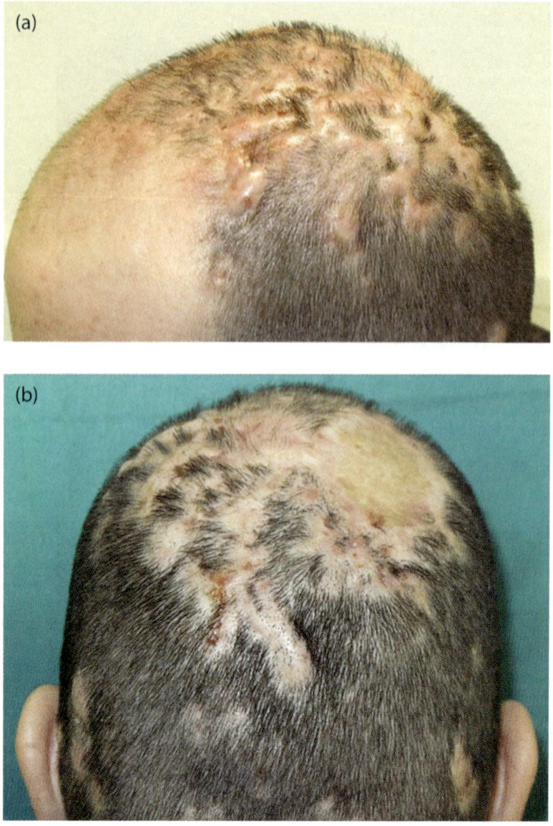

Figure 11.15 Dissecting folliculitis affecting the vertex (a) and occiput (b). Initial lesions consist on confluent pustules that form fluctuating or firm nodules, with painful suppurative follicular orifice and abscess formation, which eventually lead to scarring alopecia with sinus tracts and keloids production.

MIXED SCARRING ALOPECIA

This category includes folliculitis or acne keloidalis nuchae (AKN), acne necrotica, and erosive pustular dermatosis of the scalp.

ACNE KELOIDALIS NUCHAE

Acne keloidalis is an inflammatory process affecting predominantly the occipital hairline of young males, predominantly black. The hypertrophic or keloidal scarring has been attributed to ingrowing hairs in the past, but this has not been confirmed. It begins as follicular papulopustules that soon get umbilicated, leaving a crust with tufted hair accumulation, usually accompanied by itching and pain.[7] The papules tend to coalesce into keloidal plaques or nodules. The differential diagnosis includes FD or bacterial folliculitis. Histologically, a perifollicular lymphoplasmacytic infiltrate is observed, being more evident in the isthmus and the lower portion of the infundibulum, with lamellar fibroplasia and thinning of the follicular epithelium at the isthmus level, disappearance of the sebaceous glands, and eventual destruction of the hair, giving rise to granulomas around residual hair fragments. Acneiform follicular dilatation is an early finding and persists.[47]

ACNE NECROTICA

This condition usually affects adults. It is characterized by erythematous follicular papules that affect the frontal hair line and are found in the parietal area of the scalp undergoing central necrosis, resulting in small patches of alopecia (Figure 11.16). It is a chronic condition and recurs at irregular intervals. The lesions are described as painful and pruritic. Histopathological findings reveal an initial follicular dilatation with a composed infiltrate (lymphocytes and neutrophiles) around and in the follicular infundibulum, with a subsequent individual cell necrosis of keratinocytes within the external root sheath and surrounding epidermis.[10]

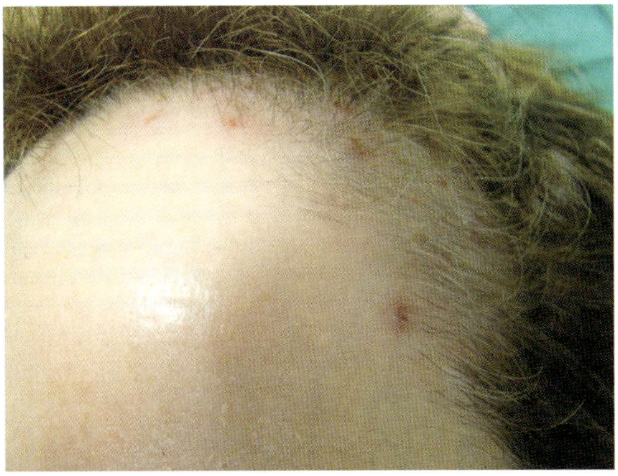

Figure 11.16 **Acne necrotica is characterized by erythematous follicular papules that affect frontal hair line and in the parietal area of the scalp undergoing central necrosis resulting in small patches of alopecia.**

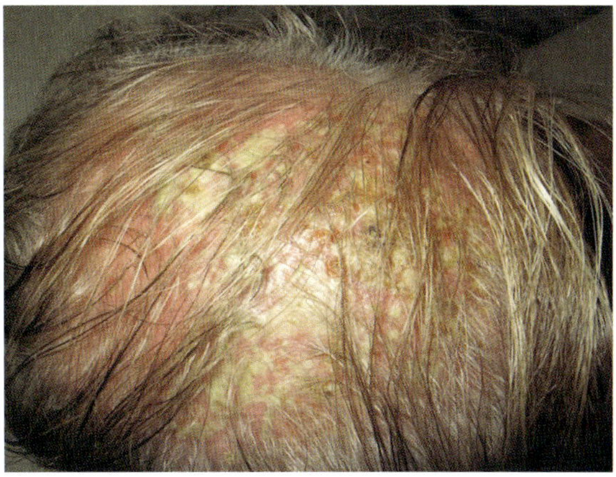

Figure 11.17 **Erosive pustular dermatosis of the scalp is characterized by the presence of pustules and erosions over an erythematous base that lead to scarring alopecia, usually in elderly women.**

EROSIVE PUSTULAR DERMATOSIS OF THE SCALP

This condition is an idiopathic chronic, relapsing amicrobial dermatosis that affects the scalp and is characterized by the presence of pustules and erosions that lead to scarring alopecia, usually in elderly women. There is usually a local trigger such as bruises, sunburn, cryotherapy, or topical application of drugs (5% fluorouracil, tretinoin). Clinically, you can see a large symptomatic, well-demarcated, superficially crusted plaque that is easily unroofed to reveal red, exudative erosion with discrete or coalescent flaccid pustules beneath. Untreated lesions undergo episodic pustular flares, with slow enlargement over years. Cicatricial alopecia is the cardinal feature of advanced disease (Figure 11.17). Histology is unspecific, observing changes in the epidermis that can include erosion, atrophy, acanthosis, parakeratosis, and subcorneal pustules. In the dermis it can be observed as dense, mixed, chronic inflammatory infiltrate, with a variable decrease in follicular units.[10]

PSEUDOPELADE OR NONSPECIFIC CICATRICIAL ALOPECIA

Today, pseudopelade is a broad term that currently includes a number of noninflammatory and idiopathic irregular scarring alopecias. It is a slowly progressive process, during which the hair follicle destruction leads to permanent alopecia. The term *pseudopelade* implies a nonspecific scarring alopecia, which can be a much more understandable term. It is likely that the scarring results from an autoimmune process. In general, there is an insidious increase in this type of scarring process that apparently is not inflammatory.[2] This phenomenon likely results due to the fact that many diseases that gradually cause scarring alopecia burn out and become indistinguishable from each other. The common end result is an irregular scar on the scalp without any distinct clinical and histological feature. The correct diagnosis may be suggested by the initial clinical or histological characteristics, but often this information is not available.

The nonspecific scarring alopecias are not uncommon. In recent studies, it is becoming one of the commonest, if not the most common, form of PCA. It affects mainly middle age women, starting generally at the vertex, but can start anywhere. Clinically, it is characterized by circular or oval, flat, smooth lesions, skin color, somewhat atrophic patches, without clinical evidence of activity in either the center or the periphery, while others tend to form irregular patches that tend to coalesce. It may have an extremely variable course and may in some cases have a rapid extension; occasionally, the patient progresses to fully bald in a few years. At the histopathological study, what is observed in many cases is an evolved scarring process with low or no inflammatory infiltrate, although sometimes you can observe some inflammatory component that is totally nonspecific or insufficient to make a diagnosis. Within the differential diagnosis are CDLE, LPP, FD, and other rare causes of scarring alopecia. Some claim that 90% of cases of pseudopelade result from LPP, although others put the percentage at only 15%.[2,3,22,31]

DIAGNOSTIC TOOLS

Dermoscopy of hair (trichoscopy)

The loss of follicular ostia, which is the most characteristic feature of PCA, may not be clinically evident in some cases, but could be clearly visualized under dermoscopy of the scalp (trichoscopy). This is where we want to emphasize the importance of trichoscopy for the study of scalp disease, and specifically for PCA, because besides allowing the physician to examine the macro- and microscopic morphology of the PCA (e.g., perifollicular erythema or scale hair tufting), by trichoscopy we can also identify subtle clinical signs, confirm diagnoses made by the naked eye, and guide the scalp biopsy to optimize the results, improving in that way the accuracy of the diagnosis, and assess the disease activity and response to the treatment. Thus, trichoscopy should be routinely performed when PCA are considered in the differential diagnoses (Table 11.3) (Figure 11.18).[48–50]

Histopathological examination

Scalp biopsy enables an accurate diagnosis in the majority of cases of PCA, especially if a correct biopsy technique is used, and the pathologist is familiar with the histopathology of the scalp. It allows us to confirm the cicatricial process and determine the predominant infiltrate for classification. This is why a proper scalp biopsy is crucial for the diagnosis of PCA, so it should be performed in the initial presentation of the disease, or shortly after, taking a sample from the active edges of the affected area (where inflammation is seen). This procedure increases the chance to establish the diagnosis by enhancing the probability of finding more inflammatory infiltrate rather than fibrosis (end stage), and initiating an appropriate treatment, improving the chance to respond to it. However, the pathological interpretation may be nondiagnostic if it is not biopsied in the right place. This is particularly relevant in the PCA as the disease may be focal, and the disease activity difficult to see with the naked eye.[12,22,31,51]

Following the above topic, trichoscopy gives a great opportunity to perform the biopsy in the right place. This was corroborated by Tosti et al.[52] in a study with 80 patients with PCA, where biopsies were selected based on the dermoscopic findings, reaching a definitive diagnosis in 95% of cases, being a fast and accurate method even for identifying individually affected follicles in focal PCA or in early stages (Figure 11.19). Trichoscopy findings for PCA are shown in Table 11.3.

Regarding the histological section used to analyze scalp biopsies, there is no consensus. Some advocate for the transverse section (allowing a quantitative and qualitative analysis), while others prefer to use a vertical classic section, or both techniques. However, multiple biopsies could burden the patients with greater medical costs and morbidity. Recently, a new technique has been proposed, the "HoVert" technique, for obtaining transversal and vertical sections from a single punch biopsy.[53]

DIRECT IMMUNOFLUORESCENCE (DIF)

While clinical differentiation between different PCAs may be difficult, particularly with regard to LPP and CDLE (and also PB if it is considered as a specific clinicopathologic

Table 11.3 Trichoscopy Findings in Primary Cicatricial Alopecia

Disease	Dermoscopy Findings
Scarring alopecia (all types)	• White patches: Well-demarcated, white patches (absence of follicular openings)
Lichen planopilaris	• Peripilar casts (hair with peripilar concentric white scales and or peripilar erythema) • Keratotic plugs (keratotic masses plugging follicular ostia) • Blue–gray dots (target pattern) • Interfollicular simple red loops
Frontal fibrosing alopecia	• Peripilar casts • Blue–gray dots (target pattern) • Interfollicular simple red loops
Chronic cutaneous lupus erythematosus	• Peripilar casts • Follicular red dots (erythematous polycyclic, concentric structures regularly distributed in and around the follicular ostia) • Keratotic plugs • Blue–gray dots (speckled pattern) • Arborizing red lines
Folliculitis decalvans	• Hair tufting: Six or more hairs emerging from the same ostium surrounded by white-yellowish scales and crust • Twisted red loops: Multiple red dots at low magnification (×10, ×20) and polymorphous beaded lines and circles at high magnification (× ≥ 40)
Central centrifugal cicatricial alopecia	Peripilar white halo: one or tw o hairs emerging together, surrounded by white–gray halo
Dissecting cellulitis	Black dots

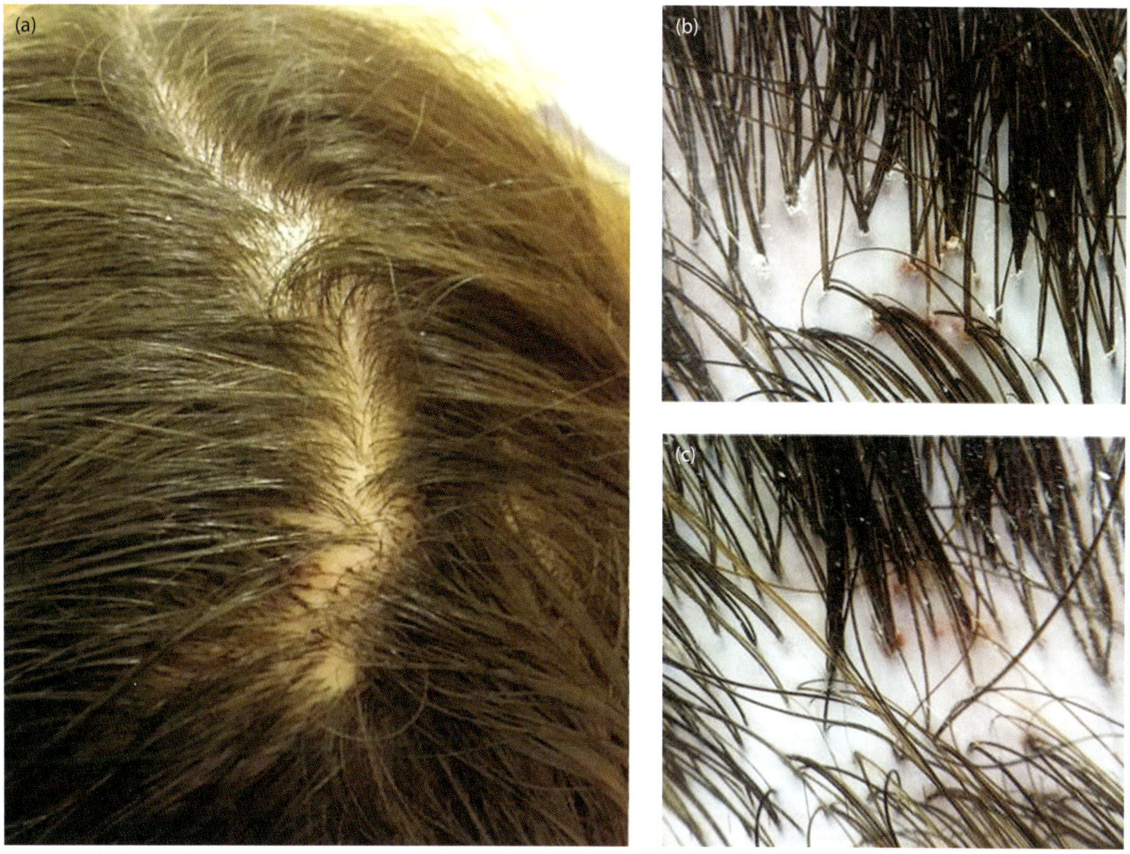

Figure 11.18 **(a) An early small patch of folliculitis decalvans that with naked eyes the characteristic features could not be recognized. (b) and (c) With trichoscopy we could identify subtle clinical signs such us tufted hairs, pustules, and crust.**

entity), specific immunopathologic patterns are discernible by direct immunofluorescence (DIF) in both LPP and CDLE. The most characteristic DIF finding in LPP consists of grouped globular deposits of IgM (cytoid or colloid bodies), adjacent to the follicular epithelium or at the dermoepidermal junction, and heavy deposits of fibrin at the dermal–epidermal junction. In CDLE, DIF studies most commonly demonstrate granular deposits (or sometimes in the band) of immunoglobulin (IgG and IgM) and C3 at the dermoepidermal junction where they, in the presence of IgA, are rare. In PB, DIF is negative or occasionally demonstrates IgM (Figure 11.20).[10]

It is not well established when you have to use DIF to establish the diagnosis. Some authors suggested that both histopathologic examination and DIF studies are always necessary for an accurate diagnosis, while others advocate performing it when you get an inconclusive result in the routine histopathological study. In most series the diagnosis is usually sufficient with a routine histological study (through clinical and histological studies, correct diagnosis is achieved in most cases), diagnosing only 6% of the LPP and 7% of DCLE exclusively with DIF. The sensitivity of this technique for the LPP is 34% and specificity is 95%, and for CDLE a sensitivity of 83% and specificity of 93% are described. So it can be concluded that the DIF can be a useful tool for diagnosing and/or differentiating various causes of PCA and can be of value in the diagnosis of CDLE, but has a low performance for diagnosis of LPP, so it should not be performed on a routine basis on all scalp biopsies, only in histopathologically inconclusive cases.[54,55]

IN VIVO REFLECTANCE CONFOCAL MICROSCOPY

In vivo reflectance confocal microscopy (RCM) is a noninvasive, infinitely repeatable technique for real-time, en face microscopic imaging of the superficial layers of the skin down to the superficial reticular dermis, with resolution at the cellular level that is close to conventional histopathology. In a preliminary study performed by Agozzino et al., they conclude that RCM is useful for the management of patients affected by cicatricial alopecia. RCM is a noninvasive, high-resolution imaging

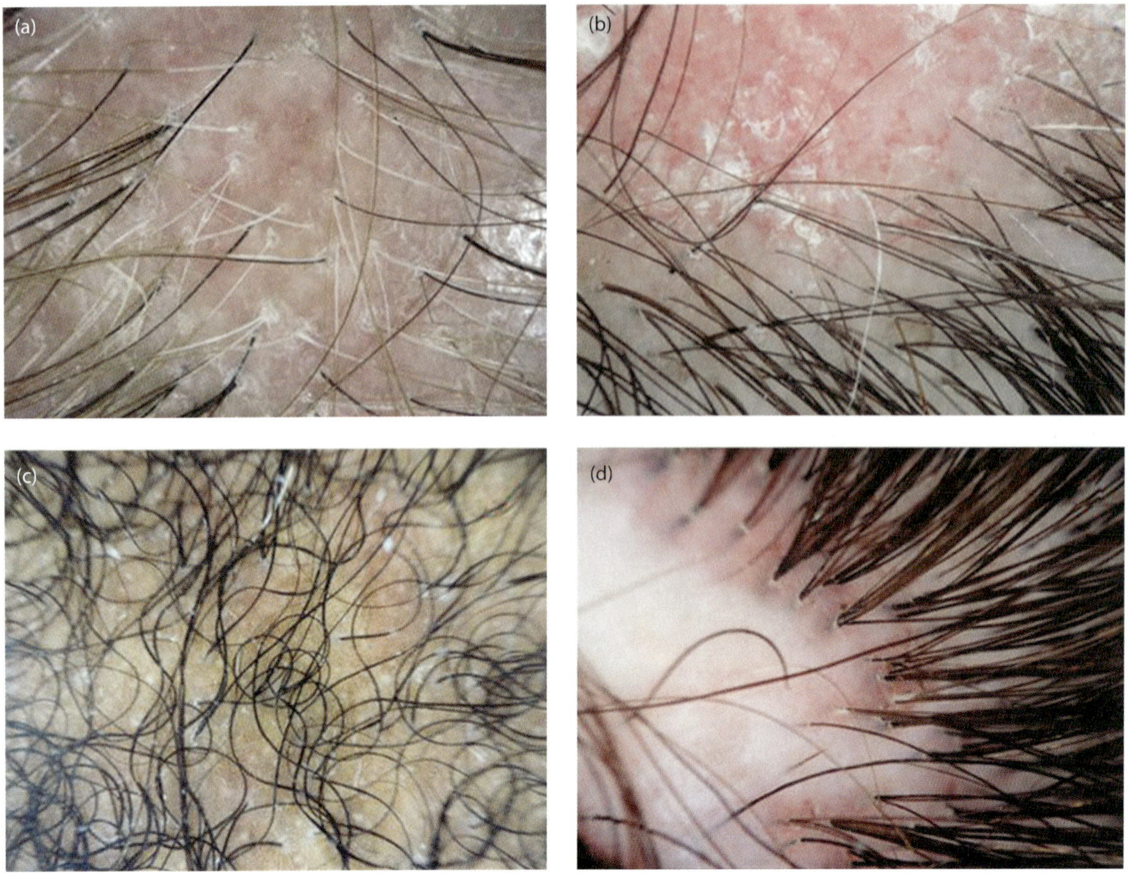

Figure 11.19 Trichoscopy findings in primary cicatricial alopecia. (a) Lichen planopilaris: peripilar casts, keratotic plugs and blue–gray dots. (b) Chronic cutaneous discoid lupus erythematosus: peripilar casts, follicular red dots, and arborizing red lines. (c) Central centrifugal cicatricial alopecia: peripilar white halo (one or two hairs emerging together, surrounded by white–gray halo). (d) Folliculitis decalvans: hair tufting (six or more hairs emerging from the same ostium).

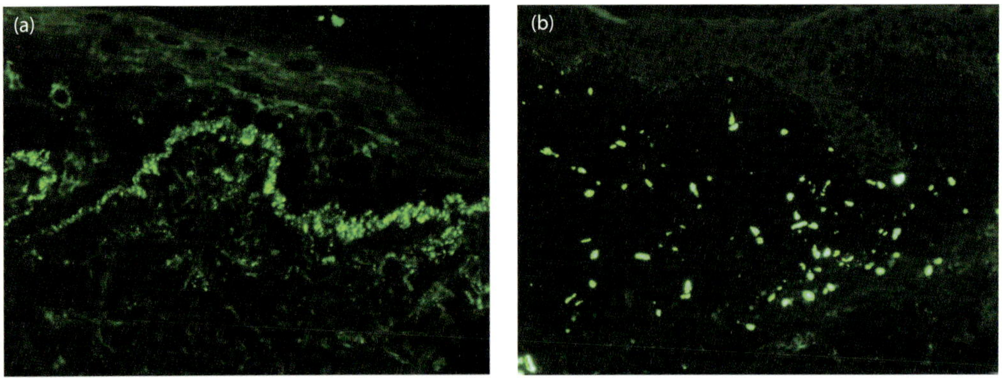

Figure 11.20 Direct immunofluorescence. (a) Chronic cutaneous discoid lupus erythematosus: granular deposits of immunoglobulin (IgG and IgM) and C3 at the dermoepidermal junction. (b) Lichen planopilaris: grouped globular deposits of IgM (cytoid or colloid bodies), adjacent to the follicular epithelium or at the dermoepidermal junction.

Table 11.4 Primary Cicatricial Alopecia Treatment

Disease	Topical Treatment	Systemic Treatment	Algorithm
Lichen planopilaris and its variants	• Clobetasol propionate 0.1% or betamethasone dipropionate 0.05% BID ± topical minoxidil 5% • Intralesional triamcinolone acetonide 4–10 mg/mL every 4–6/weeks • Topical calcineurin inhibitors BID for 8 weeks • Topical cyclosporin (oily solution BID for 3 months and once daily for futher 3 months • Wig/cosmetic camouflage/ eyebrow tattoo	• Hydroxychloroquine 400 mg/d for 6 months • Tetracycline antibiotics (Doxycycline 100 mg) • Prednisone: 0.5–1 mg/kg • Ciclosporin: 4–5 mg/kg/d for 4–6 months • Acitretin 10–20 mg/d • Thalidomide: 100–150 mg/d for 2–6 months • Mycophenolate mofetil (500–1000 mg BID) • 5α reductase inhibitors Finasteride 2.5 mg/d Dutasteride 0.5 mg/d	*First line* • Potent topical and/or intralesional corticosteroids Results are assessed until 8 weeks. If no response shift to next level • Oral corticosteroids (if progression is rapid) *Second line* • 5α reductase inhibitors (for FFA) • Oral esteriods • Antimalarials • Oral cyclosporin • Tetracyclines • Topical cyclosporin *Third line* • Oral retinoids • Thalidomide • Others: Griseofulvin, low molecular weight heparin (S/c injections 3 mg once weekly), 308 nm excimer laser New therapies: PPARγ agonist like thiozolidinediones
Brocq pseudopelade	Same as LPP	Same as LPP	Not established. No randomized trials
Alopecia mucinosa	• Clobetasol propionate 0.1% or betamethasone dipropionate 0.05% BID • Intralesional: Triamcinolone acetonide 4–10 mg/mL every 4–6 weeks	• Minocycline • Oral Indometacin • Sistemic steroids • Isotretinoin • Antimalarials • PUVA • Interferon α-2b + Interferon γ • Superficial x-rays	*First line* • Potent topical corticosteroids *Second line* • I/L triamcinolone • Minocyclin • Oral Indometacin • Dapsone *Third line* • Sistemic steroids • Isotretinoin • Antimalarials • PUVA • Interferon α-2b + Interferon γ • Superficial x-rays
Chronic cutaneous lupus erythematosus	• Sun protection • Clobetasol propionate 0.1% or betamethasone dipropionate 0.05% BID • Intralesional triamcinolone acetonide 4–10 mg/mL every 4–6 weeks • Topical calcineurin (0.1% tacrolimus ointment BID for 12 weeks; 1% pimecrolimus cream BID for 8 weeks Others: Topical 5-FU, topical tazarotene, imiquimod	• Hydroxychloroquine 200–400 mg/d • Oral corticosteroids: 1 mg/Kg, for initial actively progressing disease, tapered over 8 week) Oral retinoids • Isotretinoin: Initial regimen: 1 mg/kg/d Maintenance regimen: 10–40 mg/d • Acitretin 10–25 mg/d • Thalidomide: 50–300 mg/d Others: Oral vitamine E, dapsone, oral gold, mycophenolate mofetil, methotrexate, azathioprine, clofazimine, systemic IFNα2, monoclonal anti-CD4 antibodies	*First line* Topical corticosteroids Results are assessed untill 8 weeks. If no response shift to next level *Second line* • Antimalarials Oral corticosteroids Oral retinoids *Third line* • Thalidomide, Topical immune modulators, oral vitamine E, dapsone, oral gold, mycophenolate mofetil, methrotexate, azathioprine, clofazamine, systemic IFNα2, monoclonal anti-CD4 antibodies, topical 5-FU, topical tazarotene, imiquimod

(*Continued*)

Table 11.4 (*Continued*) Primary Cicatricial Alopecia Treatment

Disease	Topical Treatment	Systemic Treatment	Algorithm
Central centrifugal cicatricial alopecia	• Class I or II potent Topical corticosteroids: Clobetasol propionate 0.1% or betamethasone dipropionate 0.05% BID (cream, gel, lotion, foam) I/L Triamcinolone acetonide 3–10 mg/mL every 4–6 weeks	Tetracyclines: • Tetracycline hydrochloride 500 mg/12 h • Doxycycline 100 mg/12 h	*First line* • Minimize practices causing local trauma *Second line* • Potent topical or intralesional corticosteroids • Tetracyclines
Alopecia Mucinosa	I/L Triamcinolone acetonide 3–10 mg/mL every 4–6 weeks	Treatment of underlying lymphoproliferative disease if present	Not established. No randomized trials
Folliculitis decalvans	Topical antibiotics • Fusidic acid • Mupirocin • Indomethacin Gel 3%	• Oral antibiotics: • Rifampicin (300 BID) + clindamycin (300 mg BID) for 10 weeks • Rifampicin + (doxycycline/ciprofloxacin/clarithromycin) • Fusidic acid 500 mg/d for 3 weeks • Minocycline 100 mg BID • Azithromycin 500 mg for three days monthly • Trimetoprim/sulfametoxazol 1 g/d for 1–2 m • Dapsone 100 mg/d • Oral isotretinoin • Oral zinc	*First line* • Oral (minocycline/Azithromicine) ± topical antibiotics *Second line* • Oral rifampicin + clindamicin • Rifampicin + other antibiotic • Rifampicina + topical antibiotics *Third line* • Oral Isotretinoin • Oral fuscidic acid • Oral zinc • Dapsone • Others: Laser epilation, radiotherapy, human immunoglobulin, photodinamic therapy
Dissecting folliculitis	• Topical antibiotics (Clindamycin gel 1%) • Topical retinoid • Intralesional triamcinolone acetonide 3–10 mg/mL every 4–6 weeks	• Isotretinoin: 1 mg/kg/d for 4 months, followed by 0.75 mg/kg/d for an additional 6 months—In cases of intolerance, 10 mg/d continuously • Oral antibiotics (same as FD)	*First line* • Oral isotretinoin ± I/L triamcinolone acetonide *Second line* • Oral antibiotics ± topical antibiotics/topical retinoids *Third line* • Low dose corticosteroids • Colchicine • Dapsone • Others: Excision and skin grafting, laser and radiotherapy, adalimumab 40 mg every other week
Acne keloidalis nuchae	• Clobetasol 0.05% lotion or foam • Intralesional triamcinolone acetonide 10 mg/mL monthly • Antibacterial shampoos (such as povidone-iodine)	• Oral antibiotics BID • Clindamycin • Minocycline • Doxycycline • Cefadroxil • Surgical excision • CO_2 laser • Diode laser hair epilation • Radiotherapy • Isotretinoin	*First line* • Potent topical corticosteroids • Oral antibiotics + topical steroids/intralesional triamcinolone *Second line* • Surgical excision • CO_2 laser • Diode laser hair epilation *Third line* • Radiotherapy • Isotretinoin
Acne necrotica	Monthly injections of triamcinolone acetonide 10 mg/mL	Oral antibiotics (same as AKN) Oral isotretinoin	Not established No randomized trials

(*Continued*)

Table 11.4 (*Continued*) Primary Cicatricial Alopecia Treatment

Disease	Topical Treatment	Systemic Treatment	Algorithm
Erosive pustular dermatosis of scalp	• Topical potent corticosteroids • Topical calcineurin inhibitors • Calcipotriol cream	Oral isotretinoin	Not established No randomized trials
Keratosis follicularis spinulosa decalvans	Potent topical corticosteroids ± keratolytics	Dapsone Oral retinoids Laser epilation	Not established No randomized trials

Source: Adapted from Dogra S, Sarangal R. *Indian J Dermatol Venereol Leprol.* 2013;79:576–590; Darwich E, Muñoz-Santos C, Mascaró Jr JM. *Arch Dermatol.* 2011;147:252–253.

Note: BID, twice a day; FFA, frontal fibrosing alopecia; PPARγ, peroxisome proliferator-activated receptors gamma; 5-FU, fluorouracil; FD, folliculitis decalvans; AKN, acne keloidalis nuchae.

technique that may be helpful in the diagnosis and follow-up of scarring alopecia. Moreover, RCM could be used for choosing the biopsy site for more informative histology. Also, they identified a series of RCM features of scalp on LPP and CDLE correlating with the histopathological evaluation. During the treatment follow-up of the cases, RCM was shown to be sensitive for the identification of therapeutic response. Although RCM is an emerging technique in this area, it could be very promising in the future for both diagnosis and monitoring of these patients.[56–58]

TREATMENT

The treatment of PCA is difficult due to the delay in treating patients when irreversible scarring has already occurred. Moreover, the variety of treatments may reflect the current little evidence that exists for PCA. There are limited data sources and published literature on treatments, with low levels of evidence, having no randomized clinical trials, so that we can base only on case series and personal experiences. Since the causes are mostly unknown, therapy has remained empiric and nonspecific. The goal of treatment of PCA is to stop the scarring process, reduce follicular inflammation, and stop irreversible destruction of the follicle. However, the treatment of all types of PCA may be very difficult, since there are no consistent markers to trace the treatment progress. The therapeutic approach should be based on the severity and extent of the disease, the type of inflammatory infiltrate, the final diagnosis, and the patient's tolerance to the treatment, both topical and systemic treatments being valid. Often it is necessary to aggressively treat to prevent progression of the disease. In general, local treatment should be used for limited disease, and systemic modalities should be reserved for cases of rapidly progressive and refractory extensive local treatment. A general rule followed is to treat lymphocytic PCA with immunosuppression and neutrophilic PCA with antimicrobials or dapsone (Table 11.4).[59–81]

REFERENCES

1. Williamson DG, Gonzalez M, Finlay AY. The effect of hair loss on quality of life. *Eur Acad Dermatol Venereol.* 2001;15:137–139.
2. Whiting DA. Cicatricial alopecia: Clinico-pathological findings and treatment. *Clin Dermatol.* 2001;19:211–215.
3. Tan E, Martinka M, Ball N et al. Primary cicatricial alopecias: Clinicopathology of 112 cases. *J Am Acad Dermatol.* 2004;50:25–32.
4. Templeton SF, Solomon AR. Scarring alopecia: A classification based on microscopic criteria. *J Cutan Pathol.* 1994;21:97–109.
5. Harries MJ, Paus R. The pathogenesis of primary cicatricial alopecias. *Am J Pathol.* 2010;177:2152–2162.
6. Ohyama M. Primary cicatricial alopecia: Recent advances in understanding and management. *J Dermatol.* 2012;39:18–26.
7. Camacho FM, Ledo A, Moreno JC. Alopecias cicatriciales adquiridas. *Monogr Dermatol.* 2006;19:74–84.
8. Griffin LL, Michaelides C, Griffiths CE, Paus R, Harries MJ. Primary cicatricial alopecias: A UK survey. *Br J Dermatol.* 2012;167:692–705.
9. Moure ER, Romiti R, Machado MC et al. Primary cicatricial alopecias: A review of histopathologic findings in 38 patients from a clinical university hospital in Sao Paulo, Brazil. *Clinics (Sao Paulo).* 2008;63:747–752.
10. Ross EK, Tan E, Shapiro J. Update on primary cicatricial alopecias. *J Am Acad Dermatol.* 2005;53:1–37.
11. Harries MJ, Meyer KC, Chaudhry IH, Griffiths CE, Paus R. Does collapse of immune privilege in the hair-follicle bulge play a role in the pathogenesis of primary cicatricial alopecia? *Clin Exp Dermatol.* 2010;35:637–644.
12. Harries MJ, Trueb RM, Tosti A et al. How not to get scar(ed): Pointers to the correct diagnosis in patients with suspected primary cicatricial alopecia. *Br J Dermatol.* 2009;160:482–501.
13. Baima B, Sticherling M. Apoptosis in different cutaneous manifestations of lupus erythematosus. *Br J Dermatol.* 2001;144:958–966.

14. Pablos JL, Santiago B, Galindo M, Carreira PE, Ballestin C, Gomez-Reino JJ. Keratinocyte apoptosis and p53 expression in cutaneous lupus and dermatomyositis. *J Pathol.* 1999;188:63–68.
15. Nakajima M, Nakajima A, Kayagaki N, Honda M, Yagita H, Okumura K. Expression of Fas ligand and its receptor in cutaneous lupus: Implication in tissue injury. *Clin Immunol Immunopathol.* 1997;83:223–229.
16. Zheng Y, Eilertsen KJ, Ge L et al. Scd1 is expressed in sebaceous glands and is disrupted in the asebia mouse. *Nat Genet.* 1999;23:268–270.
17. Sundberg JP, Boggess D, Sundberg BA et al. Asebia-2J (Scd1(ab2J)): A new allele and a model for scarring alopecia. *Am J Pathol.* 2000;156:2067–2075.
18. Stenn KS. Insights from the asebia mouse: A molecular sebaceous gland defect leading to cicatricial alopecia. *J Cutan Pathol.* 2001;28:445–447.
19. Karnik P, Tekeste Z, McCormick TS et al. Hair follicle stem cell-specific PPARγ deletion causes scarring alopecia. *J Invest Dermatol.* 2009;129:1243–1257.
20. Olsen EA, Bergfeld WF, Cotsarelis G et al. Summary of North American Hair Research Society (NAHRS)-sponsored Workshop on Cicatricial Alopecia, Duke University Medical Center, February 10 and 11, 2001. *J Am Acad Dermatol.* 2003;48:103–110.
21. Sullivan JR, Kossard S. Acquired scalp alopecia. Part I: A review. *Australas J Dermatol.* 1998;39:207–219.
22. Sperling LC. Scarring alopecia and the dermatopathologist. *J Cutan Pathol.* 2001;28:333–342.
23. Stefanato CM. Histopathology of alopecia: A clinicopathological approach to diagnosis. *Histopathology.* 2010;56:24–38.
24. Chieregato C, Zini A, Barba A, Magnanini M, Rosina P. Lichen planopilaris: Report of 30 cases and review of the literature. *Int J Dermatol.* 2003;42:342–345.
25. Llambrich A, Moreno JA, Mascaró-Galy JM et al. Liquen plano pilar y mucositis bipolar. In: Ferrando J, ed. *Casos Clínicos en Tricología.* Madrid, Spain: Aula Médica; 2005:76–81.
26. Kossard S. Postmenopausal frontal fibrosing alopecia. Scarring alopecia in a pattern distribution. *Arch Dermatol.* 1994;130:770–774.
27. Donati A, Molina L, Doche I et al. Facial papules in frontal fibrosing alopecia: Evidence of vellus follicle involvement. *Arch Dermatol.* 2011;147:1424–1427.
28. Annessi G, Lombardo G, Gobello T, Puddu P. A clinicopathologic study of scarring alopecia due to lichen planus: Comparison with scarring alopecia in discoid lupus erythematosus and pseudopelade. *Am J Dermatopathol.* 1999;21:324–331.
29. Dawn G, Holmes S, Moffatt D, Munro C. Postmenopausal frontal fibrosing alopecia. *Clin Exp Dermatol.* 2003;28:43–45.
30. Sperling LC, Solomon AR, Whiting DA. A new look at scarring alopecia. *Arch Dermatol.* 2000;136:235–242.
31. Sperling LC, Cowper SE. The histopathology of primary cicatricial alopecia. *Semin Cutan Med Surg.* 2006;25:41–50.
32. Braun-Falco O, Imai S, Schmoeckel C et al. Pseudopelade of Brocq. *Dermatologica.* 1986;172:18–23.
33. Amato L, Massi D, Berti S, Moretti S, Fabbri P. A multiparametric approach is essential to define different clinicopathological entities within pseudopelade of Brocq: Reply from authors. *Br J Dermatol.* 2002;146:532–533.
34. Amato L, Mei S, Massi D et al. Cicatricial alopecia; a dermatopathologic and immunopathologic study of 33 patients (pseudopelade of Brocq is not a specific clinico-pathologic entity). *Int J Dermatol.* 2002;41:8–15.
35. Blattner C, Polley DC, Ferritto F et al. Central centrifugal cicatricial alopecia. *Indian Dermatol Online J.* 2013;4:50–51.
36. Cerroni L, Fink-Puches R, Back B, Kerl H. Follicular mucinosis: A critical reappraisal of clinicopathologic features and association with mycosis fungoides and Sézary syndrome. *Arch Dermatol.* 2002;138:182–189.
37. Domenéch P, Ferrando J, Corretger M et al. Queratosis espinulosa folicular decalvante (Síndrome de siemens) asociadas a otras anomalias. *Med Cutan Iber Lat Am.* 1985;13:175–181.
38. Oosterwijk JC, Nelen M, van Zandvoort PM et al. Linkage analysis of keratosis follicularis spinulosa decalvans, and regional assignment to chromosomes Xp21.2-p22.2. *Am J Hum Genet.* 1992;50:801–807.
39. Castori M, Covaciu C, Paradisi M et al. Clinical and genetic heterogeneity in keratosis follicularis spinulosa decalvans. *Eur J Med Genet.* 2009;52:53–58.
40. Paus R, Olsen E, Messenger A. Hair growth disorders. In: Wolff K, Goldsmith LA, Katz SI, Gilchrest BA, Paller AS, Leffell DJ, eds. *Fitzpatrick's Dermatology in General Medicine*, 7th ed. New York, NY: McGraw-Hill; 2008:753.
41. Sinclair RD. Acquired cicatricial alopecia. In: Burns T, Breathnach SM, Cox N, Griffiths CE, eds. *Rook's Textbook of Dermatology.* 8th ed. Oxford, UK: Wiley-Blackwell; 2010:66.38–66.52.
42. Powell JJ, Dawber RP. Successful treatment regime for folliculitis decalvans despite uncertainty of all aetiological factors. *Br J Dermatol.* 2001;144:428–429.
43. Brooke RC, Griffiths CE. Folliculitis decalvans. *Clin Exp Dermatol.* 2001;26:120–122.
44. Camacho F, Moreno D, Rodríguez Rey E. Alopecias cicatriciales adquiridas con entidad propia. II. Alopecias con infiltrado neutrofílico, mixto e inespecífico. *Monogr Dermatol.* 2006;19:133–150.
45. Zribi H, Descamps V. Folliculites décalvantes du cuir chevelu. *Ann Dermatol Venereol.* 2006;133;1021–1029.
46. Ljubojevic S, Pasic A, Lipozencic J, Skerlev M. Perifolliculitis capitis abscedens et suffodiens. *J Eur Acad Dermatol Venereol.* 2005;19:719–721.

47. Sperling LC, Homoky C, Pratt L, Sau P. Acne keloidalis is a form of primary scarring alopecia. *Arch Dermatol.* 2000;136:479–484.
48. Kose OK, Gulec T. Clinical evaluation of alopecias using a handheld dermatoscope. *J Am Acad Dermatol.* 2012;67:206–214.
49. Micali G, Lacarrubba F. Possible applications of videodermatoscopy beyond pigmented lesions. *Int J Dermatol.* 2003;42:430–433.
50. Miteva M, Tosti A. Hair and scalp dermatoscopy. *J Am Acad Dermatol.* 2012;67:1040–1048.
51. Mirmirani P, Willey A, Headington JT. Primary cicatricial alopecia: Histopathologic findings do not distinguish clinical variants. *J Am Acad Dermatol.* 2005;5:637–643.
52. Miteva M, Tosti A. Dermoscopy guided scalp biopsy in cicatricial alopecia. *J Eur Acad Dermatol Venereol.* 2013;27:1299–1303.
53. Nguyen JV, Hudacek K, Whitten JA. The HoVert technique: A novel method for the sectioning of alopecia biopsies. *J Cutan Pathol.* 2011;38:401–406.
54. Trachsler S, Trueb RM. Value of direct immunofluorescence for differential diagnosis of cicatricial alopecia. *Dermatology.* 2005;211:98–102.
55. Stavrianeas NG, Kanelleas AI, Toumbis-Ioannou E. Evaluation of histopathological examination and direct immunofluorescence in the diagnosis of cicatricial alopecia. *Dermatology.* 2006;212:400.
56. Rudnicka L, Olszewska M, Rakowska A. *In vivo* reflectance confocal microscopy: Usefulness for diagnosing hair diseases. *J Dermatol Case Rep.* 2008;4:55–59.
57. Agozzino M, Tosti A, Barbieri L et al. Confocal microscopic features of scarring alopecia: Preliminary report. *Br J Dermatol.* 2011;165:534–540.
58. Dogra S, Sarangal R. What's new in cicatricial alopecia? *Indian J Dermatol Venereol Leprol.* 2013;79:576–590.
59. Abal-Díaz L, Soria X, Casanova-Seuma JM. Scarring alopecia. *Actas Dermosifiliogr.* 2012;103(5):376–387.
60. Jessop S, Whitelaw D, Jordaan F. Drugs for discoid lupus erythematosus. *Cochrane Database Syst Rev.* 2001;CD002954.
61. Harries MJ, Sinclair RD, Macdonald-Hull S et al. Management of primary cicatricial alopecias: Options for treatment. *Br J Dermatol.* 2008;159:1–22.
62. Ruzicka T, Sommerburg C, Goerz G et al. Treatment of cutaneous lupus erythematosus with acitretin and hydroxychloroquine. *Br J Dermatol.* 1992;127:513–518.
63. Shornick JK, Formica N, Parke AL. Isotretinoin for refractory lupus erythematosus. *J Am Acad Dermatol.* 1991;24:49–52.
64. Wu JJ, Huang DB, Pang KR, Hsu S, Tyring SK. Thalidomide: Dermatological indications, mechanisms of action and side effects. *Br J Dermatol.* 2005;153:254–273.
65. Kang H, Alzolibani AA, Otberg N, Shapiro J. Lichen planopilaris. *Dermatol Ther.* 2008;21:249–256.
66. Rácz E, Gho C, Moorman PW et al. Treatment of frontal fibrosing alopecia and lichen planopilaris: A systematic review. *J Eur Acad Dermatol Venereol.* 2013;27:1461–1470.
67. Chieregato C, Zini A, Barba A et al. Lichen planopilaris: Report of 30 cases and review of the literature. *Int J Dermatol.* 2003;42:342–345.
68. Assouly P, Reygagne P. Lichen planopilaris: Update on diagnosis and treatment. *Semin Cutan Med Surg.* 2009;28:3–10.
69. Cevasco NC, Bergfeld WF, Remzi BK et al. A case-series of 29 patients with lichen planopilaris: The Cleveland Clinic Foundation experience on evaluation, diagnosis, and treatment. *J Am Acad Dermatol.* 2007;57:47–53.
70. Tzung TY, Liu YS, Chang HW. Tacrolimus vs. clobetasol propionate in the treatment of facial cutaneous lupus erythematosus: A randomized, double-blind, bilateral comparison study. *Br J Dermatol.* 2007;156:191–192.
71. Otberg N, Kang H, Alzolibani AA et al. Folliculitis decalvans. *Dermatol Ther.* 2008;21:238–244.
72. Chandrawansa PH, Giam YC. Folliculitis decalvans—A retrospective study in a tertiary referred centre, over five years. *Singapore Med J.* 2003;44:84–87.
73. Powell JJ, Dawber RP, Gatter K. Folliculitis decalvans including tufted folliculitis: Clinical, histological and therapeutic findings. *Br J Dermatol.* 1999;140:328–333.
74. Gemmeke A, Wollina U. Folliculitis decalvans of the scalp: Response to triple therapy with isotretinoin, clindamycin, and prednisolone. *Acta Dermatovenerol Alp Panonica Adriat.* 2006;15:184–186.
75. Stites PC, Boyd AS. Dissecting cellulitis in a white male: A case report and. review of the literature. *Cutis.* 2001;67:37–40.
76. Bolz S, Jappe U, Hartschuh W. Successful treatment of peri folliculitis capitis abscedens et suffodiens with combined isotretinoin and dapsone. *J Dtsch Dermatol Ges.* 2008;6:44–47.
77. Callender VD, Young CM, Haverstock CL et al. An open label study of clobetasol propionate 0.05% and betamethasone valerate 0.12% foams in the treatment of mild to moderate acne keloidalis. *Cutis.* 2005;75:317–321.
78. Shah GK. Efficacy of diode laser for treating acne keloidalis nuchae. *Indian J Dermatol Venereol Leprol.* 2005;71:31–34.
79. Petiau P, Cribier B, Chartier C et al. Acne necrotica varioliformis; resolution with isotretinoin. *Eur J Dermatol.* 1994;4:608–610.
80. Van Exel CE, English 3rd JC. Erosive pustular dermatosis of the scalp and nonscalp. *J Am Acad Dermatol.* 2007;57:S11–S14.
81. Darwich E, Muñoz-Santos C, Mascaró Jr JM. Erosive pustular dermatosis of the scalp responding to acitretin. *Arch Dermatol.* 2011;147:252–253.

12 Management of definitive alopecia in African Americans

Pierre Bouhanna

INTRODUCTION

The hair and scalp for African Americans, because of their anatomical, histological, and physiological characteristics, have a specific pathology based on the fragility of the hair shaft and the inflammatory hyperreactivity of the scalp tissue. Some types of hairstyles practiced in this ethnic group can also cause disorders, manifesting in types of folliculitis, in traction alopecia, or in hypertrophic scars or keloids. These multiple clinical varieties must be distinguished from diseases common to all ethnic groups. The cosmetic, surgical, and medical treatments must be adapted to the etiology and also to specific ethnic considerations.

CHARACTERISTICS OF AFRICAN AMERICAN HAIR

Between the three main ethnic groups (Caucasian, East Asian, Black) there are few differences in biochemical structure and no differences in the composition of amino acids or proteins.

In contrast, the hair and scalp of African Americans have specific structural, anatomical, and physiological characteristics: the shaft has a helical and spiral appearance[1]; in cross section it is flattened or elliptical; there are curved roots (Figure 12.1); there is hair density 20% lower than that of Caucasians; and there is a growth rate 30% lower than that of Caucasians.

The parameters of hair growth were compared in 38 African patients born in Africa (19 women and 19 men) with those of Caucasians of the same age (27 ± 10 years).[2] The hair of Africans, compared to Caucasian hair, has a lower density (190 ± 40 vs. 227 ± 55 hair/cm^2), slower hair growth (256 ± 44 vs. 396 ± 55 μm/day), and a higher percentage of telogen hair (18 ± 9 vs. 14 ± 11%).[1]

Often, patients will have a biracial or multiracial character, rather than pure African heritage.

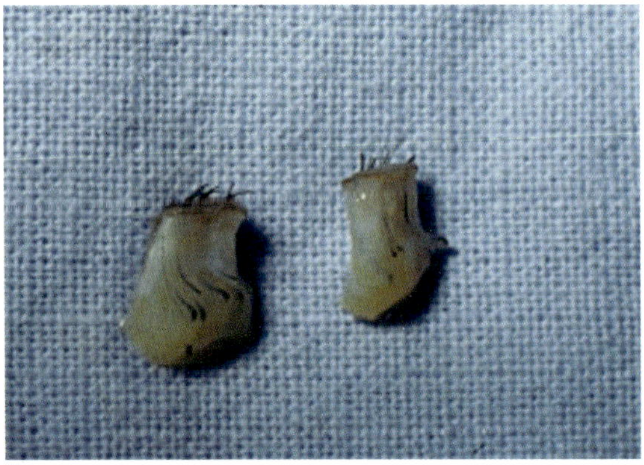

Figure 12.1 Specific anatomical features of African American hair (spiral shafts and curved bulbs) visible on the fragments of the scalp.

DISEASES COMMON TO ALL ETHNIC GROUPS

1. Alopecia areata: There are several types to be distinguished—patchy, ophiasis, total, and universal—for which the diagnosis, prognosis, and treatment are similar to those of other ethnic groups (Figure 12.2).[3,4]

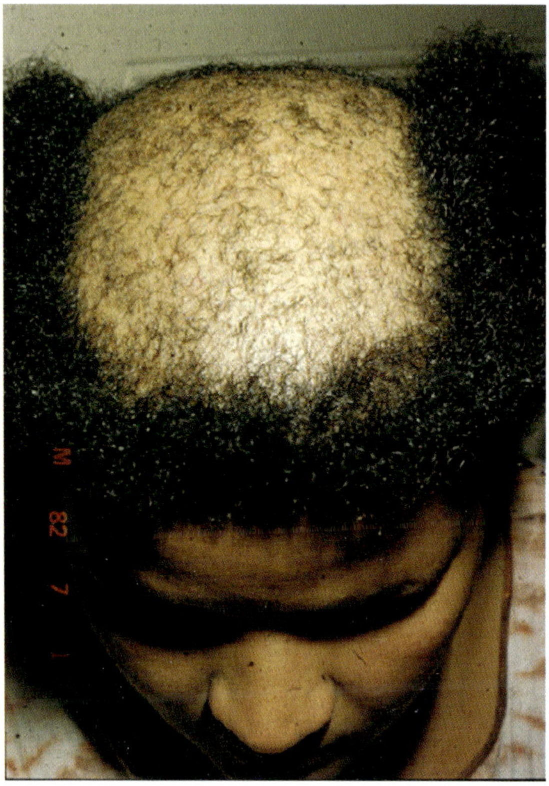

Figure 12.2 Alopecia of the vertex, which appeared suddenly in a woman after severe stress (the kidnapping of her child).

2. Male and female androgenetic alopecia[5] have the same topography and are of the same prognosis in African Americans as in other ethnic groups, but the therapeutic approach and treatments are not always the same.
   a. Lotions of 2% for female and 5% minoxidil for male have better cosmetic acceptance among African Americans than among Caucasians and East Asians, due to the "greasing" effects of propylene glycol on the hair shafts. The prescription advice and information are similar.
   b. Finasteride is indicated almost identically as in other ethnic groups.
   c. Hair transplantation in men and in women is similar to that of other ethnic groups. The peculiarities of transplantations among African American patients are essentially.
      i. Harvesting a graft in the midoccipital donor zone to prevent a hypertrophic or keloid scar (Figure 12.3).
      ii. Preparation of grafts in follicular units of two to four hairs rather than micrografts of one hair, harvesting of follicular units is possible with follicular unit extraction (FUE) or with strip segmentation (follicular units for long hair [FUL] or follicular unit transplantation [FUT]).
      iii. In men, a design of a flatter frontal line than in other ethnic groups (Figure 12.4).
      iv. In women, a more rectilinear design by combining frontal and temporal reconstruction (Figure 12.5).
3. Trichotillomania[5] is observed in both children and adults. Clinical and psychological aspects are similar to those in other ethnicities. One should always look out for other types of additional traction, particularly in African American patients.
4. Scarring alopecia in children and adults[6]: Scarring alopecia is defined as the destruction of hair follicles, replaced by fibrous tissue. The diagnosis is clinical, with diagnostic confirmation coming from histological examination with direct immunofluorescence. There are multiple causes. We can distinguish congenital scarring alopecia (hereditary syndromes, localized forms, and diffuse forms) from primary or secondary scarring acquired alopecia:
   a. Acquired primary scarring alopecia acquired with lymphocytic infiltrate (discoid lupus erythematosus, lichen planus pilaris, pseudopelade of Brocq, follicular degeneration syndrome, mucinous alopecia).
   b. Acquired primary scarring alopecia with neutrophilic infiltration (decalvans folliculitis,

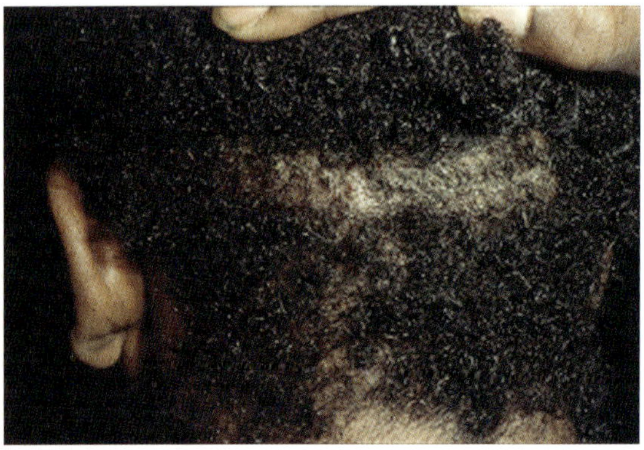

Figure 12.3 **Area of harvesting of a graft (in the midoccipital region) a few days after closure of the suture.**

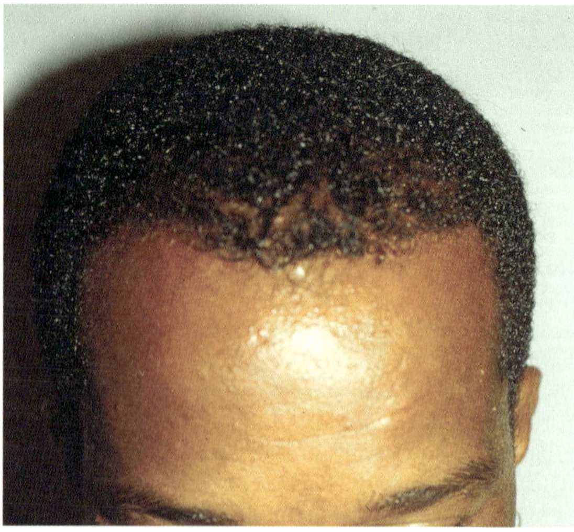

Figure 12.4 **Male frontal hair line (flatter than in other ethnic groups).**

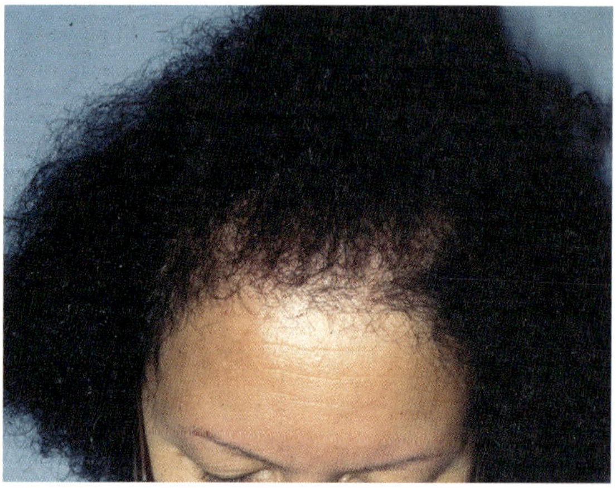

Figure 12.5 **Female frontal hair line (more rectilinear than in other ethnic groups).**

ringworm, dissecting cellulitis of the scalp, acne keloid, necrotic acne, folliculitis in clumps).
   c. Acquired secondary scarring alopecia of physical origin (Figure 12.6) or of tumor-induced or infectious origin.
5. Seborrheic dermatitis: As with other ethnic groups, there are aggravating effects to cosmetic products often used by African Americans: lanolin oil, soybean oil, wheat germ, lecithin, squalene, and castor oil. Stopping use of the product is essential. Rather than frequent washing, it is better to advocate a weekly shampoo with the aid of a low-strength cortisone lotion or shampoo.

SPECIFIC CONDITIONS TO AFRICAN AMERICANS

Traction alopecia

These occur in patients of all ages, due to the various types of hair-stylings practiced in this ethnic group such as ponytails, braids (Figures 12.7 and 12.8), brushing, curlers, and hairpieces (Figure 12.9). Of basically frontotemporal location, clinical signs vary between perifollicular inflammation, reversible alopecia, and permanent alopecia. Treatments include stopping traction and applying

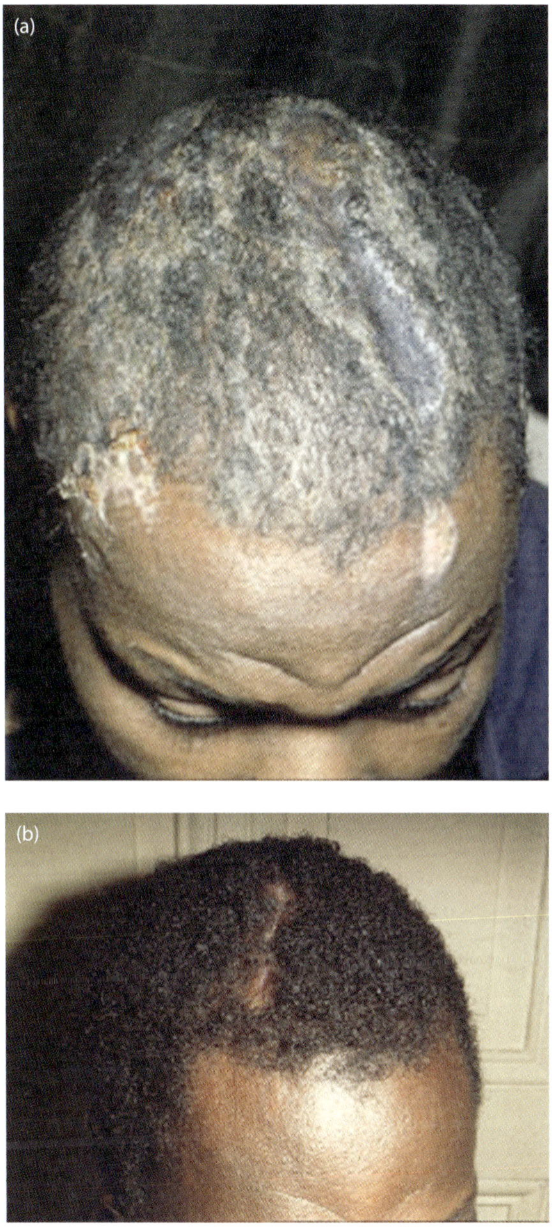

Figure 12.6 **A burn with caustic soda before (a) and after (b) good spontaneous healing without any treatment.**

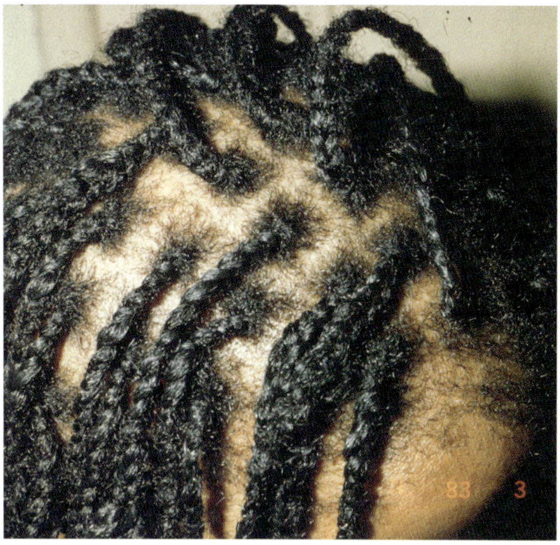

Figure 12.7 **Early definitive traction alopecia following styling with braids.**

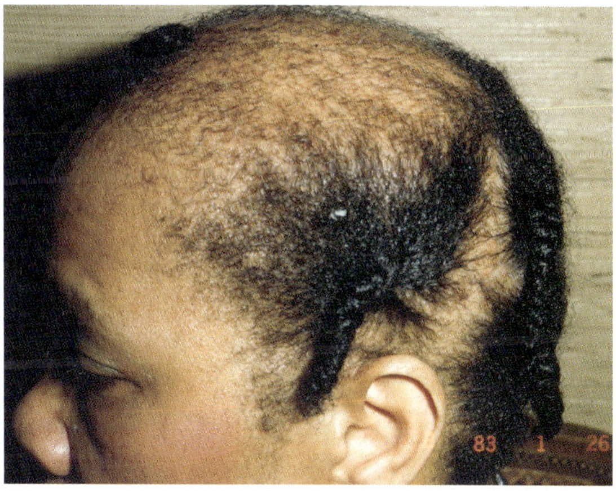

Figure 12.8 **Advanced traction alopecia, following styling with braids.**

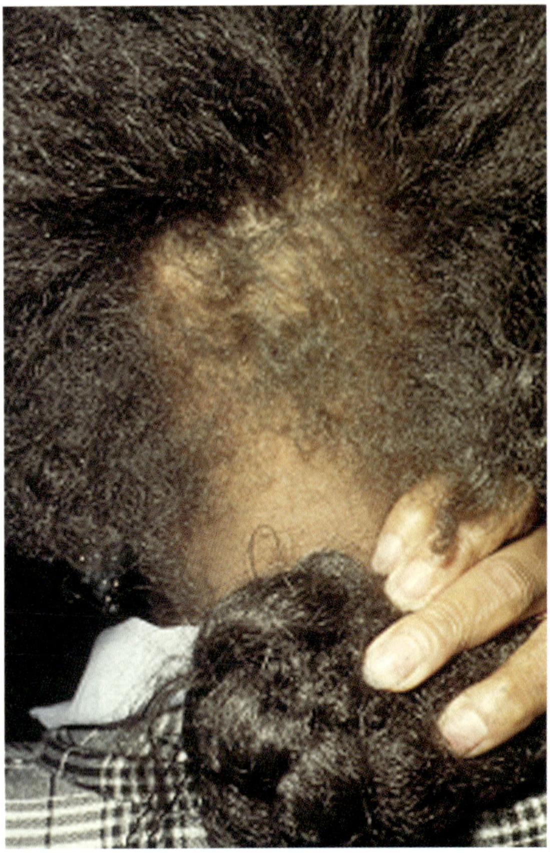

Figure 12.9 **Occipital traction alopecia following wearing a hairpiece.**

minoxidil 2% lotion. Hair transplants are recommended on patches of alopecia remaining after 6 months of treatment (Figures 12.10 and 12.11).[7–13]

"Hot comb" alopecia (follicular degenerative syndrome of Sperling)

Most often caused by a combination of hot oil and a hot or a curling iron comb, "hot comb" alopecia is sometimes idiopathic. It is a smooth and permanent alopecia with loss of follicular orifices, localized preferentially to the vertex. One sees islands of hair and scar patches, and sometimes there is polytrichia (Figures 12.12 and 12.13). Preventive treatment is to stop the hair manipulation taking place and to stop also the excessive use of heat. The definitive treatment is then provided by hair transplantation or the use of a hairpiece (Figure 12.14).[14–16]

Folliculitis and pseudo-folliculitis

These are the result of skin inclusion by the curved hair shaft (after scalp shaving in men or after traction hair alopecia in women), which causes the formation of papules, follicular papules and pustules, perifollicular papules or pustules, or foreign body granulomas. Severe scarring may result. Preventive treatment is to stop shaving or hair traction with tweezers and to advocate waxing, using depilatory creams or lotions, or using special shavers (with triple blade or an electric shaver with adjustable length) or permanent hair removal. The treatment of lesions consists of administering topical or oral (erythromycin, cyclin) antibiotics locally (topical erythromycin) or orally (Figure 12.15).[3,5,17]

Keloid folliculitis

Located mainly on the neck, keloid folliculitis is a chronic inflammatory and potentially scarring process characterized histologically by a preliminary papule (inflammation of the infundibulum and isthmus) and a granulomatous

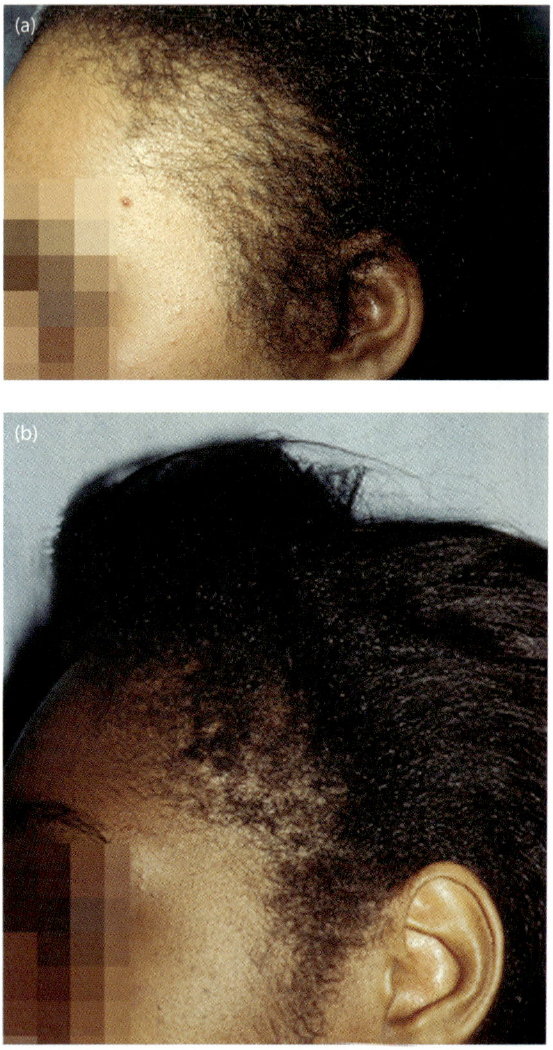

Figure 12.10 **Definitive traction alopecia (6 months after stopping traction), (a) before and (b) after a session of follicular unit long (FUL) hair grafts.**

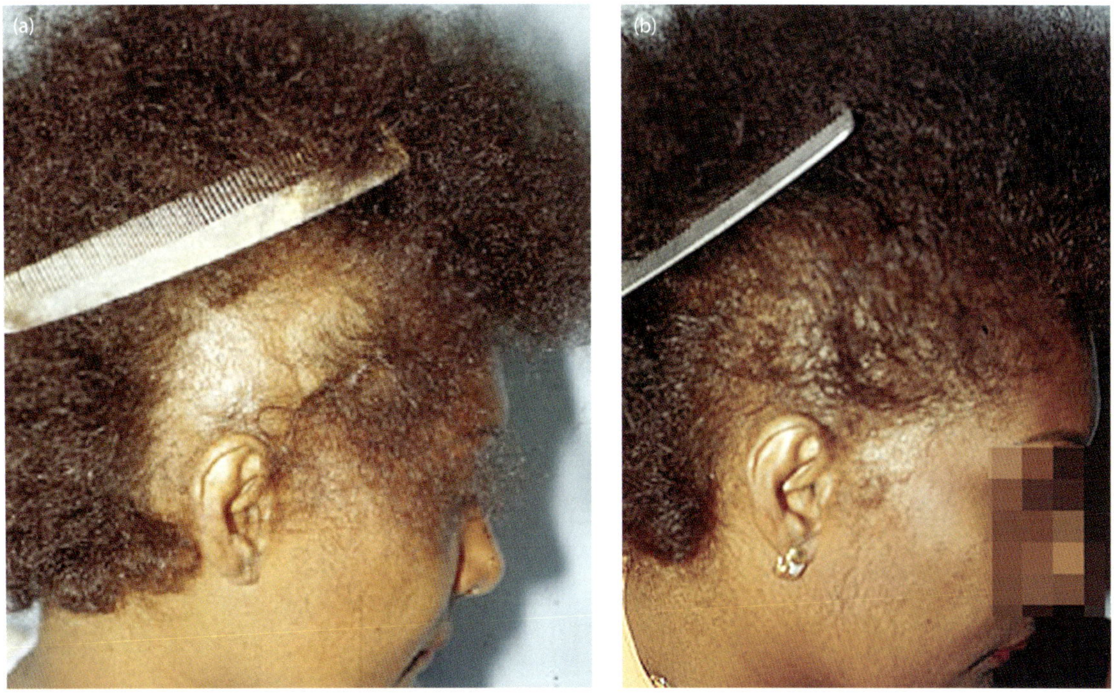

Figure 12.11 Definitive traction alopecia (6 months after stopping traction), in a postmenopausal woman (a) before and (b) after a session of follicular unit grafts.

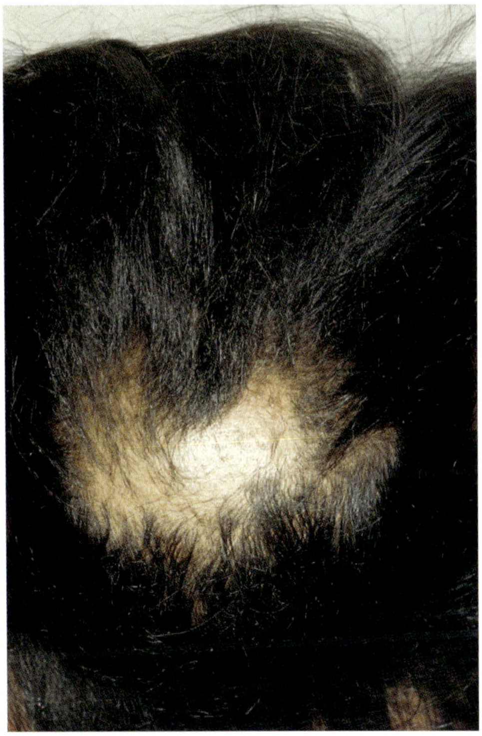

Figure 12.12 "Hot comb" alopecia caused by a combination of hot oil and heated comb.

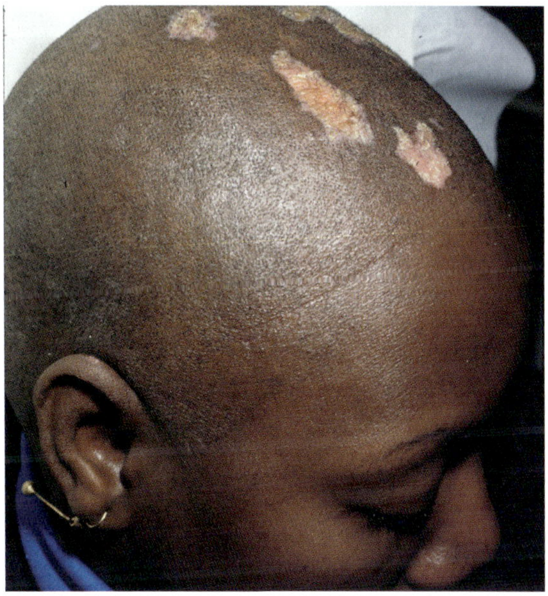

Figure 12.13 Burning after using a "hot comb."

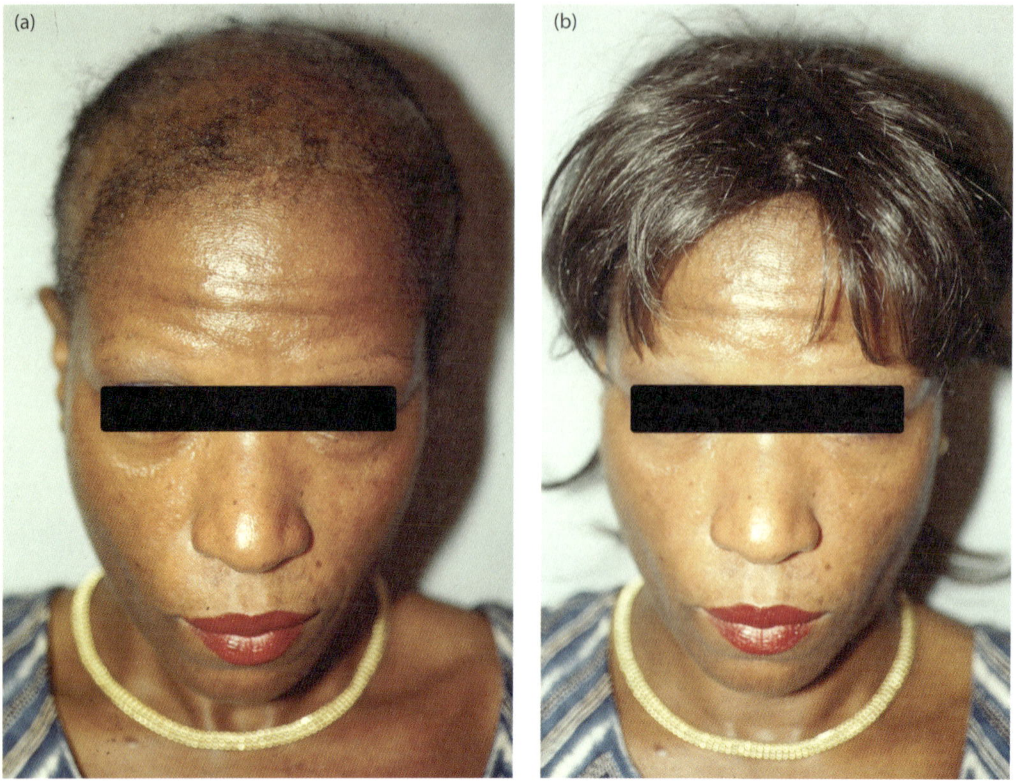

Figure 12.14 "Hot comb" alopecia, (a) before and (b) after correction by the use of a wig.

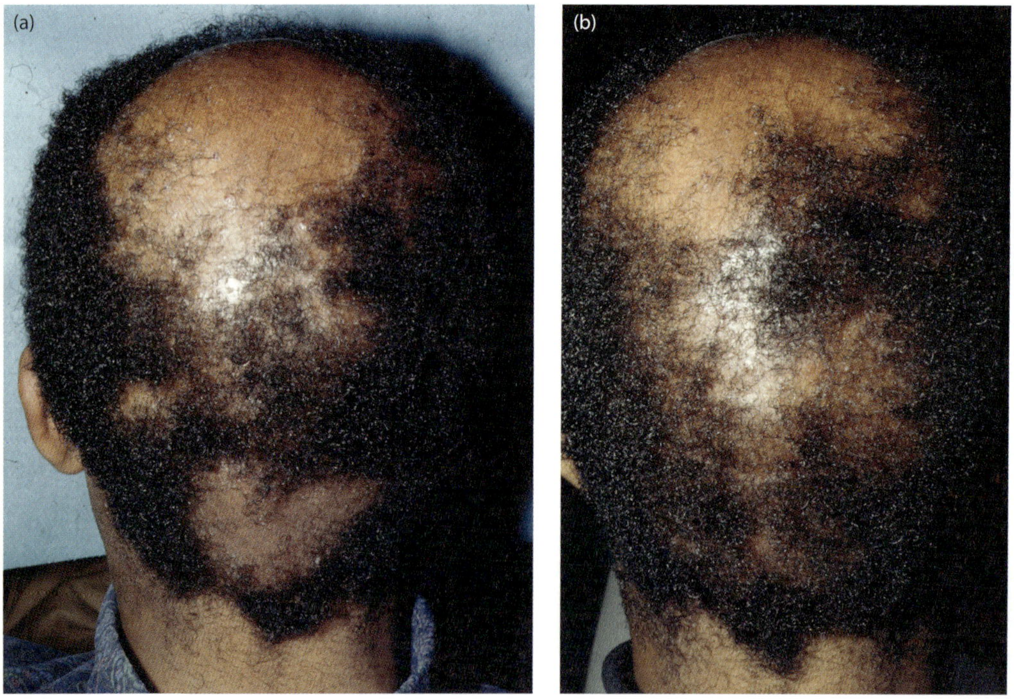

Figure 12.15 (a) Folliculitis before treatment, (b) scar appearance after healing of inflammation by antibiotic therapy.

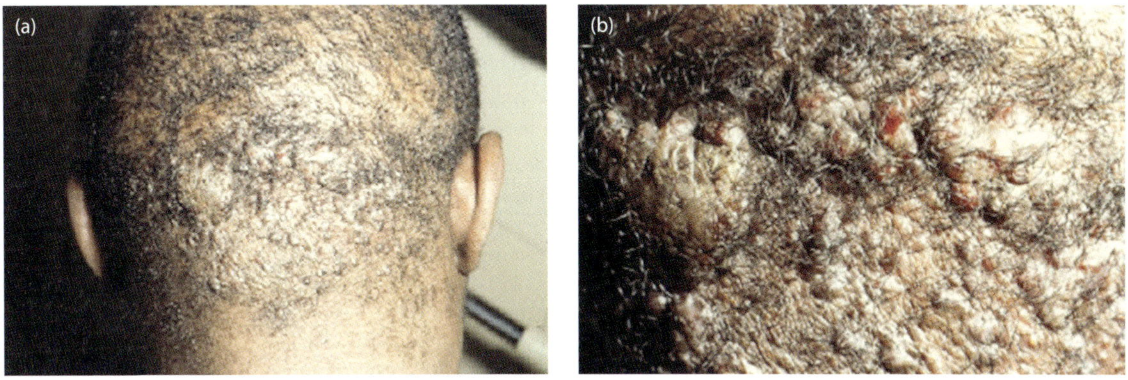

Figure 12.16 **(a,b) Folliculitis and keloid papules of the neck.**

infiltrate (at the deep end), then by a scar plate (Figure 12.16). Mainly in African American men, the lesions are distributed in areas where a razor is used to shave the hairline. Do not shave the area, and treat with antibiotics locally and orally (cyclin), intralesional corticosteroids (1 time per month), and surgical excision (performed with caution).[3,5,8]

Dissecting cellulitis of the scalp (perifolliculitis capitis abscedens and suffodiens)

Of poorly defined etiology, dissecting cellulitis of the scalp is a mixture of follicular occlusion, acne conglobata, and hidradenitis suppurativa. Observed especially in men, it presents clinically with multiple abscesses sometimes coalescing, follicular occlusion, scarring alopecia, hypertrophic scars, or keloids (Figure 12.17). Bacteriological tests are negative (for *Staphylococci*). Various treatments can be applied: corticosteroids and oral antibiotics, surgical excision, isotretinoin (40 mg/d), zinc sulfate (400 mg orally), cephalosporin (500 mg) + rifampicin (600 mg/d), or incision/drainage for fluctuating abscesses.[3,5,8,18]

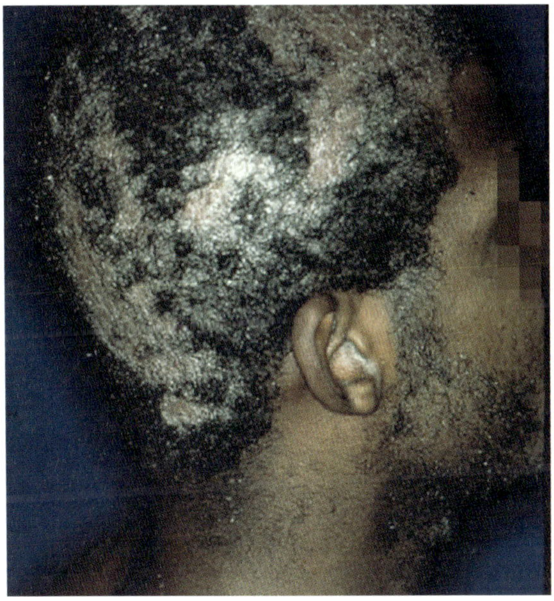

Figure 12.17 **Dissecting cellulitis of the scalp.**

SPECIFIC THERAPEUTIC CONSIDERATIONS FOR THE AFRICAN AMERICAN SCALP AND HAIR

Treatments also will need to be adapted to these ethnic differences.

Cosmetologic treatments

The particular cosmetic features among African Americans are related to dryness and brittleness of hair shafts. The best cosmetologic advice will then aim to prevent and correct these ongoing structural abnormalities of the hair.[3,5,6,11]

Shampoos

Excessive dryness will result if those of African descent shampoo their hair too frequently. Shampoos that contain anionic agents are particularly drying to the hair. Their hair needs shampoos that contain humectants and milder cleansing agents, such as amphoteric and nonionic blends (Table 12.1).

Oils and pomades

African Americans often employ some type of heavy emollient or oil to assist in grooming their hair or to treat a dry, scaly scalp. Castor oil, wheat germ oil, olive oil, and mineral oil are some of the most popular oils used (Table 12.2). Jojoba oil does not appear to aggravate dandruff or seborrheic dermatitis.

Pomades consist primarily of petrolatum, lanolin, mineral oil, olive oil, and perfume, whereas solid *brillantines* are vegetable or mineral oils stiffened with waxes. Both of these agents coat the hair, thereby reducing the static electric charges between the hairs and allowing for ease of combing and styling.

Table 12.1 Hair Grooming Products for African American Hair

Uses of Product	Brand Name
Dry brittle hair, natural or curly perm, hot-pressed or chemically relaxed hair	Black Alive Moisturizing Shampoo Black Alive Curl Shampoo Optimum Care Moisture Shampoo
Hard-to-comb hair, any style	Crème of Nature Shampoo Black Alive Curl Shampoo
Chemically relaxed hair	Optimum care Mizani Nexus
Split ends, hair chemically dramaged from relaxers	Optimum care Mizani Nexus
Unusually dry hair with breakage from chemicals and dryes	Pure karite Nexus Humectress Optimum Care Black Alive Curl Revitalizer Moisture Max Luster's Pink Lotion Mizani Cholesterol
For those with seborrheic dermatitis: free of lanolin and other contributing agents	Murray's Superior Hair Dressing White petrolatum Black Alive Line Jojoba oil Mineral oil

Moisturizers

Moisturizers contain humectants that attract and hold water in the keratin fibers. Hair that has been chemically curled or waved will require more moisturizing than non-chemically treated hair. Most of the moisturizers contain lanolin (Table 12.1), glycerin, and propylene glycol.[3,5,8,18]

Activators

Activators are products specifically designed for curls. They contain surface active agents such as proteins, cationic agents, and/or plant oils (soybean and wheat germ oil) (Table 12.1).

Conditioners

Hair conditioners enhance manageability of the hair. A conditioner may be simply an emollient or a very complex mixture of proteins, quaternary ammonium compounds, oils, gums, and humectants (Table 12.1).

Styling gels and spritzes

The gels contain carbomer 940 and hydrolyzed animal protein: this combination forms a thick, tacky gel that dries on the hair, leaving it very stiff and fixed in the style sculptured into the hair. The spritzes usually contain a copolymer of polyvinyl–pyrrolidone and vinyl acetate.

Table 12.2 Oils and Pomades

Ingredients	Products Containing
Petrolatum, mineral oil, fragrance	Murray's Superior Hair Dressing Pomade
Petrolatum, olive oil, fragrance	Royal Crown Hair Dress
Petrolatum, mineral oil, lanolin, fragrance	Dax-Wave and Groom Hair Dress
Petrolatum, lanolin, lecithin, mineral oil, fragrances, D&C green No. 6, D&C violet No. 2	Blue Magic Conditioner Hair Dress
Petrolatum, coconut oil, castor oil, mineral oil, fragrance	Dax-Short and Neat
Petrolatum, lanolin, mineral oil, fragrance, D&C green No. 6, D&C violet No. 2	Blue Magic Pressing Oil
Petrolatum, lanolin, olive oil, lecithin; fragrances, isopropyn myristate, D&C yellow No. 11, D&C green No. 6	Blue Magic Bergamot Hair and Scalp Conditioner Queen Bergamot Hair and Scalp Conditioner
Petrolatum, mineral oil, lanolin, aluminium stearate, microcrystalline wax, fragrance, lauric acid, propylparaben, D&C green No. 6	Ultra Sheen Conditioner and Hair Dress

Medical treatments

The specific medical treatments are based upon the prevention effort, antibiotherapy, and anti-inflammatory prescriptions (Table 12.3). Medical treatments will be selected primarily to stop the inflammation that has occurred despite prevention efforts (Table 12.3).[3,5,6,10]

Surgical treatments

Surgical treatments need to be specific to African Americans because of the nature of the curly shafts, the curvature of the roots, the risk of hypertrophic scarring or keloid scars, and the risk of hyperpigmentation or hypopigmentation. They should always be selected based on the location of the surgery to best prevent the risk of excessive or discolored scarring. The surgical techniques themselves (resections, flaps, grafts, etc.) must be adapted to the particular features of the African American scalp.[9] As with any dermatologic surgery of the scalp, the indications are guided by many factors, such as the nature, extent, and location of the alopecia; the sex, age, and individual characteristics of the patient; and finally, the development of alopecia. This surgery follows three main technical principles: autologous hair transplantation in the form of follicular unit grafts, or transposition flaps, or assisted excision by placing an expander.[19–21]

Table 12.3 Specific African American Hair Diseases and Therapy

African American Specific Pathologies	Advice	Medical Treatments
Traction alopecia	Stop the traction Hair transplant (in some cases)	2% minoxidil lotion for 6 months
Hot comb alopecia	Stop the hair traction Hair transplant in some cases Hairpieces (in some cases)	
Folliculitis and pseudo-folliculitis	Stop shaving or hair traction	Local antibiotherapy Oral antibiotherapy
Keloid folliculitis	Stop shaving Excision (with caution)	Local antibiotherapy Oral antibiotherapy Intralesional corticosteroids
Dissecting cellulitis of the scalp	Incision/drainage Fluctuating abcesses Excisions (with caution)	Oral antibiotherapy Oral corticosteroids Isotrétinoïn (40 mg/d) Zinc sulfate (400 mg *per os*)

- The follicular unit (FU) graft technique consists of harvesting small fragments of the scalp in the mid-occipital donor area.

  The intradermal curl follicles are associated with higher transection rates. This rate can be lowered with certain surgical modifications. The use of tumescent solution prior to donor harvesting reduces transection by separating follicles and by partially straightening their curled intradermal elements.

  Schematically two procedures are selected (see Chapter 15):

  - The strip harvesting technique has a closure with sutures or staples and a segmentation onto 1–4 hours FU. It is called the follicular unit technique (FUT) if the scalp is previously shaved and follicular unit long hair (FUL)[22] if the scalp is unshaved. These procedures are the most commonly indicated (Figure 12.18 through 12.21).
  - The follicular unit extraction (FUE) consists of harvesting on a scalp previously shaved follicular unit with manual or automated rotated punches of 0.8–1 mm diameter. The FUE are then extracted manually with forceps. The very small round scars are nearly invisible. Follicular unit extraction (FUE) might be an appropriate

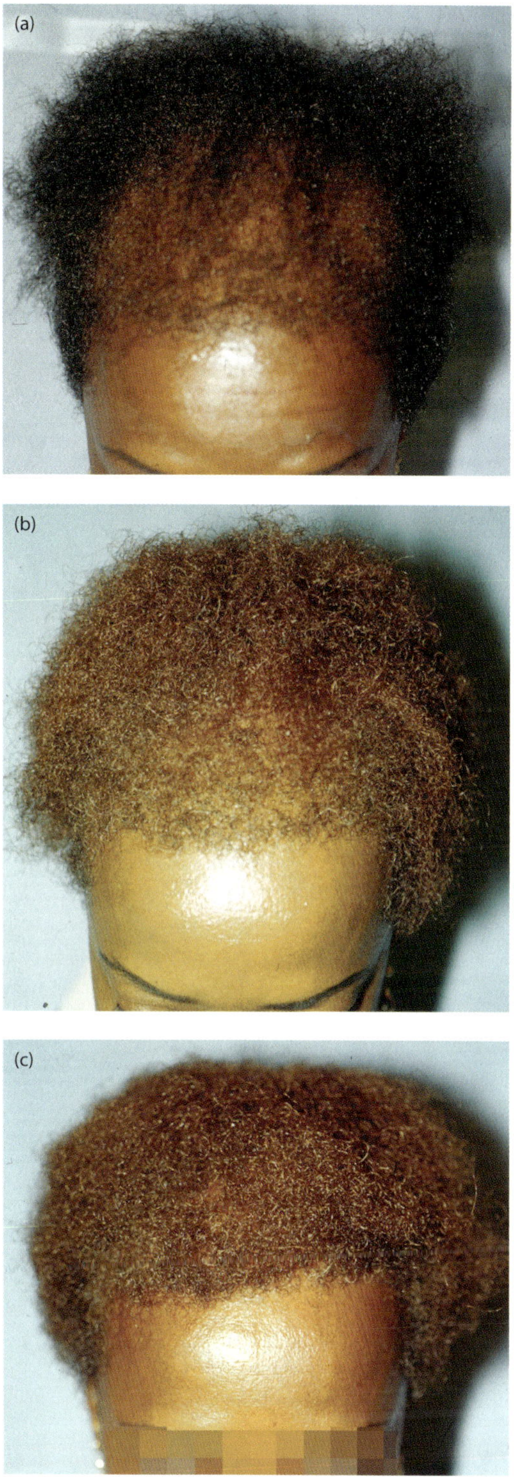

Figure 12.18 Definitive traction alopecia, (a) 6 months after stopping any traction; (b) appearance after the first session; (c) and after a second session of follicular unit long (FUL) hair transplantation.

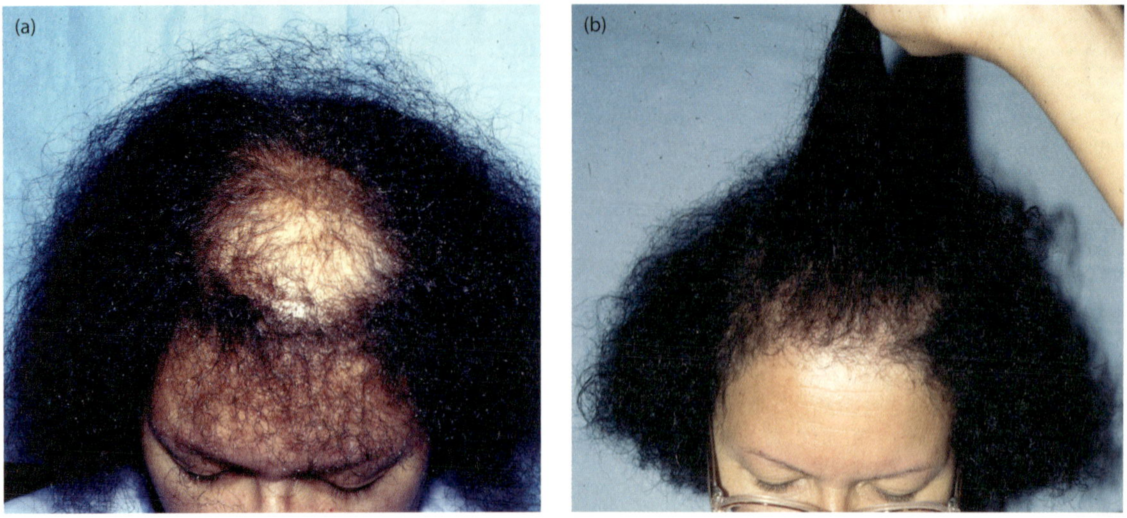

Figure 12.19 Female androgenetic alopecia, Ludwig type II, (a) before and (b) after correction by one session of follicular unit long (FUL) hair grafts.

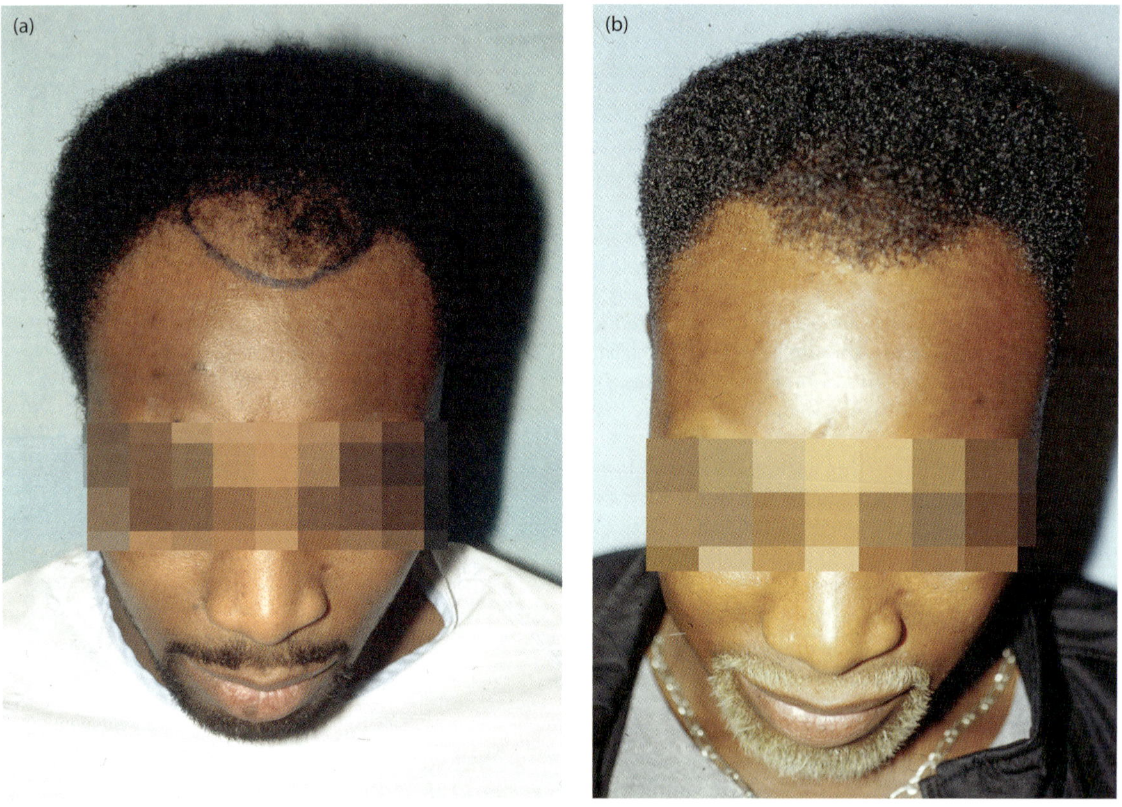

Figure 12.20 Male androgenetic alopecia (a) before and (b) 10 years after correction by one session of follicular unit transplantation (FUL).

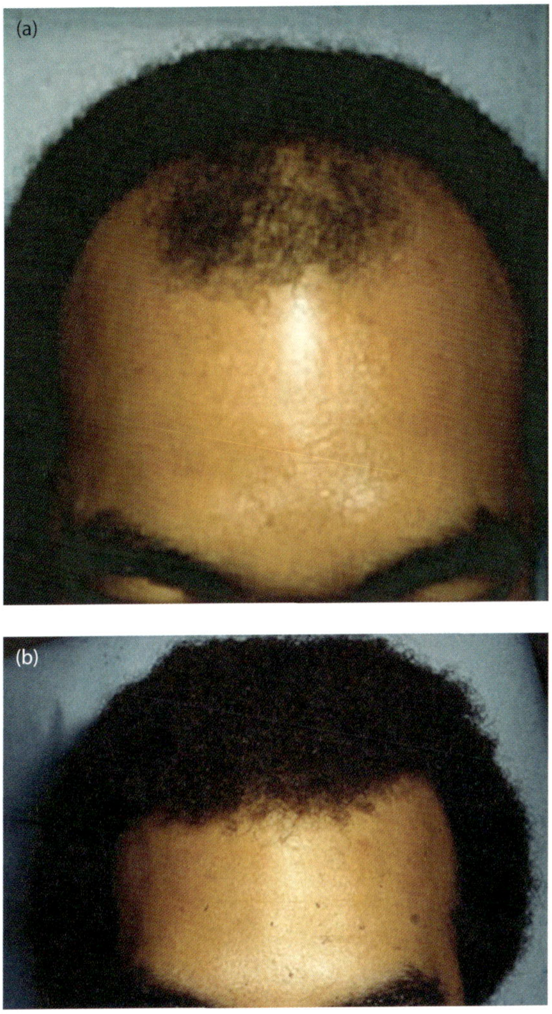

Figure 12.21 **Male androgenetic alopecia (a) before and (b) after correction with two small vertical flaps on the frontal area.**

method of graft harvesting in the minority of black patients. It relies on blind excision, and given the follicle curl, the risk of intradermal transection is extremely high.

- All the FU harvested are then inserted with forceps in each slit incision done with needles or microsurgery blades in the recipient area (see Chapter 15).

The goal is to create hair density and a natural aspect of the frontal hairline through the best selection of FU according to their caliber, shape, and color shaft. The pattern and type of grafts used in patients of African heritage is different compared with other ethnicities. The hairline for most black patients is flatter than is seen for Caucasians, but not as flat as is seen for Asians.

- Surgical correction of male pattern baldness was initiated early in the twentieth century by the development of flaps. In the technique of vertical flaps,[23] a strip of scalp of variable size is taken at the crown, placed on the bald area, and sutured; the hair is left long and the band of scalp retains its vascularization via a rotation pedicle. This process should be proposed to correct stable male frontal baldness (Hamilton stages IV and V). It allows you to recreate a natural frontal hairline, with a reduction of the frontotemporal recession, and hair orientated obliquely forward and coming through the anterior thin scar line to help obscure it.
- Scalp excision[23] consists of removing part of the bald area, following a variable design, then putting together and suturing the hairy regions. Excision may be facilitated by prior distension of hairy areas of the crown with an expander (a balloon inflated progressively, with saline injections). These prostheses are set in position, after local anesthesia in the separated galeotic membrane, to cause additional laxity of the surface to be excised; a wide bald zone can be removed after 1 month of distension.

CONCLUSION

The hair and scalp pathology of African Americans presents, in addition to those disorders common to the other main ethnic groups, particular genetic characteristics, particular sociocultural characteristics (such as types of hairstyles), particular chemical characteristics of the hair (such as a dry shaft), and peculiarities of scalp tissue (the inflammatory responses).

Treatment and prevention advice will be essentially guided by the fragility of the hair shaft, the risks of folliculitis, and the risk of poor wound healing, and will aim to try to change some traditional styling habits.

REFERENCES

1. Bernard BA. Hair shape of curly hair. *J AM Acad Dermatol.* 2003;48(suppl 6):S120–S126.
2. Loussouarn G. African hair growth parameters. *Br J Dermatol.* 2001;145:294–297.
3. Bouhanna P, Reygagne P. *Pathologie du cheveu et du cuir chevelu.* Paris, France: Masson; 1999.
4. Halder RM. Pseudofolliculitis barbae and related disorders. *Dermatol Clin.* 1988;6:407–412.
5. Bouhanna P. La pathologie des cheveux Afro-Américains: spécificités diagnostiques et thérapeutiques. In: *Les alopécies-de la clinique au traitement. Collection Guide Pratique de Dermatologie.* Paris, France: Med'Com; 2004.
6. Scott DA. Disorders of the hair and scalp in blacks. *Dermatol Clin.* 1988;6:387–395.
7. Olsen EA, ed. *Disorders of Hair Growth—Diagnosis and Treatment.* New York, NY: McGraw-Hill; 1994.

8. Bouhanna P. Pathologie des cheveux afro-américains: spécificités diagnostiques et thérapeutiques. *BEDC*. 2004;12(4):74–77.
9. Callender V. African-American scalp disorders and treatment considerations. *Skin Aging*. 2002;10:12–14.
10. Petit A, Reygagne P. Alopécies particulières aux femmes noires. *Ann Dermatol Venereol*. 2006;133:891–898.
11. Fitoussi C. Cosmétologie des cheveux antillais. *EMC, Cosmétol Dermatol esthétique*. 2007;50-220-I-20.
12. Khumalo NP, Jessop S, Gumedze F, Ehrlich R. hairdressing and the prevalence of scalp disease in African adults. *Br J Dermatol*. 2007;157:981–988.
13. Yang A, Lorizzo M, Vincenzi C, Tosti A. Hair extensions: A concerning cause of hair disorders. *Br J Dermatol*. 2009;160:207–209.
14. Sperling LC, Sau P. The follicular degeneration syndrome in black patients: "Hot comb alopecia" revisited and revised. *Arch Dermatol*. 1992;128:68–74.
15. Lopresti P, Papa CM, Kligman AM. Hot comb alopecia. *Arch Dermatol*. 1968;98:234–238.
16. Gathers RC, Lim HM. Central centrifugal alopecia: Past, present, and future. *J Am Acad Dermatol*. 2008;60:660–668.
17. Halder RM. Hair and scalp disorders in blacks. *Cutis*. 1983;32:378–380.
18. Schewach-Millet M, Fiv R, Shapira D. Perifolliculitis capitis abscedens et suffodiens treated with isotretinoin (13 cis-retinoic acid). *J Am Acad Dermatol*. 1986;15:1291–1292.
19. Bouhanna P. Chirurgie du cuir chevelu par micro-greffes. Traité cosmétologie et dermatologie esthétique. *EMC*. 2013;8(1):1–14.
20. Bouhanna P. Les greffes de cheveux chez les patients afro-américains. *Dermatol Pratique*. 2010;344:12–13.
21. Ozcelik D. Extensive traction alopecia attributable to ponytail hairstyle and its treatment with hair transplantation. *Aesthetic Plast Surg*. 2005;29:325–327.
22. Bouhanna P. Greffes à cheveux longs immédiats. [Grafts with immediate long hair.] *Nouv Dermatol*. 1989;8:418–420.
23. Bouhanna P. Newer techniques in hair replacement. In: Roenigk RK, Roenigk H, eds. *Surgical Dermatology, Advances in Current Practice*. Vol. 51. London, UK: Martin Dunitz; 1993:527–553.

13 Management of definitive hair alopecia in Asians

Damkerng Pathomvanich

INTRODUCTION

Hair loss affects both Asian men and women; however, the incidence and severity of the baldness are less than in Caucasians.[1,2] Hair transplantation in the Asian population has been increasing in popularity over the past decade, but is associated with unique demands. The International Society of Hair Restoration Surgery (ISHRS) practice census results in 2013 showed there were 102,702 hair transplantation cases being performed in Asia, ranking the highest in the world, a 10% increase from 2010. There were 54,343 procedures in Europe and 88,340 procedures in the United States.[3] It is paramount to understand the Asian culture, knowing the difference in hair character, skull and facial features, before performing hair transplantation surgery, to achieve optimal results and avoid litigation.

ASIAN FEATURES

Anatomy

The Asian skull has less frontal and occipital projection than the more oblong Caucasian skull, and therefore appears round (Figure 13.1). The Asian face also appears round, with less frontal projection, to almost flat in some Asians, posing a special challenge for hairline placement.

Hair character

Asians in general have coarser, straight, black hair in contrast to many different color shades found in Caucasians; however, variations exist among Asian ethnicities. There are many studies on hair density in Asians, with biopsy results confirming low hair density compare to Caucasians (Figure 13.2). In one study by Jui-Hung Ko, Yu-Huei Huang, and Tseng-Tong Kuo, the average hair

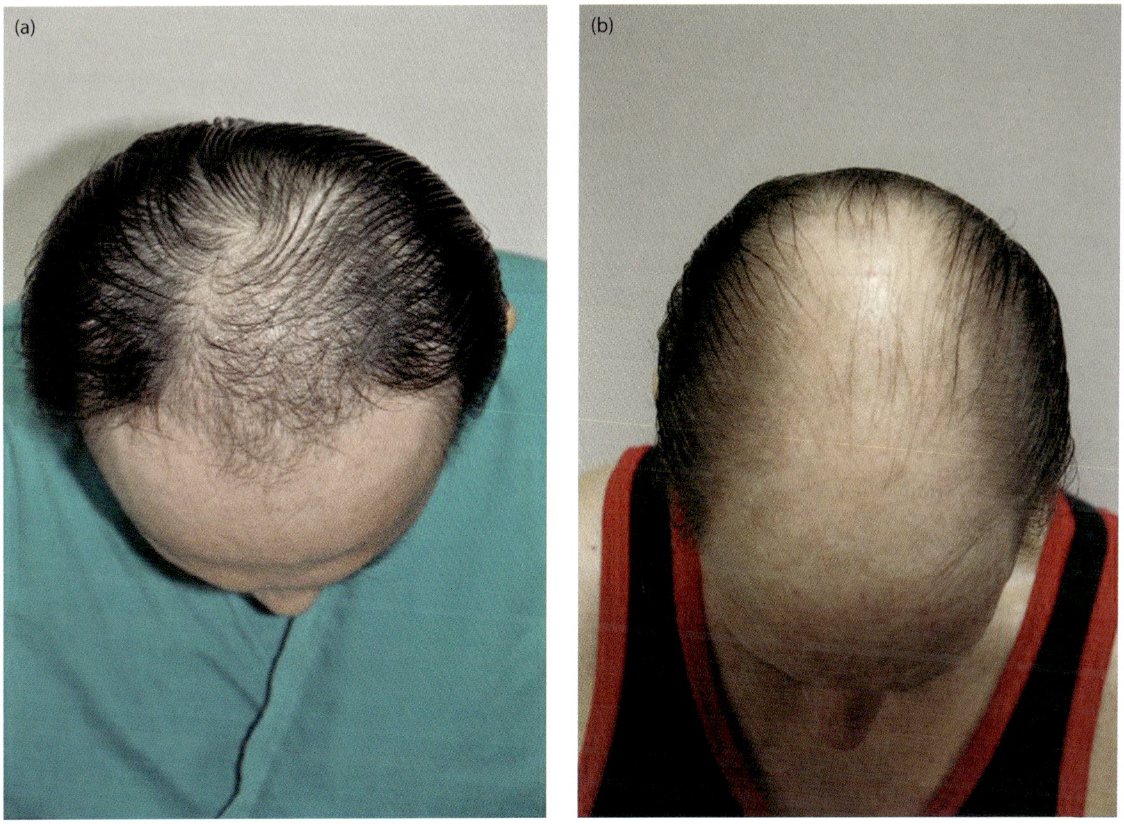

Figure 13.1 **(a) Rounder head with less frontal projection in an Asian patient, compared with (b) a typical Caucasian.**

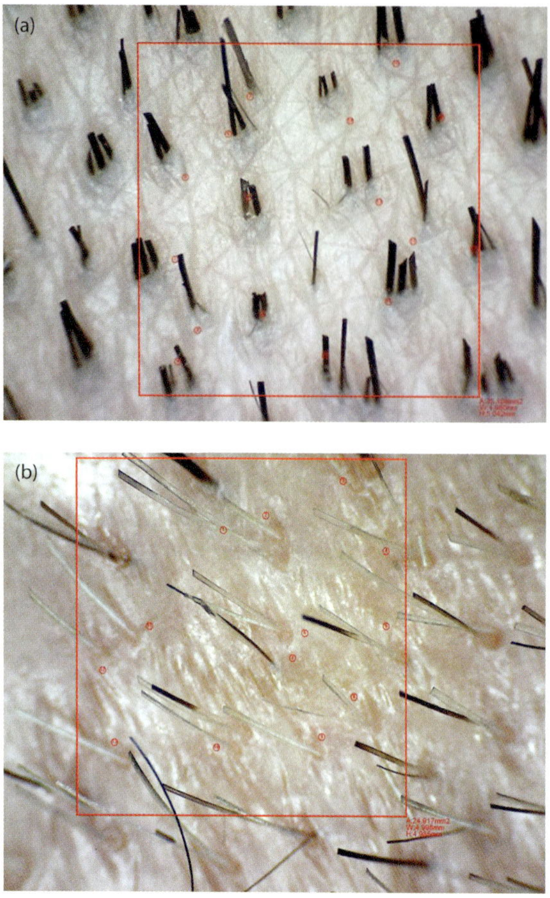

Figure 13.2 **(a) Picture from digital VDO microscope 65×; the density can be counted precisely with the red marker and also can identify any lesions. Gray hairs are visualized well in (b) and are easy to count. Patient identity including the picture can be recorded on the chart.**

counts of total hairs = 21.3, terminal hairs = 20.5, vellus hairs = 0.8, and follicular units = 9.4 by 4 mm punch biopsy. The mean ratio of anagen hair to telogen hair was 91.6:8.4 and of terminal hair to vellus hair was 25.3:1. The average density of hair follicles was 1.69 mm. The mean counts of terminal hairs, total hairs, follicular units, and hair follicles/mm^2 were significantly different between different age groups.[4]

Imagawa studied androgenic alopecia in Japan and found at the midocciput, Asians have 80–90 FU/cm^2 or 170 hairs/cm^2, while in the temporal zone; they have 55–70 FU/cm^2 or 100–127 hairs/cm^2. This represents 1.8 hairs per follicular unit (FU). Caucasians have a similar density of FUs, but have 2.3 hairs per FU, and therefore a greater total number of hairs. Studies of donor zone hair shafts in androgenic alopecia revealed an average diameter of 71 μm, and a range of 63–79 μm. In Asians, the average follicle length from epidermis to dermal papilla is 5.5 mm compared to 4.5 mm in Caucasians; therefore, it has a higher transection rate during the follicular unit extraction (FUE) procedure as well as strip.[5] Kim reported density in Korean hair at midocciput = 120 hairs/cm^2 and 100 hairs/cm^2 at the temporal region. It is interesting to see variation density in people from different Asian countries. Kim reported 45% of one hair follicular unit and 42 hairs follicular unit and 7% of three hairs follicular unit that will challenge Korean hair surgeons in performing hair transplantation.[6]

Most Asians have black hair and light skin, which creates a contrast rarely seen in Caucasians. This can become a concern in individuals with wide scars. In addition, Asian skin is more prone than Caucasian skin to keloid or hypertrophic scarring, hyperpigmentation, and hypopigmentation, but to a lesser extent than African skin. The problematic scars most commonly occur at the donor site, especially at the mastoid region.

Medical treatment

The two medications that the U.S. Food and Drug Administration (FDA) has approved to treat male pattern hair loss are oral finasteride and topical minoxidil.[7,8] Finasteride is a competitive inhibitor of type II 5AR. The recommended dosage of finasteride is 1 mg/day; however, due to its side effect of erectile dysfunction (ED) with reports of irreversible ED, many Asian men have shied away from this drug. Many experienced hair surgeons have cut down the dosage to 0.5 mg/day or every other day or even only 2–3 times per week. Some even lower the dosage to 0.3 mg/day and note fewer side effects, but still give the patient the overall same result. However, there is no scientific report to document that low-dose finasteride is effective to treat male pattern baldness. Since the change in dose is not approved as standard medical treatment, most physicians stick to finasteride 1 mg/day. In my experience the side effects of this drug in Asians tend to be higher than in Caucasians. Before prescribing the drug, we routinely check prostate-specific antigen (PSA) in men older than age 40.

Topical minoxidil has not been popular in Asia because the weather is warmer, and patients commonly complain of sticky scalp, no time to apply, as well as being itchy and irritating to the scalp. In this practice, 5% minoxidil lotion is used in both men and women. Rogaine foam is not available worldwide and claims to have less irritation to the scalp. In some Asian countries concentrations of minoxidil at 10%–15% or higher are available, but no study regarding the efficacy of these concentrations compares with 5% minoxidil.

We instruct most patients with genetic hair loss to consider the following two drugs despite some negative side effects.

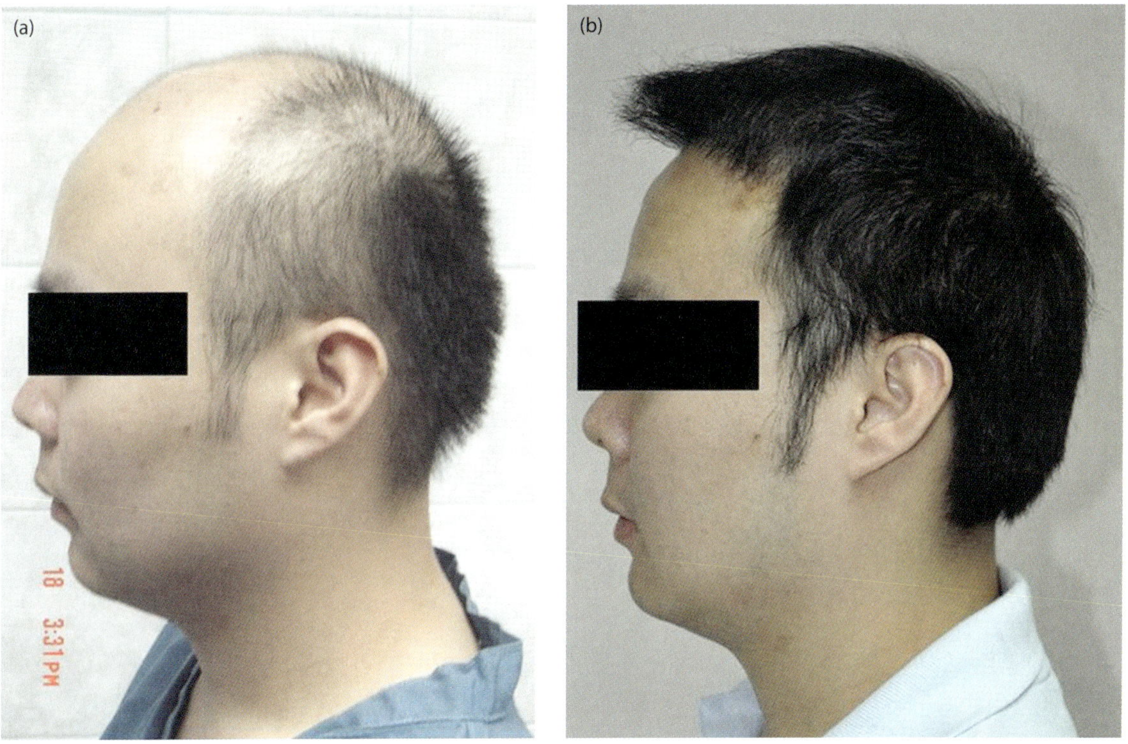

Figure 13.3 **(a) Before and (b) after—oral minoxidil grows hairs at temples, the humps, and fringe and made hair transplantation possible at front and top.**

Dutasteride (*Avodart*) is a potent inhibitor of type I and type II 5AR. It is not yet FDA approved to be used in male pattern baldness. Dutasteride improved male pattern hair loss in a randomized study in identical twins.[9] I have limited experience using this drug but did not see consistency of hair growth when a patient switched from finasteride to dutasteride, but I did note an increased incidence of ED over the finasteride group.

There are many over the-counter drugs in the Asian market, especially a product named 101 from China with no documented proof to stop hair loss.

I have conducted research on growth factor application to the scalp with dermal roller for thinning hair for 6 months with no improvement of hair loss (oral presentation at ISHRS regional live surgery workshop in Bangkok 2010).

For those patients who have extensive baldness or are poor candidates for hair transplantation and want to proceed with hair restoration surgery, I give a trial of low-dose minoxidil tablets. Since the drug is not FDA approved to use in hair loss, the patient will need to be informed of the off-label use and sign consent. Of the reported side effects, salt retention and hypertrichosis are the most common side effects encountered. If the patient responds to the drug without side effects, he or she needs to maintain use for life and needs yearly blood tests and electrocardiogram (ECG). Oral minoxidil treatment can make previously thought impossible hair transplantation become possible (Figure 13.3).

Low-level laser light therapy has been in the market for many years to treat hair loss. Laser comb from Hair Max is FDA approved; however, patient-reported feedback has been negative, without documented hair growth or the stopping of further hair loss.[10]

CORRECTION OF MALE PATTERN BALDNESS IN ASIANS

At consultation, basic history and physical examination plus in-depth history of the patient's hair loss, including hair loss in family members (both maternal and paternal), are very important notes for the surgeon to evaluate prior to surgery. Any medical problems found need to be treated by appropriate specialists. The length and width of permanent donor hair are measured, donor density is counted in different zones with video (VDO) microscope. Test for scalp laxity, measure recipient and donor areas,

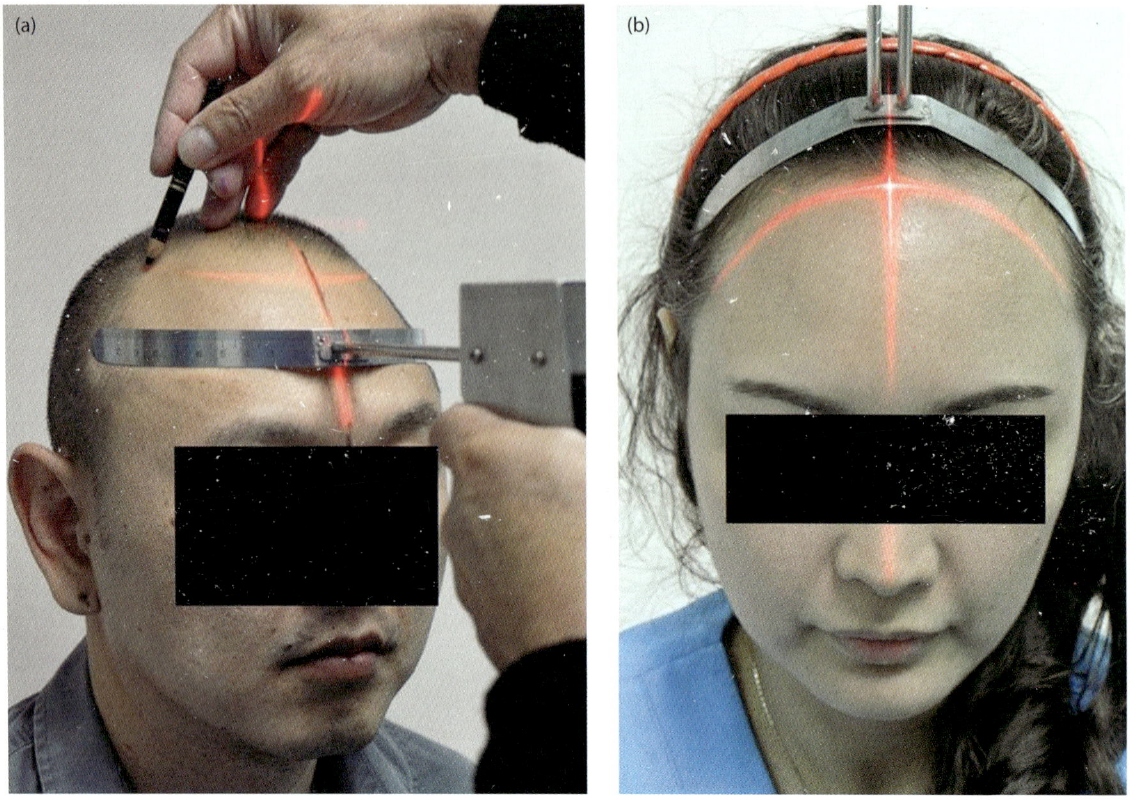

Figure 13.4 **(a,b) Rapid laser hairline device assists the surgeon to achieve symmetric hair line placement and shape.**

and examine the entire scalp for any existing lesion. The patient is then assessed as to whether he or she is a good candidate for surgery, medical therapy, or both.

Hair line design is challenging in both men and women. The majority of surgeons use visual (eyeball) or some form of measurement that is both time consuming and difficult to achieve symmetric appearance. I use a laser hair line device that I developed[11] (Figure 13.4); I then modify the shape and make irregular lines as appropriate.

I then use the modified Chang method to calculate the number of grafts to be transplanted.[12,13]

Patients need to be informed that there are two types of methods to harvest donor graft, strip (follicular unit transplantation [FUT]) and follicular unit extraction (FUE). The public often sees advertisements that "FUE is scarless and less painful" compared to the strip method with linear scars. Surgeons must inform the patient of the differences of each technique and advise what is the best method (FUT or FUE) for the patient. If the surgeon does not perform FUE and the patient insists, he or she should be referred to a surgeon who performs FUE, or vice versa.

A safe donor area is selected and marked. A long single strip or multiple strips can be performed as surgically feasible. A mega session of 3000–4000 plus grafts can be obtained for those who have both good density and scalp laxity. However, Asian hair tends to have lower density, making 3000–4000 graft mega-sessions in general more difficult compared with Caucasians.

Asian skin tends to have thicker dermis than Caucasians, more collagen density, and larger melanosomes with more melanin production. These characteristics lead to higher tendencies of developing hypertrophic scar and hyperpigmentation after skin injury. Hair follicles are longer in Asians, and the preference is to harvest by strip approach, except for patients with tight scalp or if patients want to wear the hair very short, then FUE is an excellent alternative.

FUT or strip is by far the most common technique currently used for donor harvesting in hair restoration surgery throughout the world. The ISHRS 2013 census results utilize FUT 68% compared with 32% for FUE.[3] The majority of surgeons use blind harvesting by cutting parallel to the hair follicle or scoring deep enough and then using the spreader to separate the incision. The stem cells are located just short of 1 mm deep,[14,15] and there is a

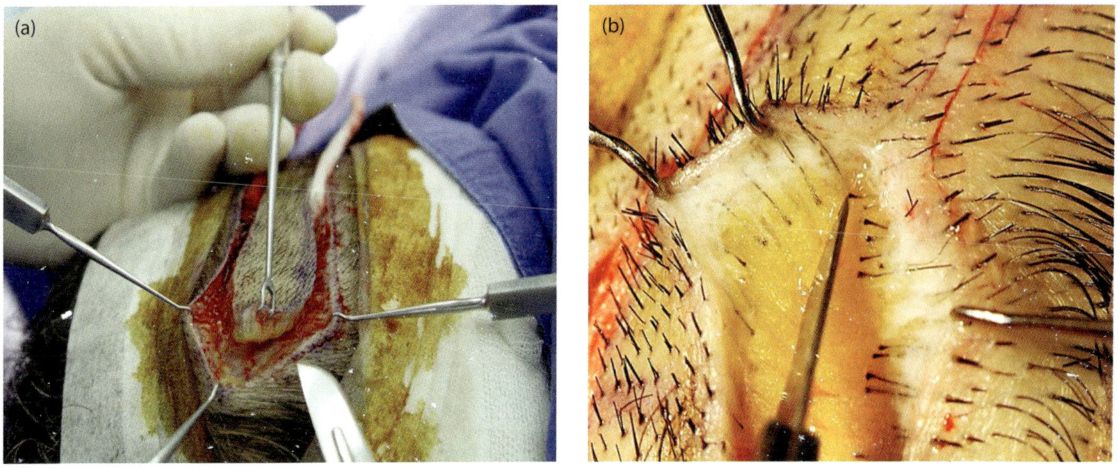

Figure 13.5 **(a,b) Donor harvesting with direct visualization assisted by skin hook to minimize transection and suction to clear blood from the field to speed dissection.**

potential for damage if blind scoring is too deep. Because Asian hairs are coarse and long and the scalp is thick, the chance for transection of the follicle is very high. To overcome this I have developed an open technique with a skin hook, thus minimizing follicular transection below 2%.[16] The technique is easy to master based on cutting under direct visualization; suction is helpful to clear the field to speed dissection (Figure 13.5).

Strip length and width are calculated, and the width must not be too wide to exceed closure without tension. The wider the strip, the greater is the potential for scar formation. I usually use the Mayer method,[17] but the laxity should be judged again at the end with an up-and-down push with the fingers before making a mark for the strip. I have found the Mayer method to be about 70% accurate. Previously, both inferior and double trichophytic closures were used, but no difference was found in the appearance of scarring and more time was wasted. Currently, I use only the inferior trichophytic closure, but the superior hanging edge is trimmed for easy closure in some patients. The wound is closed with 3/0 Nylon interrupt as retention sutures about 1.5 cm apart, and the bite is 1 cm away from the incision. The skin is then closed with running 4/0 Vicryl Rapide. In the past, a two-layered closure failed to produce minimal scarring (Figure 13.6) so I have not used it for the past 6 years.

Because slivering takes some time and desiccation might happen, especially for those surgeons who just started using this technique, I have designed a special slivering tray with a small chamber to house the normal saline solution. Medical-grade silicone is placed inside the chamber to submerge under saline solution. The strip is laid on top of silicone and also submerged in normal saline; both ends are fixed with 23G and 2–4 needles might be used to stabilize the strip for easy

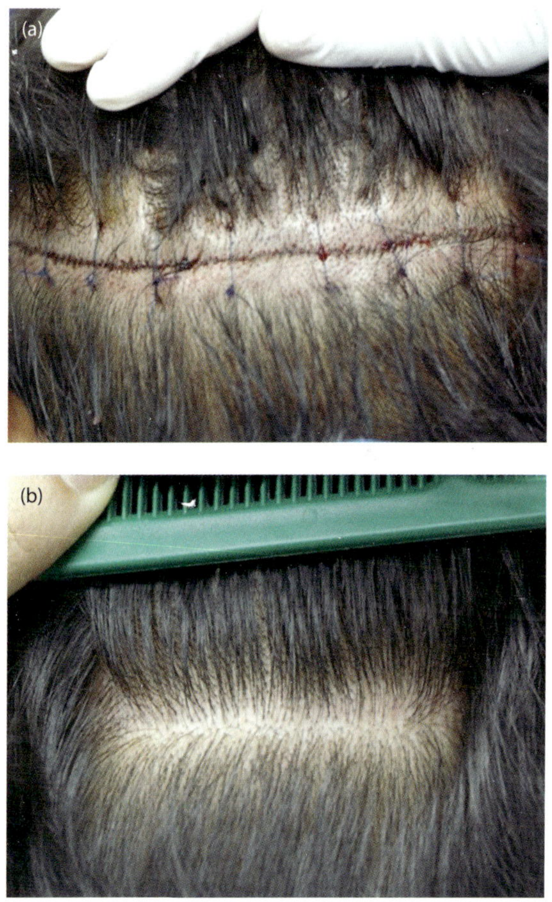

Figure 13.6 **(a) A 2 cm wide strip excision at midocciput left (b) 1 year post-op with minimal donor scar.**

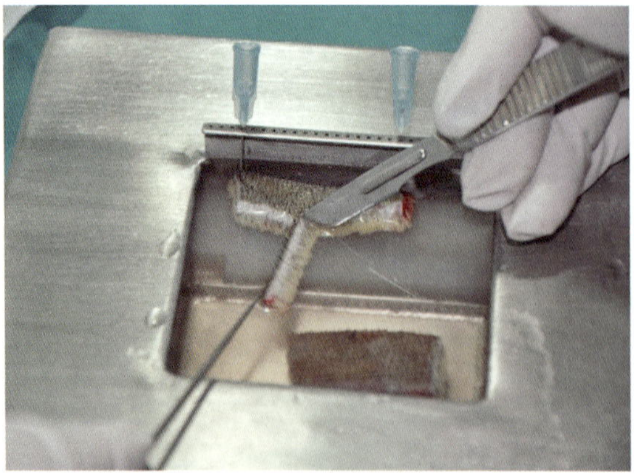

Figure 13.7 **Portion of strip is pinned at both ends with 23G for stabilization during sliver. Note the entire strip is submerged in normal saline to prevent desiccation.**

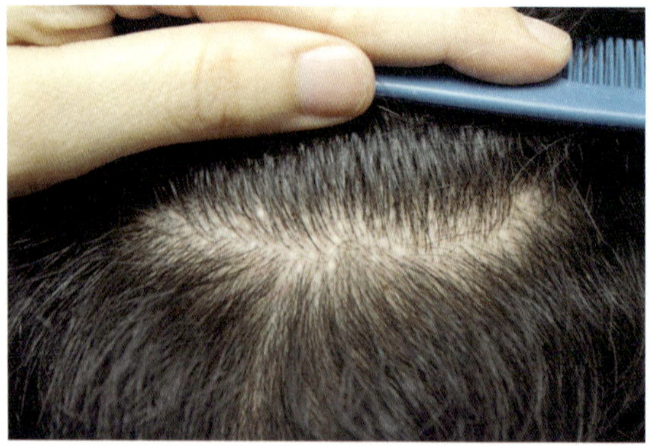

Figure 13.8 **One year post-op FUE with moth-eaten scar prominent in Asian with black hair and light color skin.**

slivering (Figure 13.7). A skin hook holds the superior edge on the end of the strip. Dissection is carried out with a 15-blade by cutting from the top to the bottom of the follicle. Abduction of the dissected strip speeds the cutting because both sides of the sliver are well visualized, thus minimizing transection.

The follicles are cut from a narrow strip under the microscope with 10 times magnification and stored in normal saline. The downside for the strip is to have a linear scar. Fortunately, for over 85% of my patients, the scars are minimal and almost undetectable. Less than 15% have a slightly wider scar, most likely due to intrinsic factors, which are many. If surgeons try to keep the excised strip at a width not to exceed 1.5 cm at midocciput and not more than 1 cm at the temporoparietal area in the first session, minimize transection, and prevent desiccation of both the skin edges when closing, the scar will be minimal most of the time. For subsequent sessions, the scar in the majority of surgeries is included.

FUE (follicular unit extraction) is increasing in demand and rising in popularity.[18–20] This technique is usually limited to 1500–2000 grafts per session depend on the individual density; however, over 3000 grafts extracted in a single session was presented at the hair meeting, but no result of growth rate and donor scar were presented. There are several automated machines available (e.g., Neografts, Bell Hand Engine, Dental machine, robotic [ARTAS]) with some doctors still using the manual punch technique. My transection rate is higher with sharp punch, so a switch was made to dull punch and less transection and chubbier grafts were noted compared with the sharp punch. My experience of FUE is limited to the automated SAFE SYSTEM which uses a dull punch for graft extraction. The punch size of 0.9 is a workhorse, except with coarse hair with large follicular units a switch is made to 1 mm. The transection rate is in the range of 10% but improving with time and experience. The healing process is rapid and almost invisible after 1 week. Most patients experience no pain or minimal discomfort. Diffuse small scars from FUE are seen throughout the donor area. The growth rates from FUE are comparable to those from FUT (Figure 13.8).

Recipient site

I routinely use a supraorbital nerve block and tumescent fluid with epinephrine 1:100,000 plus triamcinolone.[21] A pre-made incision with 22G to 18G is used, and sometimes a precut blade size 0.7–1.2 mm, depending on the size of the follicle, is used for tough skin. Hair density in Asians is not as high as in Caucasians—35 grafts/cm^2 might give a patient a good outcome in one session. In my practice I use a two-handed technique for insertion. The right dominant hand holds a very fine sharp point straight forceps to insert the graft, and the left nondominant hand holds the curve forceps to open the incision, reducing trauma during insertion; and vice versa for those with a dominant left hand. On average, two to four assistants insert the grafts at the same time, if space permits, to reduce operative time. If the patient needs more grafts and the scalp is not tight, the stitches are removed at the midocciput region about 10 cm and either the inferior or the superior edge is re-excised. Sometimes FUE is used to obtain more grafts to avoid a wide scar. Grafts are carefully checked when the procedure is over to make sure all the grafts are settled well with good direction and that there is no visible bleeding at both donor and recipient sites. A head band is used to hold the dressing at the donor area and also compress the incision for hemostasis. The patient returns the next day for shampoo and wound care. The stitches are removed in 1 week. It will take at least one and a half years to look good (Figures 13.9 and 13.10).

Platelet-rich plasma (PRP) has been used in hair restoration surgery with unpredictable results.[22,23] ACell

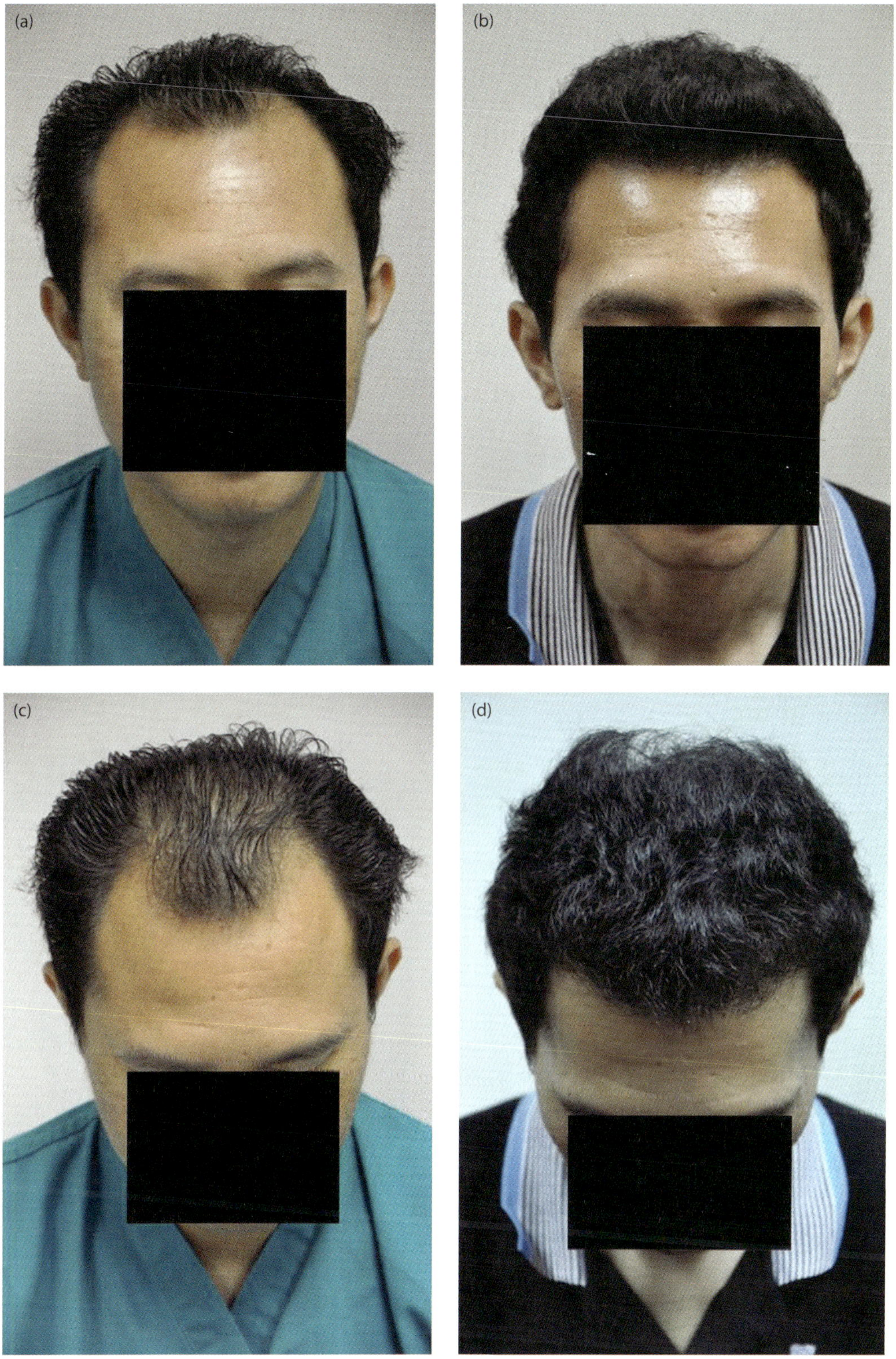

Figure 13.9 (a,c) Before and (b,d) 10 months after surgery, with weight loss and orthodontic treatment.

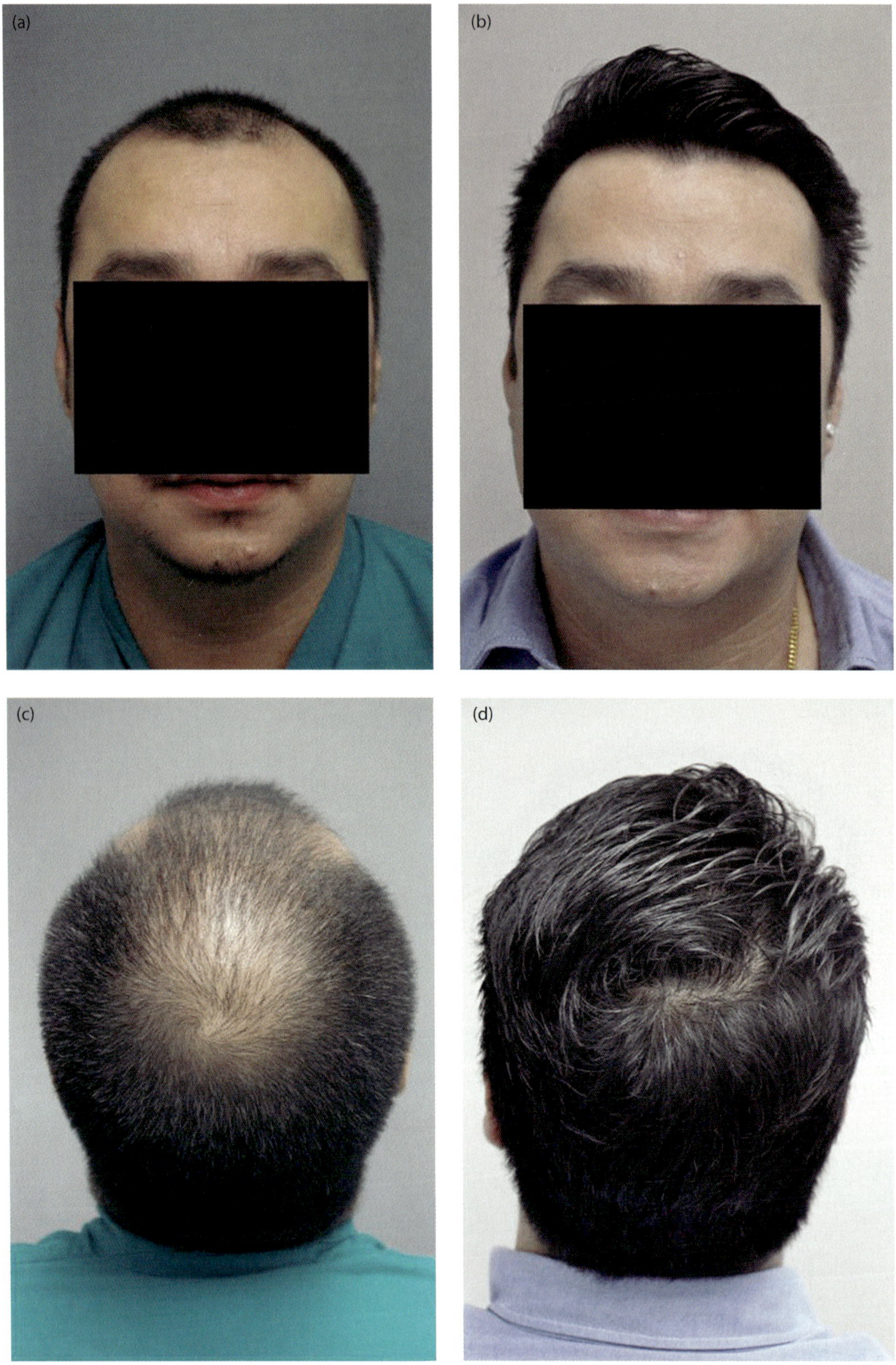

Figure 13.10 (a,c) Pre-op and (b,d) post-op 2 years 9 months; 4483 grafts were transplanted in one session.

MatriStem has also been used with no current scientific proof that it has worked in reducing donor scarring and increasing hair growth. I have no personal experience using these products and awaits the results of further studies.

For graft storage, the majority of surgeons use NSS, Ringer lactate, or Plasmalyte. We have studied with patient permission on one patient, William E medium used as storage solution on the right side and normal saline on the left side for comparison of growth rates and different times of insertion. Grafts were stored half in NSS and the other half in William E medium for 2, 4, 6, 24, and 72 hours and then planted accordingly. After 6 and 10 months there were amazing results with good growth on William E solution compared with less growth in NSS (presented at ISHRS Annual Scientific Meeting at Bahamas in 2012) (Figure 13.11).

Correction of female pattern baldness in Asians

Through the years, there has been a steady increase in Asian women seeking consultation for hair loss due to various causes and subsequently undergoing hair transplantation as a treatment option. As with women of all ethnic backgrounds, a thorough diagnostic investigation has to be done to ascertain if the cause of hair loss is amenable to hair transplantation. Medical therapy alone may be the treatment option of choice for many etiologies (e.g., telogen effluvium, alopecia areata, active cicatricial alopecia, etc.). However, for certain causes of hair loss, such as female pattern hair loss (FPHL), transplantation may be a consideration. After confirming that the hair loss etiology is amenable to hair transplantation, evaluation then has to be made as to whether the female patient is a good candidate for this procedure. In some female cases, the donor hair might not be sufficient to cover the hair loss at the recipient area. The Ludwig and Norwood types of pattern baldness seen in women are the most common conditions for which surgeries are performed.

Hair characteristics of Asian women are similar to those of Asian men, except in women there is more subcutaneous fat, and the skin is soft and easy to cut.

Approach to hair transplantation in Asian women

In *Ludwig type* baldness, the main problem is central thinning with retention of the frontal hair line; thus, the goal would be to add density over the thinning area in the

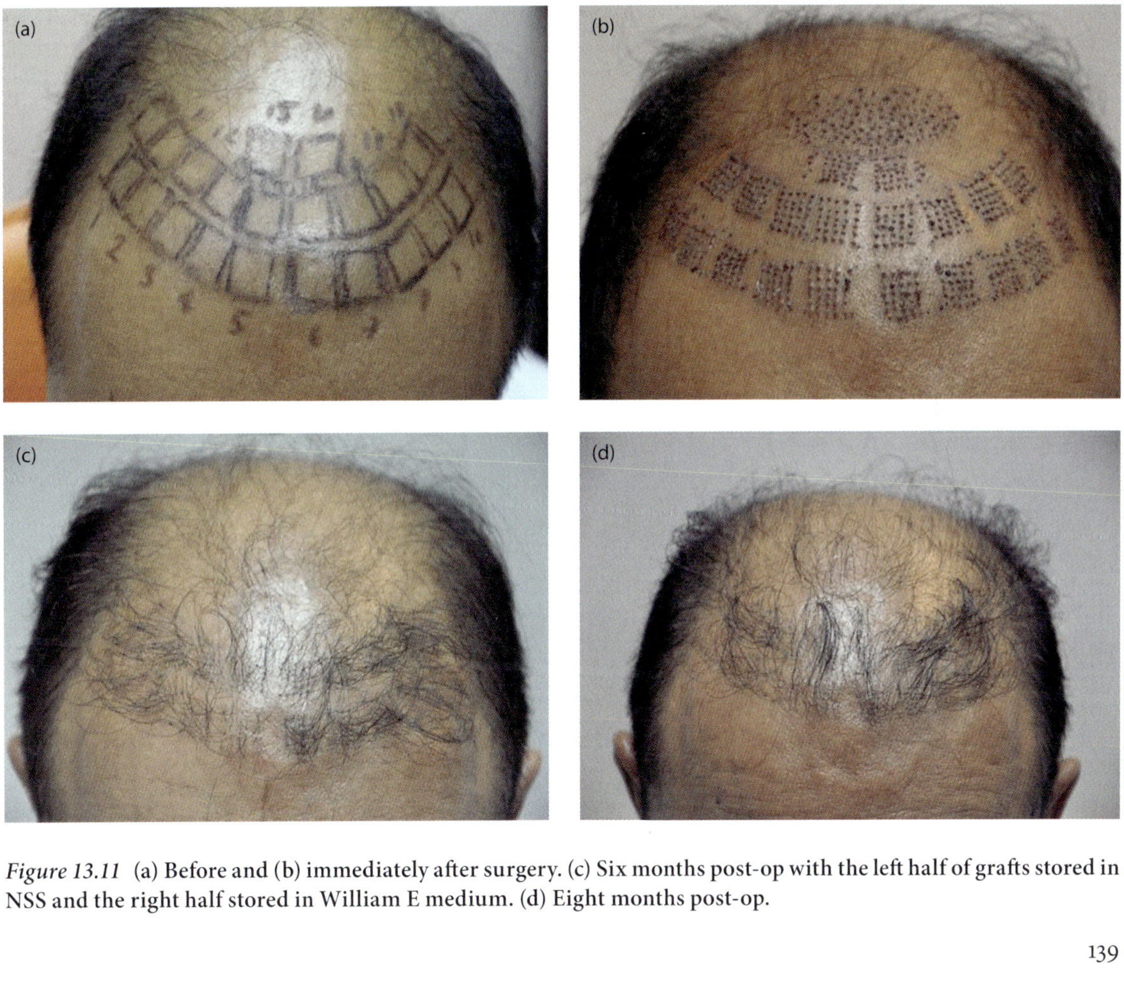

Figure 13.11 (a) Before and (b) immediately after surgery. (c) Six months post-op with the left half of grafts stored in NSS and the right half stored in William E medium. (d) Eight months post-op.

central aspect of the scalp. If the area to be transplanted has existing hair, minimizing damage to these follicles is paramount. Adjacent hair follicle injury can be lessened by following the angle and direction of the existing hair and using high-power loupes of at least 3.5 when making the incisions.[24,25] If the patient has preexisting hair, 20–25 graft/cm^2 may be appropriated. Telogen effluvium or post-op shedding may cause distress to the patient. This must be informed, recorded, and signed. Minoxidil lotion might be helpful if the patient uses it preoperatively at least a few months prior to surgery.

In Norwood–Hamilton pattern (Figures 13.12 and 13.13), hair loss is usually confined to the frontotemporal region. High forehead, deep temple recession with miniaturized hair at the gulf are more common findings in women. The goal is to restore the frontotemporal hairline. Hair line design is time consuming in women. Pattern design that is oval and heart shaped, with or without a widow's peak is drawn, and then the patient participates in observing whether the new hair line fits her face well. Because most patients have good and sufficient donor hair, high density can be achieved with 40 or even 50 graft/cm in selected patients.

The surgical technique in women is the same as in men.

Complications in hair restoration in Asians

Surgical complications can happen even in experienced hands, and surgeons need to know how to avoid and correct complications if they occur. There are significant differences between Asian skin and the skin of other ethnicities. Even within the Asian race, significant differences are apparent. In the Indian population the skin varies significantly in terms of skin color, which makes pigmentation an important scar issue.

Early complications include facial swelling, which is the most common seen in hair practice; however, with the addition of a steroid to the tumescent fluid, wearing of the headband, plus a cold compress to the forehead post-op, the incidence is dramatically improved.[21] If persistent hiccoughs occur during surgery, this can limit the ability to place the grafts. Bleeding, syncope, and infection are uncommonly seen. Post-op effluvium at recipient and donor sites are unpredictable; patients need to be warned that it may occur.

Late complications are scarring, pitting, effluvium, and poor direction and angle (Figure 13.14). Ridging and tenting are still seen in the hair practice today. Inadequate and poor growth is of concern to the patient as well as to the surgeon, and requires further investigation and assessment.

The difference between Asian and Caucasian surgery results is mostly with the donor scar; again, the wider the strip, the wider is the scar. Surgeons need to avoid tension upon closure. The scar is seen more in the younger age groups and less in elderly patients. The surgeon needs to check for Ehlers–Danlos type II which can result in a very wide scar. In case of a hypertrophic scar or keloid, a series

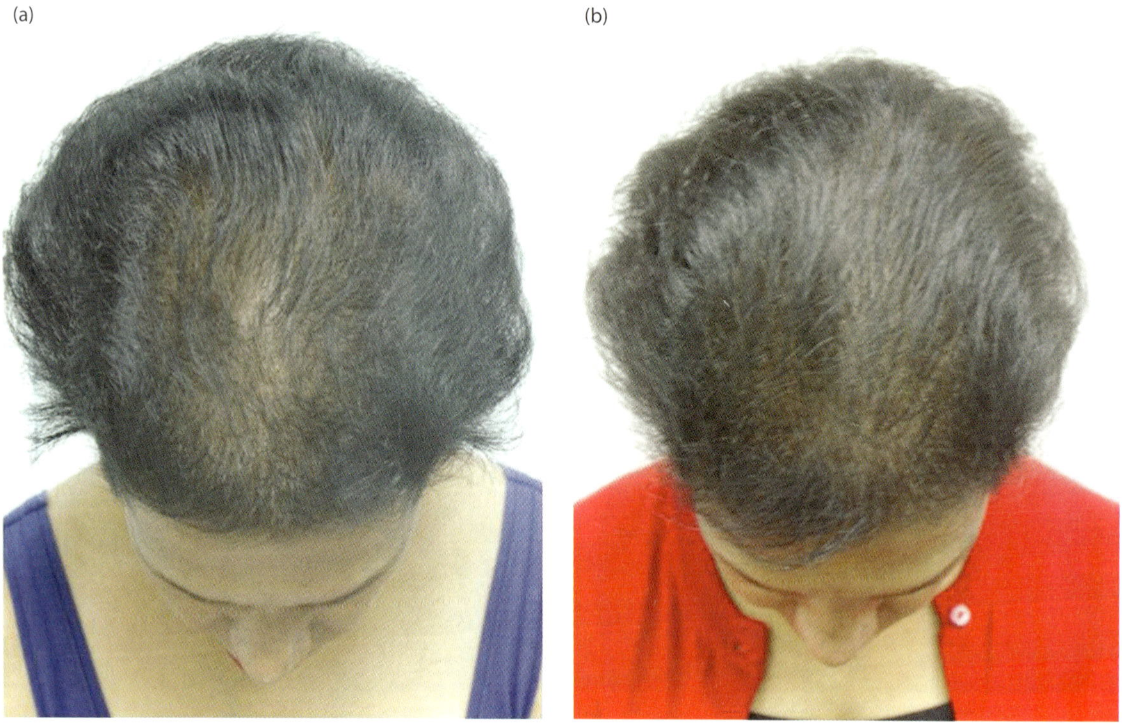

Figure 13.12 (a) Before and (b) 8 months after 3030 grafts in Ludwig II.

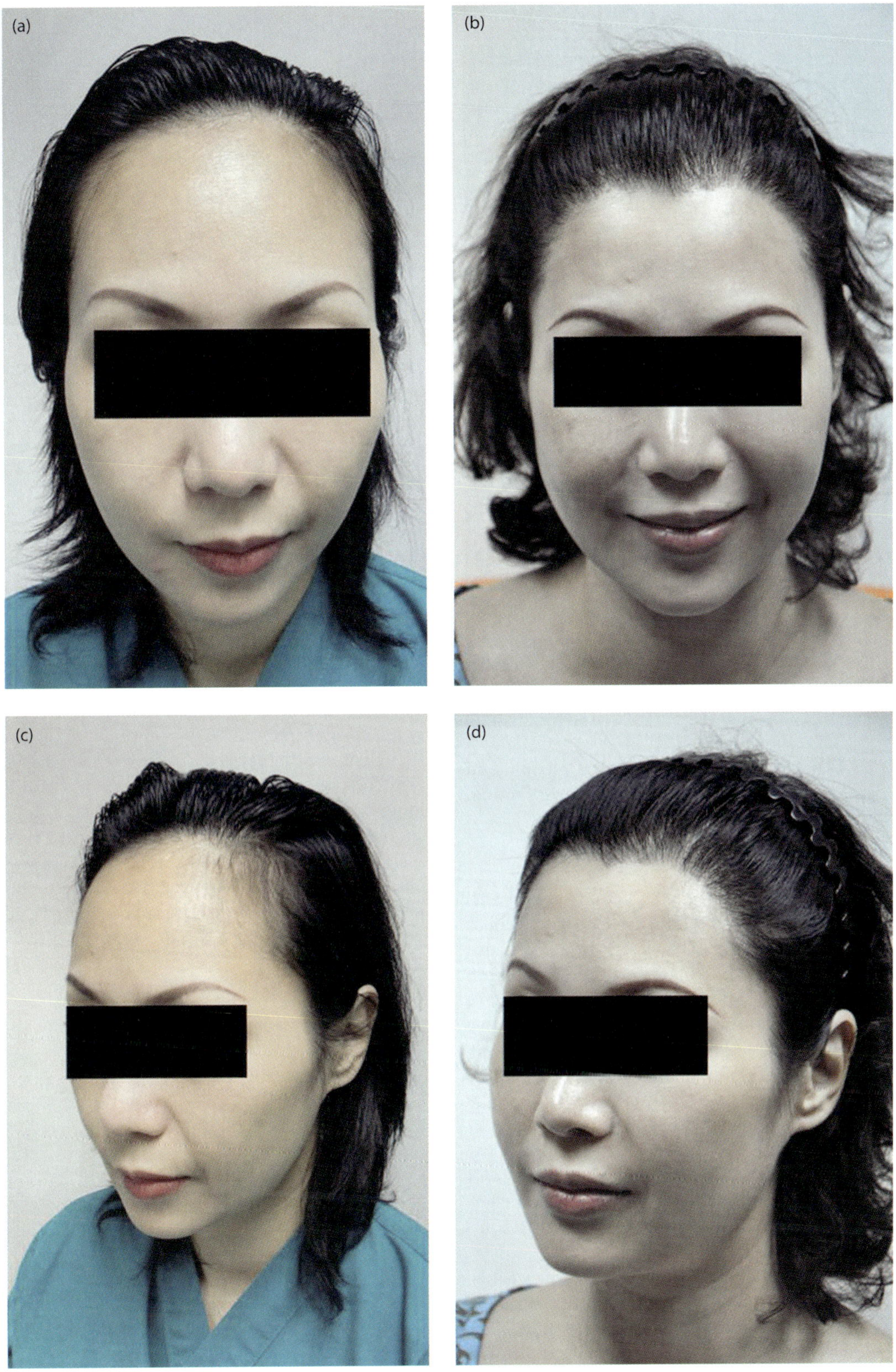

Figure 13.13 (a,c) Before and (b,d) 1 year after 2419 grafts in Norwood type of pattern baldness.

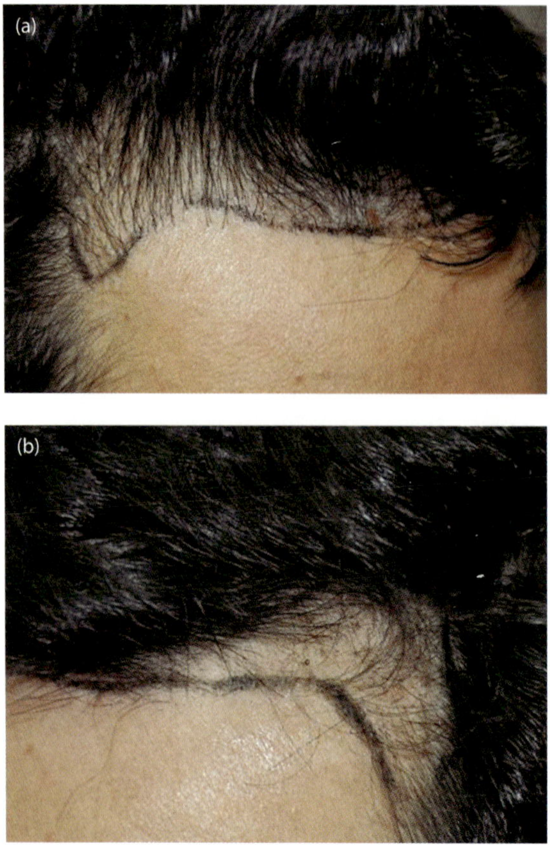

Figure 13.14 **(a) Poor hair transplant direction and angle; grafts were transplanted in posterior direction. (b) Poor growth.**

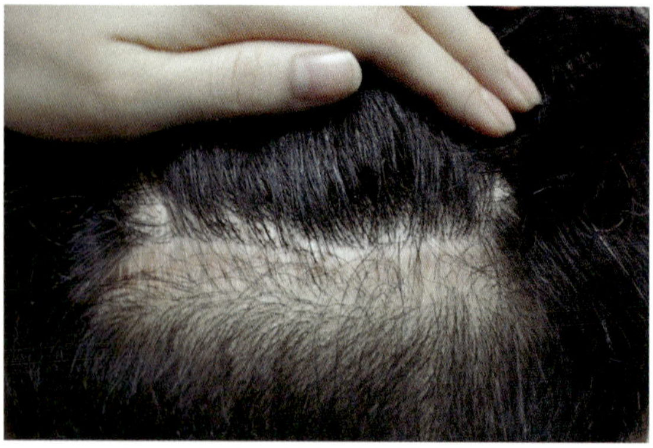

Figure 13.15 **Wide and hypertrophic scar from strip surgery after multiple sessions.**

of injections of intralesional corticosteroids (e.g., triamcinolone acetonide 10–40 mg/mL) are helpful to reduce the size or related symptoms. On average, three injections spaced at 4 and 8 weeks will markedly improve the scar. Scar revision is usually unsuccessful (Figure 13.15). I have done a few W-plasty procedures with only one acceptable result, the others having no change. The FUE planting into the scar may be helpful. Micropigmentation into the scar may be considered.

Effluvium or postoperative shock loss of existing hair might not grow back at the recipient site, especially the miniaturized hair. The effluvium at the donor area will grow back after 4 months. There is no treatment for effluvium other than to be patient. Ingrown hair is uncommonly seen and needs to be removed.

Because there is a constant influx of newcomers entering the field of hair restoration, pitting is still commonly seen in hair practice today, sometimes in conjunction with poor hair direction and angle that can be difficult to correct. The best solution may be to selectively surgically punch out the most visible grafts.

Folliculitis

Folliculitis is the most common complication occurring in practice, usually occurring about 3 weeks to 4 months postsurgery. It usually disappears spontaneously, but occasionally, a chronic recurrent form of folliculitis can develop. This may be due to a foreign body reaction of recipient dermis against the epidermal component of the transplanted hair or a small fragment of hair, as well as obstruction of a sebaceous gland, because no hair grafts have yet exited the scalp. Fortunately, this eventually clears with time and rarely reduces eventual growth, although it can be delayed. Treatment consists of wet warm compresses for 15 minutes every 4–6 hours and wiping the area with alcohol 70%. Advise use of antiseptic shampoo (Hibiscrub) twice a day, oral and topical antibiotics, and drainage of pustules if necessary (Figure 13.16). Culture of the pustule for both aerobe and anaerobe plus Gram stain is helpful so the surgeon can give the appropriate antibiotic.

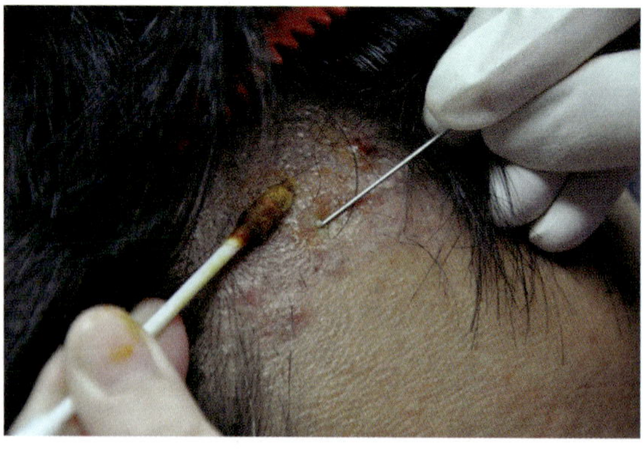

Figure 13.16 **Post-op folliculitis drains with 21G despite no pustule visible on the skin.**

As a means of prevention of folliculitis, preoperative cleansing of the scalp with shampoo reduces the colony counts in the skin, resulting in less overall risk of infection. Antiseptic shampoo pre-op is still debated because it also kills resident flora on the scalp to fight against bacterial intruders. The use of systemic antibiotics is still controversial because the scalp contains an abundant blood supply except in patients who have artificial heart valves or prostheses. However, in cosmetic surgery, most surgeons give antibiotics immediately before, during, and after surgery. Some surgeons prescribe for 5–7 days.

Poor growth is considered rare in follicular unit transplantation (FUE) by an experienced surgeon. It can be caused by follicle trauma, mishandling of the grafts during the procedure, transection, manipulation, desiccation, oxygen starvation, etc. To avoid these complications, it is important to follow each step of the protocol that may influence results.

Correction of cicatricial alopecia

Healthy scalp hair is a human characteristic that conveys aspects of self-image, identity, and perceptions of health. Hair loss from disease or other conditions may result in distorted self-perception and psychological conflicts. Cicatricial alopecia (CA) encompasses a diverse group of disorders characterized by permanent destruction of the hair follicle and irreversible hair loss. It is classified into primary (the hair follicle is the main target) and secondary (nonfollicular) disease. Dermatological disorders causing permanent hair loss such as cicatricial alopecia make immediate diagnosis and therapeutic intervention imperative. Location of biopsy is very important; it should include good hair at the border of the lesion and inside the lesion that contains the hair follicle. At least two specimens 4 mm each should be sent for horizontal and vertical sectioning and direct immunofluorescence.

Primary cicatricial alopecia is an uncommon hair loss condition seen in everyday practice. The incidence is very low. In my practice, over 20 years only six primary CA were seen, but only three were Asian. Generally speaking, at least 2 years is the safe window period to perform hair transplantation in CA; however, the longer period of waiting is better. Should biopsy be performed to make sure the disease is in remission?

I have performed hair transplantation on two patients with frontal fibrosing alopecia (FFA), one pseudopelade of Brocq, and two lichen planopilaris. The FFA patients were instructed to take dutasteride and an immunomodulator postoperatively. In my experience, 3-year follow-up is promising, with the hair grafts being maintained over this time period (Figure 13.17). However, the long-term

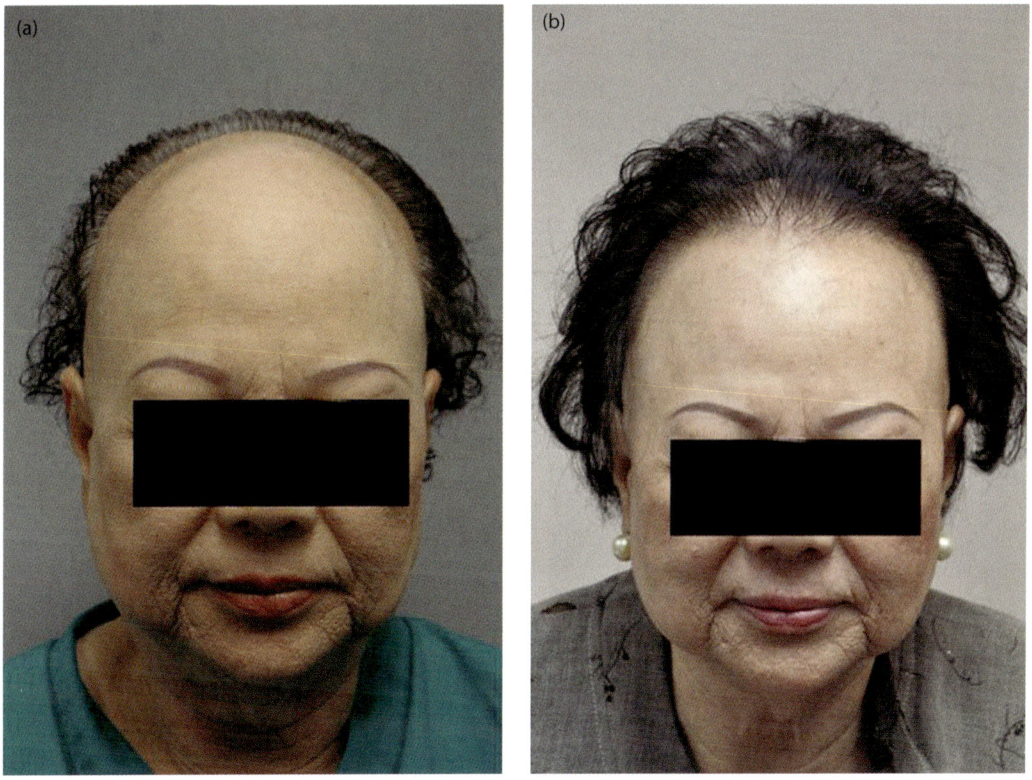

Figure 13.17 (a,c) Before and (b,d) 2 years after two sessions of 4293 grafts. *(Continued)*

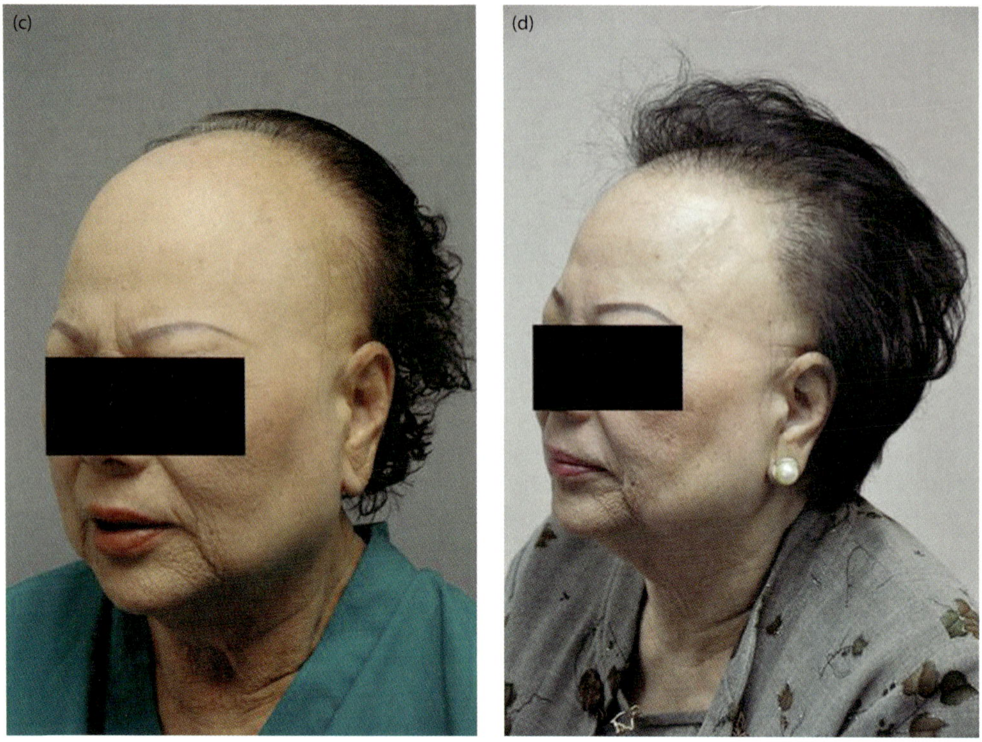

Figure 13.17 (Continued) **(a,c) Before and (b,d) 2 years after two sessions of 4293 grafts.**

results need to be verified as to whether there will be loss of grafts with medical treatment.

Jeminez and Nausbaum reported total loss of grafts in 4 years after transplant in FFA and do not recommend hair transplantation in FFA.[26,27]

Secondary cicatricial alopecia is increasingly seen—the majority from cosmetic surgery (e.g., face lift, coronal lift) (Figures 13.18 and 13.19) and some from burns and other injury to the scalp, thus resulting in hair loss.

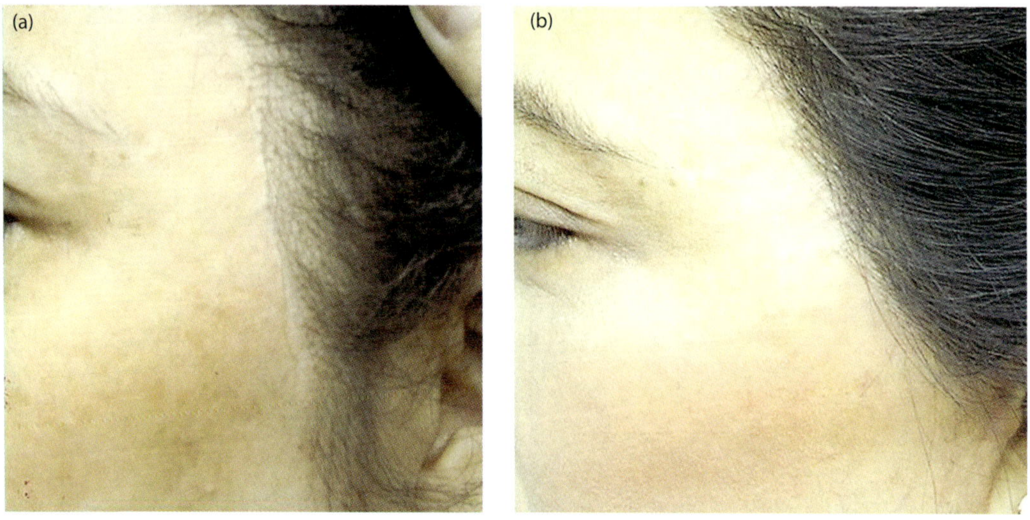

Figure 13.18 **(a) Temporal lift scar. (b) One year post-op FUT.**

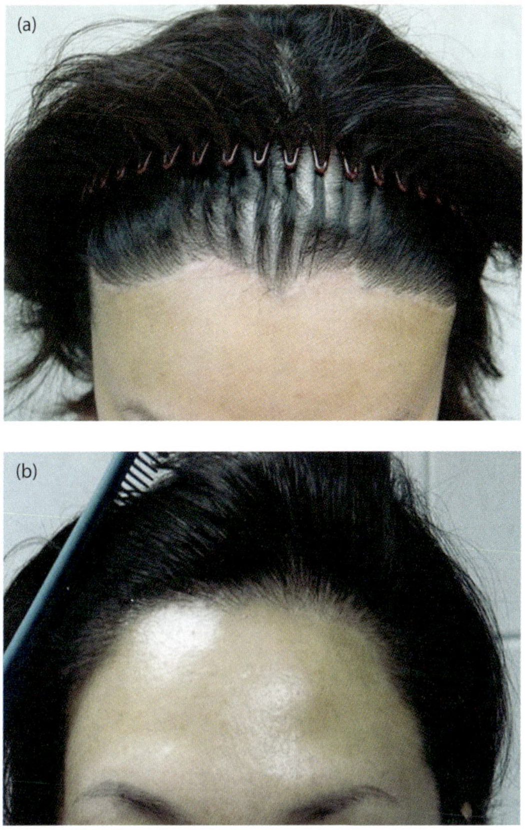

Figure 13.19 **(a) Post-op bilateral short temporoparietal flap with unsightly scar and reverse hair direction (posteriorly). (b) FUT to camouflage the scar with aesthetically pleasing new hair line and anterior direction.**

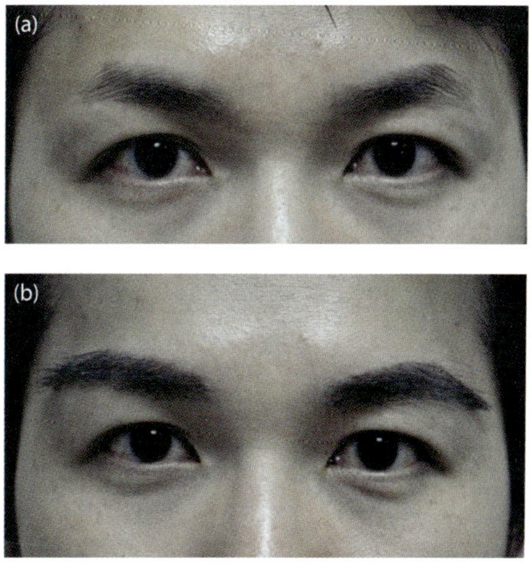

Figure 13.20 **(a,b) Eyebrow transplant 538 grafts to both sides.**

Face and body alopecia in Asians

Eyebrow transplant (Figure 13.20) is the most common surgery of all face and body alopecia, and second is from hair transplant of the scalp. The majority of East Asians do not have as much facial and body hair as do Indians and those of Middle Eastern descent. There are increasing demands of facial hair transplants, especially beard and goatee (Figures 13.21 through 13.23). However, men of Indian and Middle Eastern descent who are depleted in facial hair also want restoration to blend with their native culture. Hair transplantations for eyelashes, chest hair (Figure 13.24), pubic hair, and sideburns is still very low in demand.

The technique of surgery is different from scalp hair, and it is a more delicate and time-consuming procedure:

1. Mustache and eyebrow are coarser than scalp hair, so the surgeon needs to look for scalp donor hair of a caliber to match the beard and eyebrow.
2. A two-hairs graft might be needed to blend for density.
3. Direction and angle need to be precise, especially with eyebrow transplantation.
4. The design of the pattern needs to fit the individual's face, and the surgeon needs to communicate with the patient whether he or she is happy with the drawing.
5. The donor site can be harvest by FUE or FUT.
6. Grafts insertion can be performed using stick and place, premade incision, or implanter.

Post-op care is important to avoid lost grafts and changing hair direction, especially after eyebrow transplantation. Infection must be avoided, especially where grafts transplant surrounds the lip with potential contamination from food and saliva. Antibiotic ointment or Vaseline ointment may be applied to keep the wound moist and to seal the grafts. An oral antibiotic is also given longer than 1 week. For unknown reasons, most grafts healed without infection. Subsequent sessions might be needed to add more density.

CORRECTION OF UNSIGHTLY SCAR AND POOR AESTHETIC OUTCOME FROM PREVIOUS COSMETIC SURGERY

The FUE with large plugs in the past (Figure 13.25), post rhytidectomy, temporal lift (Figure 13.18), and bilateral temporoparietal flap (Figure 13.19) result in several cosmetic problems needing surgical correction to improve aesthetic appearance. Several sessions of FUT or FUE are often needed to provide improved density.

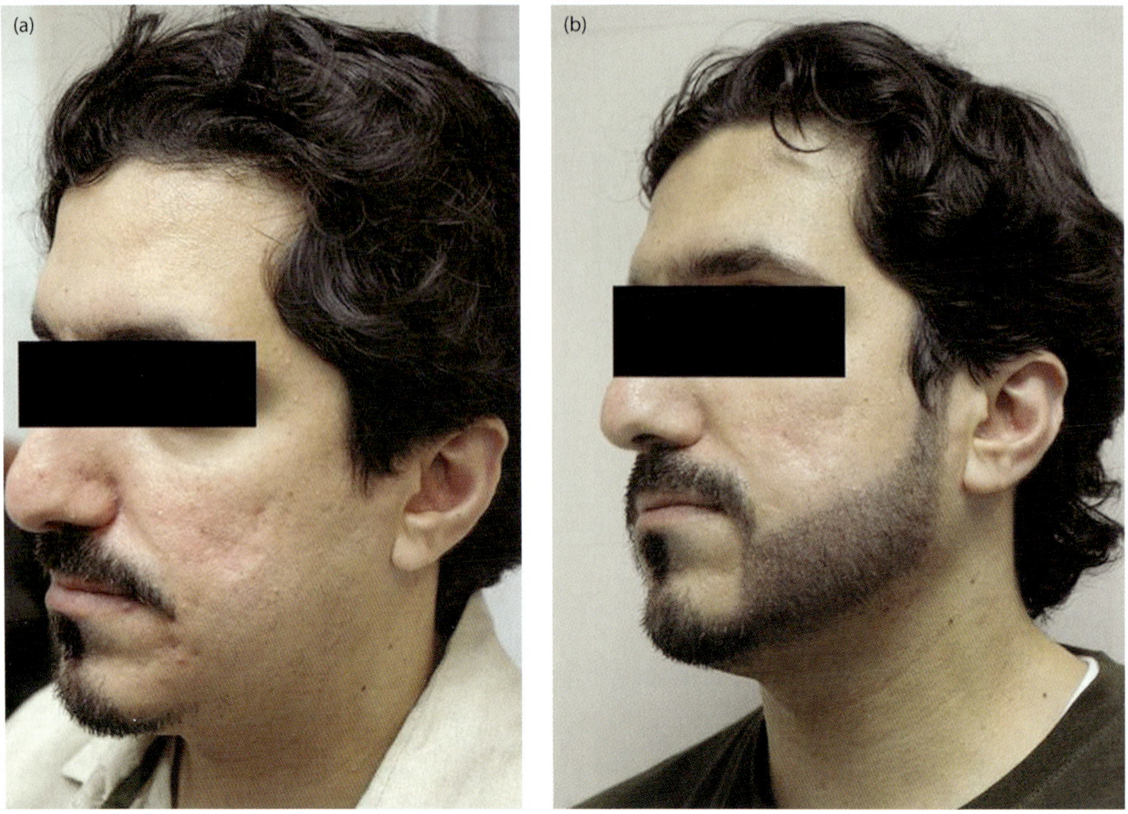

Figure 13.21 (a,b) 2700 FUG (follicular unit grafts) on both sides.

CONCLUSION

Hair transplantation in Asian male and female pattern hair loss can produce results as good as those in Caucasians in spite of the high hair and skin contrast. Finasteride and minoxidil lotion are recommended in conjunction with surgery, because the hair loss is progressive in nature. Low hair density is compensated for by larger caliber follicular grafts. A large quantity of single-hair grafts is needed for the frontal hairline to produce a pleasing aesthetic result. Special attention must be focused on the unique anatomical features of the Asian patient for optimal natural-appearing results.

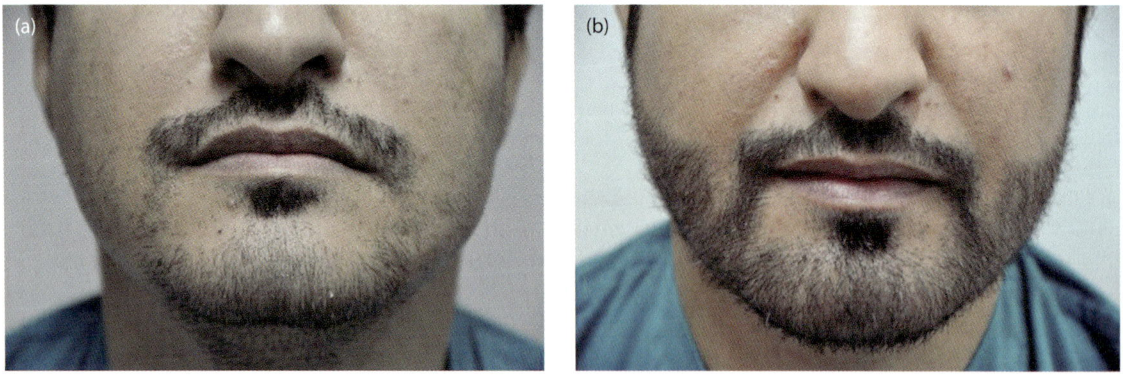

Figure 13.22 (a,c) Pre-op: hair, moustache, sideburn, and goatee. (b,d) One year post-op. *(Continued)*

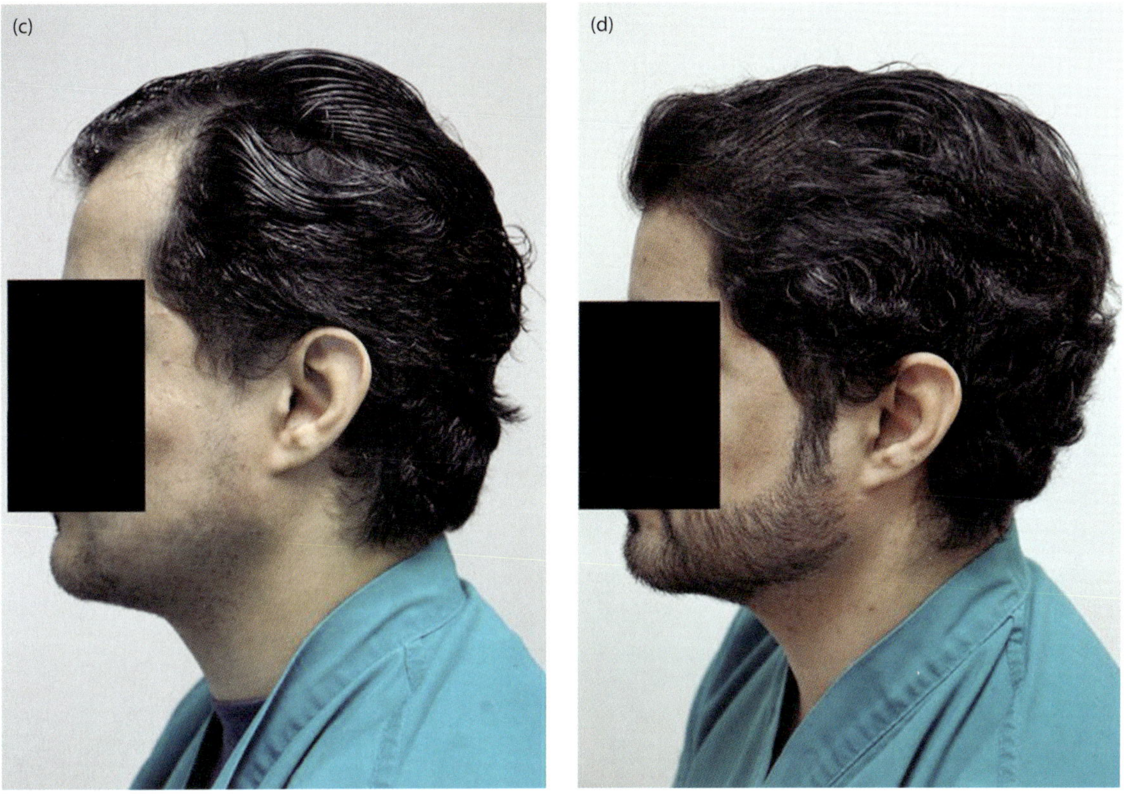

Figure 13.22 (*Continued*) (a,c) Pre-op: hair, moustache, sideburn, and goatee. (b,d) One year post-op.

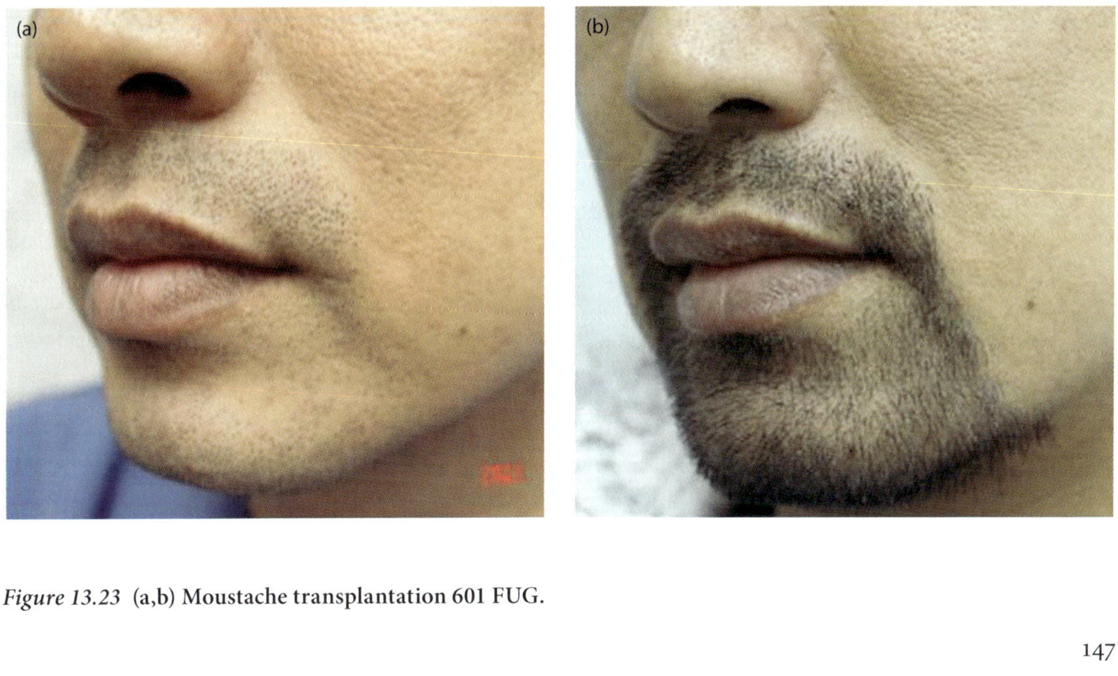

Figure 13.23 (a,b) Moustache transplantation 601 FUG.

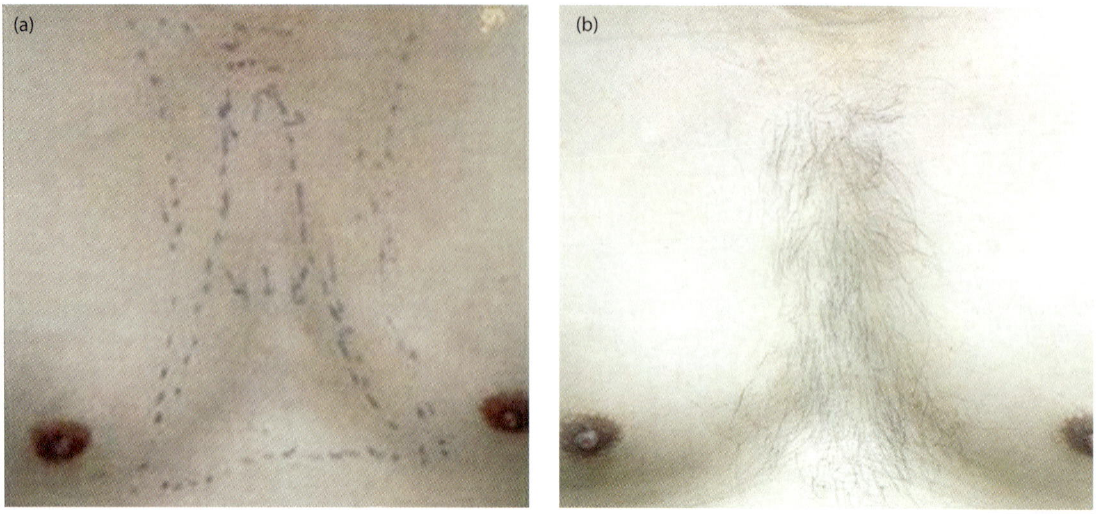

Figure 13.24 **(a) Before with different design, (b) 1 year after.**

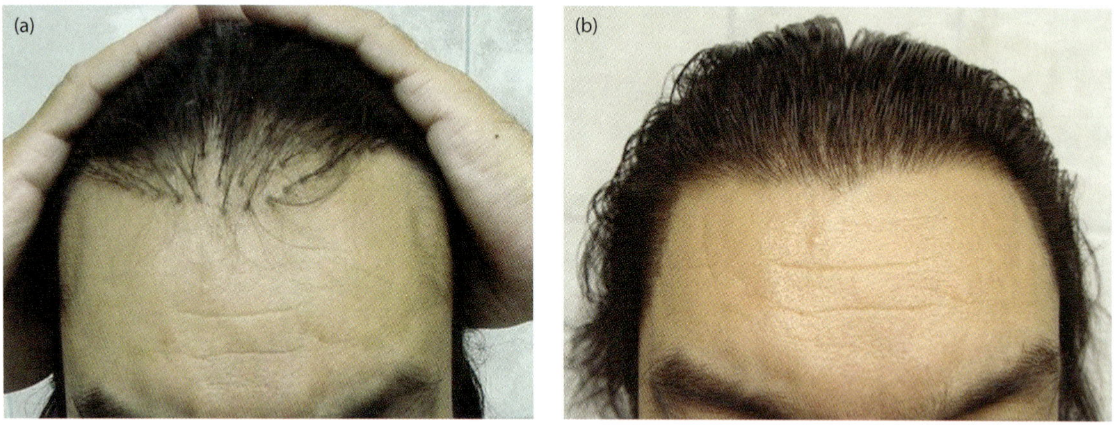

Figure 13.25 **(a) Round grafts. (b) One year after FUT.**

REFERENCES

1. Palakurthi R. The prevalence of male pattern baldness in Asian men. In: Pathomvanich D, Imagawa K, eds. *Hair Restoration Surgery in Asians.* New York, NY, Springer; 2010:11–13.
2. Pathomvanich D, Pongratanakul S, Thienthaworn P. A randomstudy of asian male androgenetic alopecia in Bangkok, Thailand. *Dermatol Surg.* 2002;28:804–807.
3. Leonard RT, Charles GM, Dorin RJ et al. *International Society of Hair Restoration Surgery: 2013 Practice Census Results*, 2013, p. 4.
4. Ko J, Huang Y, Kuo T. Hair counts from normal scalp biopsy in Taiwan. *Dermatol Surg.* 2012;38(9): 1516–1520.
5. Imagawa K. Knowing the difference in restoring the Asian look. In: Pathomvanich D, Imagawa K, eds. *Hair Restoration Surgery in Asians.* New York, NY, Springer; 2010:15–20.
6. Kim JC. Asian hair: A Korean study. In: Pathomvanich D, Imagawa K, eds. *Hair Restoration Surgery in Asians.* New York, NY, Springer; 2010:21–22.
7. Levy LL, Emer JJ. Female pattern alopecia: Current perspectives. *Int J Womens Health.* 2013;29(5): 541–556.
8. Nusbaum AG, Rose PT, Nusbaum BP. Nonsurgical therapy for hair loss. *Facial Plast Surg Clin North Am.* 2013;21(3):335–342.
9. Stough D. Dutasteride improves male pattern hair loss in a randomized study in identical twins. *J Cosmet Dermatol.* 2007;6(1):9–13.
10. Wikramanayake TC, Villasante AC, Mauro LM, et al. Low-level laser treatment accelerated hair regrowth

in a rat model of chemotherapy-induced alopecia (CIA). *Laser Med Sci*. 2013;28(3):701–706.
11. Ng B. Laser-assisted rapid hairline placement. In: Pathomvanich D, Imagawa K, eds. *Hair Restoration Surgery in Asians*. New York, NY, Springer; 2010: 41–46.
12. Calori S, Pathomvanich D, Amonpattana K, Cacas TM. Optimising the efficacy of recipient area estimation: A comparative study. *Hair Transpl Forum Int*. 2010;20(6):183–185.
13. Caroli S, Pathomvanich D, Amonpattana K, Kumar A. Current status of hair restoration surgery. *Int Surg*. 2011;96:345–351.
14. Kim JC, Choi YC. Regrowth of grafted human scalp hair after removal of the bulb. *Dermatol Surg*. 1995;21(4):312–313.
15. Jimenez F, Izeta A, Poblet E. Morphometric analysis of the human scalp hair follicle: Practical implications for the hair transplant surgeon and hair regeneration studies. *Dermatol Surg*. 2011;37(1):58–64.
16. Pathomvanich D. A refined open donor harvesting to minimize follicular transection. In: Pathomvanich D, Imagawa K, eds. *Hair Restoration Surgery in Asians*. New York, NY, Springer; 2010:109–115.
17. Mayer M, Paul T. Scalp elasticity scale. *Hair Transpl Forum Int*. 2005;15(4):122.
18. Harris J. The SAFE system: New instrumentation and methodology to improve follicular unit extraction (FUE). *Hair Transpl Forum Int*. 2004;14(4):163–164.
19. Cole JP. An analysis of follicular punches, mechanics, and dynamics in follicular unit extraction. *Facial Plast Surg Clin North Am*. 2013;21(3):437–447.
20. Ng B. Follicular unit extraction in the Asian population. In: Pathomvanich D, Imagawa K, eds. *Hair Restoration Surgery in Asians*. New York, NY, Springer; 2010:133–140.
21. Abbasi G. Hair transplant without post operative edema (Abbasi's solution). *Hair Transpl Forum Int*. 2005;15(5):149–158.
22. Li ZJ, Choi HI, Choi DK, et al. Autologous platelet-rich plasma: A potential therapeutic tool for promoting hair growth. *Dermatol Surg*. 2012;38:1040–1046.
23. Uebel CO, Silva JBd, Cantarelli D, Martin P. The role of platelet plasma growth factors in male pattern baldness surgery. *Plast Reconstr Surg*. 2006;118(6):1458–1466.
24. Pathomvanich D, Bunagan KS. Hair transplantation in Asian women. In: Unger WP, Shapiro R, Unger R, Unger M, eds. *Hair Transplantation*. 5th edn. Informa Healthcare; 2011:435–437.
25. Ludwig E. Classification of the types of androgenetic alopecia (common baldness) occurring in the female sex. *Br J Dermatol*. 1977;97:247–254.
26. Nusbaum BP, Nusbaum AG. Frontal fibrosing alopecia in a man: Results of follicular unit test grafting. *Dermatol Surg*. 2010;36:959.
27. Jiménez F, Poblet E. Is hair transplantation indicated in frontal fibrosing alopecia? The results of test grafting in three patients. *Dermatol Surg*. 2013;39:1115.

14 Hair transplantation in the reconstruction of the face and scalp

Alfonso Barrera

INTRODUCTION

We have been able to provide significant improvements in the reconstruction of the face and scalp utilizing current plastic surgical techniques, such as simple skin grafts, local and regional flaps, free tissue transfers, tissue expansion, lasers, autologous fat grafting, even face transplantation.

Follicular unit hair transplantation, however, adds a new dimension, camouflaging scarring and enhancing aesthetics in the reconstruction of the face and scalp.

In my practice, I often see patients who are seeking correction of iatrogenic alopecias (lost sideburns and temporal hairline after facelift procedures), burn alopecia, and other scarring alopecias due to tumor resections, trauma, congenital deformities, etc.[1]

Current techniques of follicular unit hair transplantation can easily be applied to the scalp area; naturally, the graft take in scarred areas is less than in nonscarred areas, due to various factors, including fibrosis and ischemia. In selected cases, autologous fat injections a few months in advance of the hair transplantation may help in preparing the recipient site, making it a better ground for the grafts.

The purpose of this chapter is to share with you my experience on these cases.

In almost all these cases, I operate under IV sedation (Midazolam and Fentanyl) and local anesthesia; only in small children do I operate under general anesthesia.

Clearly in areas of scarring alopecia, either scalp or facial, often there is fibrosis and less vascularity, and tissues are thin and often tight. It is best not to try to pack too densely the grafts, I would not exceed 30–35/cm^2; beyond that may interfere with graft take. In selected cases I will prepare the recipient site by autologous fat grafting prior to the hair grafting, and this can help in improving the quality of the recipient site and may increase the yield of hair growth.

To date we are unable to make new hair, so to be candidates for this procedure patients need to have a reasonably good amount of donor hair. We are only doing a redistribution of the patient's own hair. The supply and demand ratio most be favorable for the patient to be a good candidate. In cases where the donor supply is limited, we have to selectively favor certain areas to be grafted to give the patient a strategic redistribution to the most important areas.

It is very important to give the patient realistic expectations as to the limited density that we can accomplish with hair transplantation.

I always make sure the patient understands that very likely it will take two or three sessions of hair transplantation to get reasonable hair density, and these procedures are done a year apart. It is often not a one-shot deal.

The eyelashes with the strip graft technique (see below) may well get the desired result in one session; other areas will take at least two sessions.

TECHNIQUE

Technique for hair transplantation to the scalp

With the patient on the supine position, under IV sedation with midazolam (Versed, Dormicum) and Sublimaze (fentanyl) and occipital and supraorbital nerve blocks with 0.5% Bupivacaine (Marcaine) with epinephrine 1:200,000.

Once the area is locally well anesthetized, I use tumescence infiltration along the donor ellipse. This provides hemostasis and, I feel, assists in the graft dissection.

My tumescence solution consists of 120 cc of normal saline with 20 cc of 2% plain xylocaine plus 1 cc of epinephrine 1:1000 plus 40 of triamcinolone (Kenalog) the same solution is used to infiltrate both the donor and the recipient area. By adding Kenalog, I have found significantly less postoperative pain, and significantly less postoperative edema have been seen (Figure 14.1).

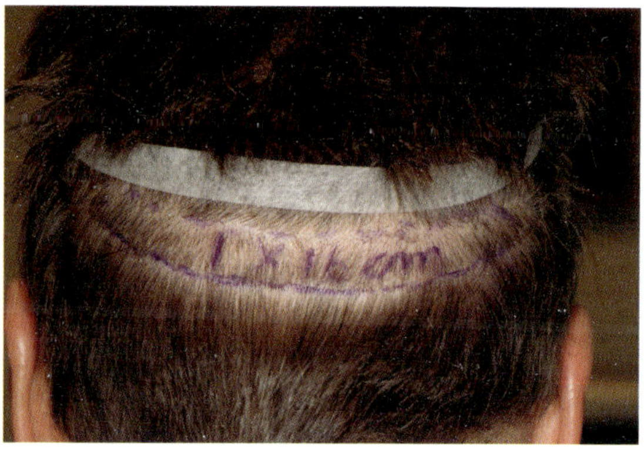

Figure 14.1 **Donor site ellipse, in this case 1 cm by 16 cm, which should yield about 1500 grafts.**

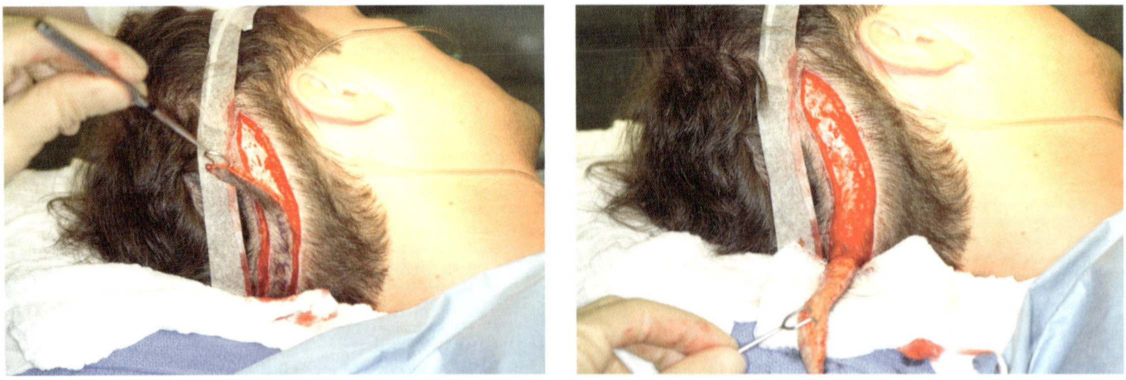

Figure 14.2 **Patient in supine position, with the head turned to the left, harvesting the right half of the donor ellipse.**

A horizontal ellipse of scalp is harvested from the occipital area, often extending to the temporal areas, frequently from above the ear on one side to above the ear on the other side.

The ellipse will vary in dimensions depending on the number of grafts planned and the density of the donor site. When planning on 2000 or more grafts, in my practice generally the ellipse will measure 25–30 cm by 1 cm in width at the midline, sometimes up to 1.5 cm gradually tapering to 1 cm over the temporal areas. It is important to make sure to have a tension-free closure as it allows for optimal donor site healing (Figures 14.2 through 14.8).

First, I have the patient's head turned to the left and I harvest the right half of the ellipse. This is then immediately dissected into 1.5 mm thick slices under the microscope at 10×. Two or three surgical technicians dissect these slices into the individual follicular unit micrografts (one to two hair grafts) and minigrafts (three to four hair grafts). This is also done usually under 3.5× loupe magnification or microscopes (10×), especially if the hair is gray or very light in color, which makes the dissection easier and safer.

As the grafts are dissected, the surgeon proceeds to close the right side of the ellipse by doing a single-layer closure with #3 "0" Prolene or Nylon, then the head is turned to the right and the left half is harvested and closed in the same fashion. Usually I find no need to undermine when harvesting these narrow and long ellipses, but undermining is done as needed.

Then, we proceed patiently to insert the grafts (Figure 14.9).

On the scalp, I use follicular unit grafting by a stick and place technique using a 22.5 Sharpoint blade or a Feather 11 blade. Often the blade is inserted at a more acute angle (20°–30° as opposed to 45°) than usual to compensate for the thinness of the tissues, allowing the graft to be sufficiently embedded into the recipient slit—that is, I make the slit and immediately my assistant inserts the graft by sliding it along the side of my blade.

To avoid the "popping out" of grafts, I insert them initially 5 mm apart from each other. Working from

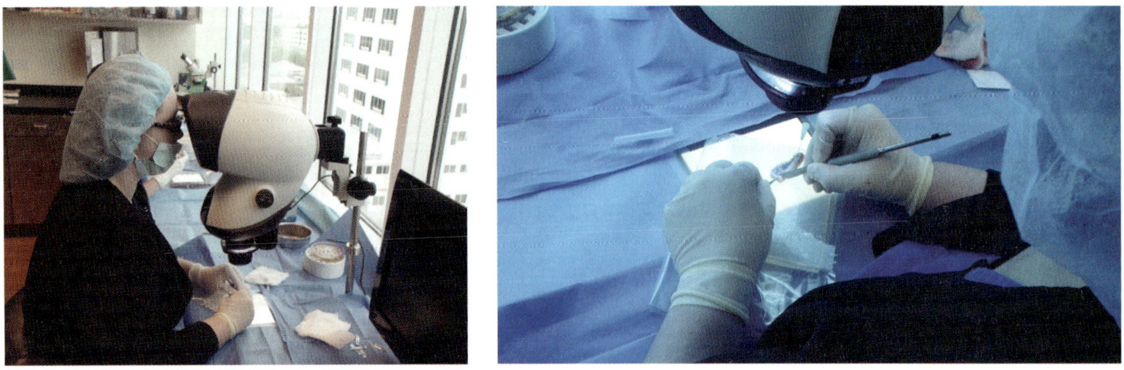

Figure 14.3 **Use of the Manthis microscope at 10× power magnification.**

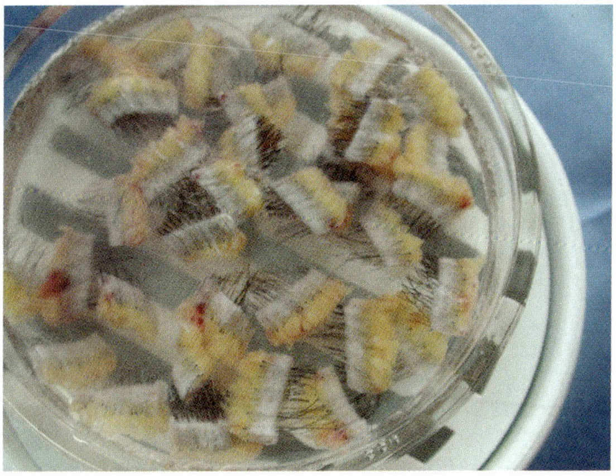

Figure 14.4 **Initial 2 mm slices on a petri dish in chilled saline solution, out of this slices the grafts are dissected.**

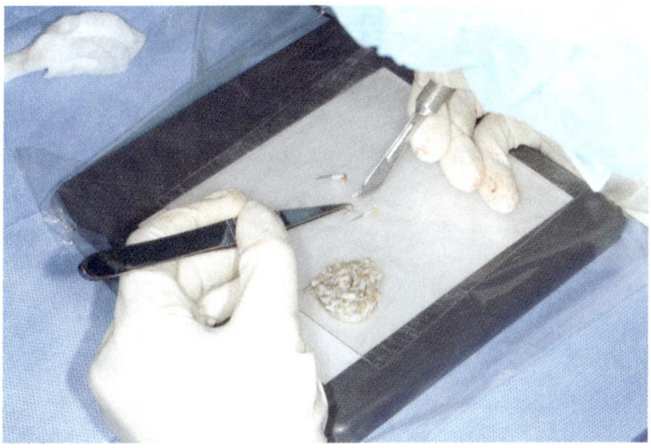

Figure 14.5 **Graft dissection. It is important to use background lighting, by translumination.**

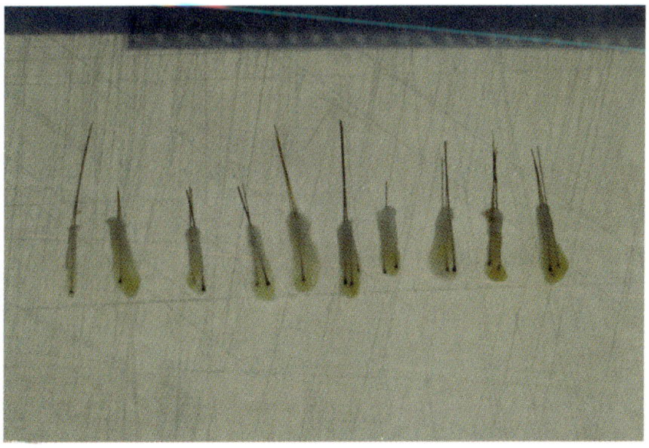

Figure 14.6 **Follicular units micrografts 1,2 hair grafts, and 3–4 hair minigrafts.**

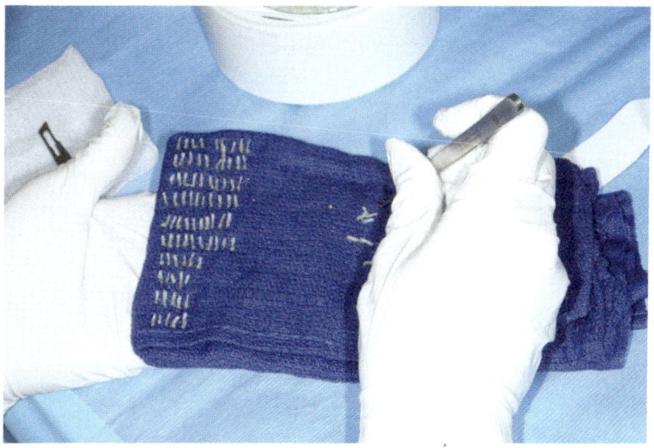

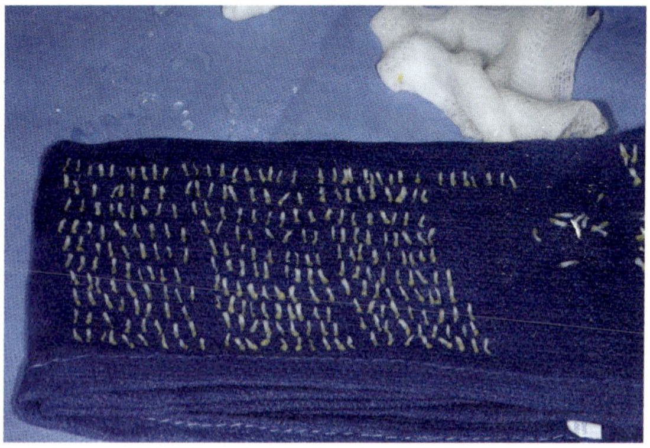

Figure 14.7 **Lining up the grafts on a wet surgical towel in groups of 10 by 10 = 100.**

anterior to posterior direction, 20–30 minutes later, I return to the anterior-most part. By then the fibrinogen has converted into fibrin, and the grafts are a bit more stable in their corresponding recipient slits. I then make slits between them, and now the grafts are about 2.5 mm from each other. The same process is repeated until all the grafts are inserted and densely packed (about 1–1.5 mm from each other).

Greater emphasis is given to the front part of the scalp than to the back, as the front is more visible and important in framing the face. The hair can always be combed back helping to cover the posterior scalp.

For dressing, I use Adaptic, Kurlex, and a 3 inch Ace bandage for the first 48 hours, and then I allow the patient to gently shampoo daily.

I remove the donor site sutures 10 days later.

A lot of the transplanted hair will go into telogen (rest phase) and will shed in the first 2–3 weeks, then at about 12–14 weeks it shifts into anagen (growth phase) and the hair begins to grow. By the third or fourth month, it becomes evident that hair begins to grow. Over the next 6–10 months, hair gains length and thickness. The final result is usually evident at 1 year postoperatively, and then if the patient desires, a second session may be done.

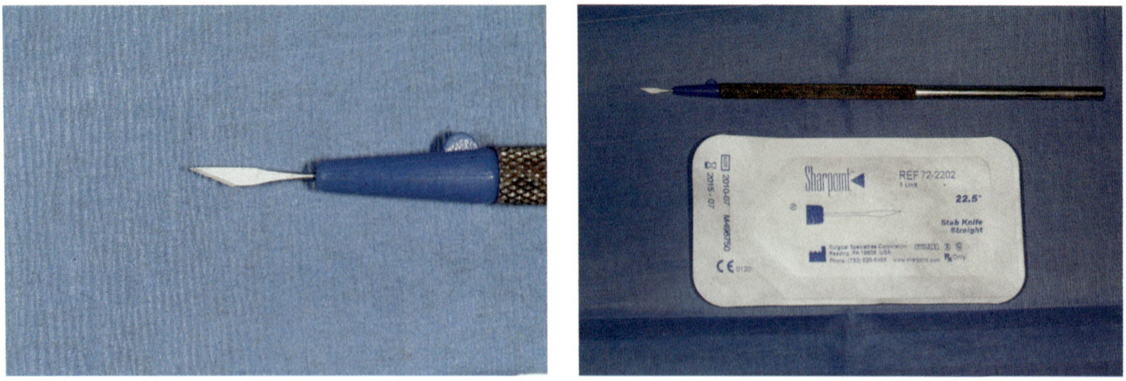

Figure 14.8 **The 22.5° Sharpoint blade, preferred for the scalp. The 15° Sharpoint blade or the 18-gauge needle preferred for the face.**

As far as mustache, beard, and eyebrows, I prefer to make the most of the recipient slits first (with 22.5° Sharpoint blade) and insert the grafts after that.

On the face there tends to be a lot more "popping out" than on the scalp, particularly with the "stick and place" technique.

On the beard and moustache, I incline the blade to get the growth in a caudal direction; again most incisions are done in a preliminary fashion, and then the grafts are inserted.

On the eyebrows, I use a 15° Sharpoint or a 22-gauge needle. Here it is crucial to incline the blade or needle as much as possible 5°–10° because they always tend to grow a lot more perpendicular to the surface than intended. We are trying to mimic nature cephalically and laterally in the medial area and laterally lateral to that.

Usually, I would do 150–200 grafts per eyebrow. As the grafts are inserted, we check that the direction of the hair shaft of each graft is the most desirable or it is turned around, making sure the curl, if any, favors the direction we need the hair to grow.

Naturally trimming will be needed, and often grooming.

On eyelash reconstruction, I prefer to use a scalp strip as opposed to individual follicular unit grafts. I harvest a strip of scalp from a retro-auricular or occipital about two rows of hair, and the length needed. I use a chalazion clamp and stabilize the lid at the same time, protecting the eye globe. Then

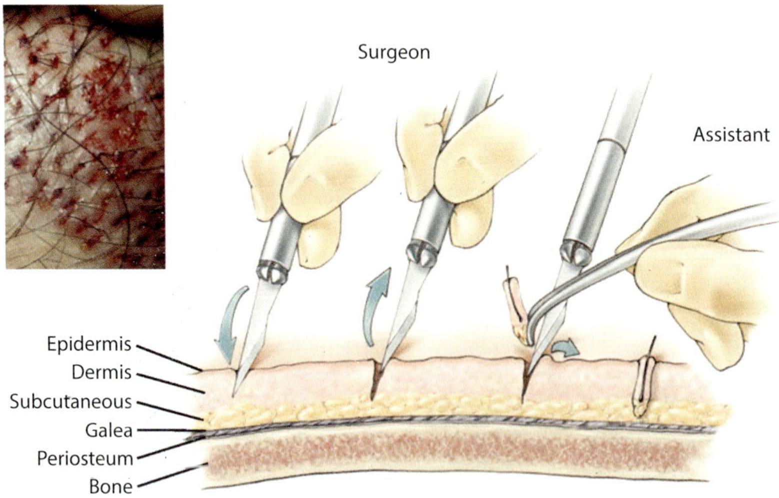

Figure 14.9 **Stick and place technique. Immediately after making the slit, the graft is inserted. (From Barrera and Uebel, *Hair Transplantation: The Art of Micrografting and Minigrafting*, 2nd edn. Boca Raton, FL: CRC Press; 2013. With permission.)**

I use a Sharpoint blade to incise at the tarsal plate free edge, opening the ciliary edge of the lid, and doing this far enough to then be able to accommodate the scalp strip. You want to see how it lays better as to the direction of the hair on the strip. Trimming will likely be needed as well as curling.

Individual single hair grafting to reconstruct the eyelashes has been nicely presented by Marcelo Gendelman of Brazil, who has great experience using a French needle and feeding the graft into the lid on the skin side and exiting at the tarsal plate.[2,3]

Most cases are done under IV sedation with Versed and Fentanyl and local anesthesia (xylocaine, Marcaine with epinephrine). Representative examples are shown in Figures 14.10 through 14.19.

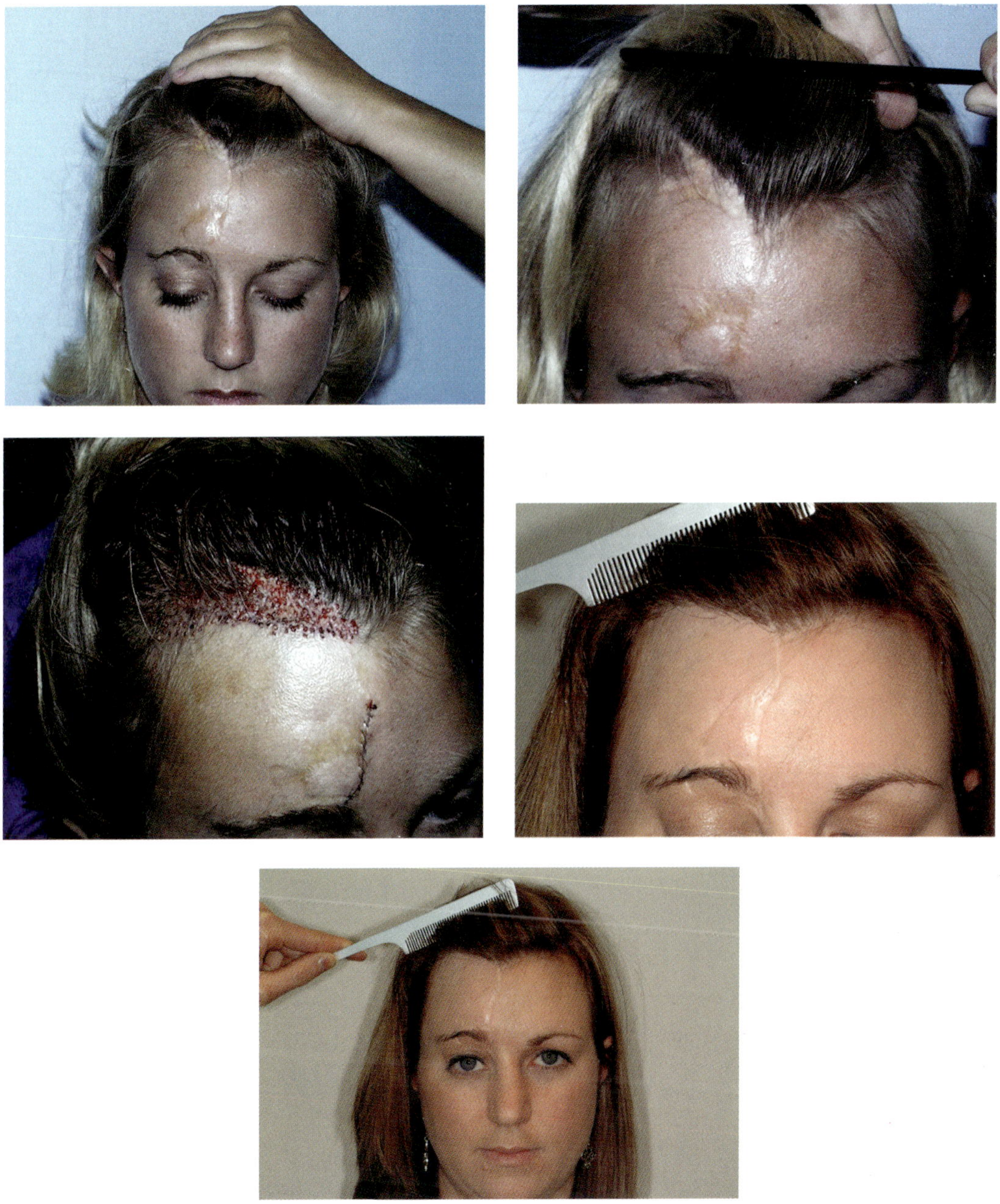

Figure 14.10 A 21-year-old female who suffered from an automobile accident resulting in scarring alopecia of the frontal scalp on the right side, shown here immediately postoperatively and a year later.

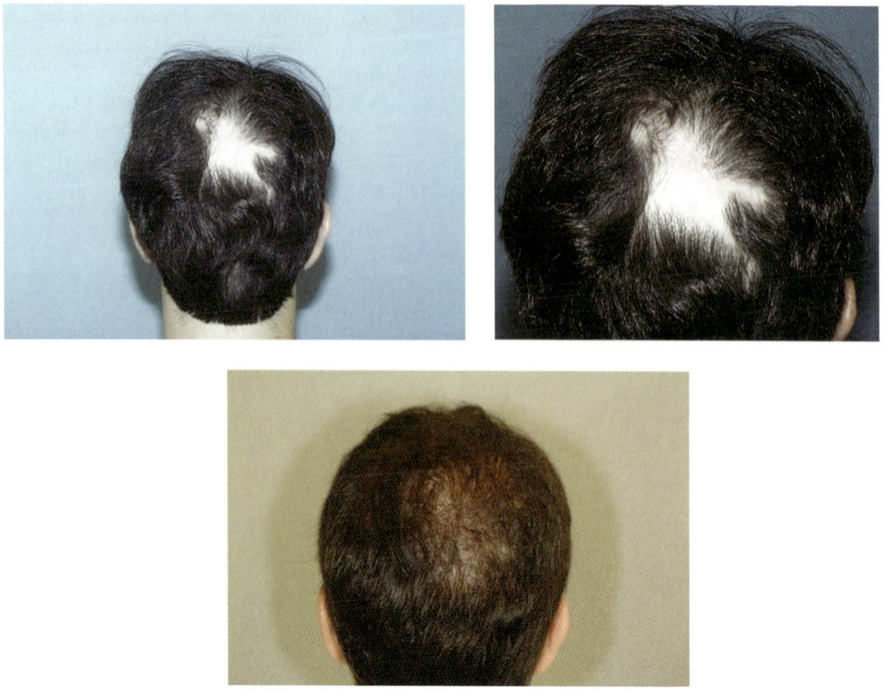

Figure 14.11 Young partially paralyzed man due to a fractured spine, here with scarring alopecia from a healed decubitus ulcer (pressure sore), shown before, and a year postoperatively.

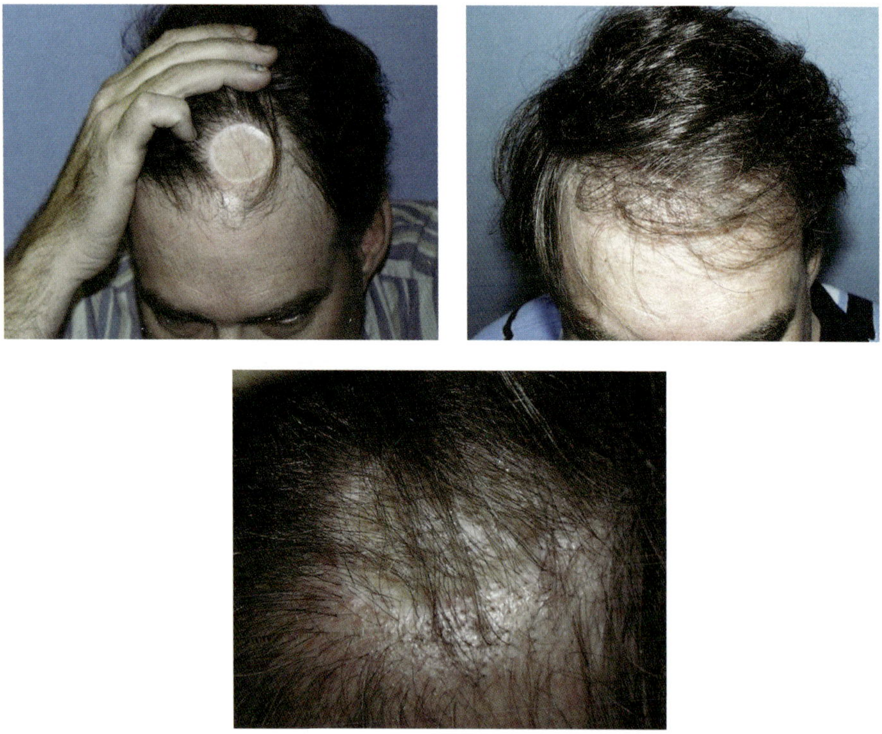

Figure 14.12 Middle-age man after resection of a melanoma from the scalp and full thickness skin graft directly on periosteum. Shown before and a year after the procedure.

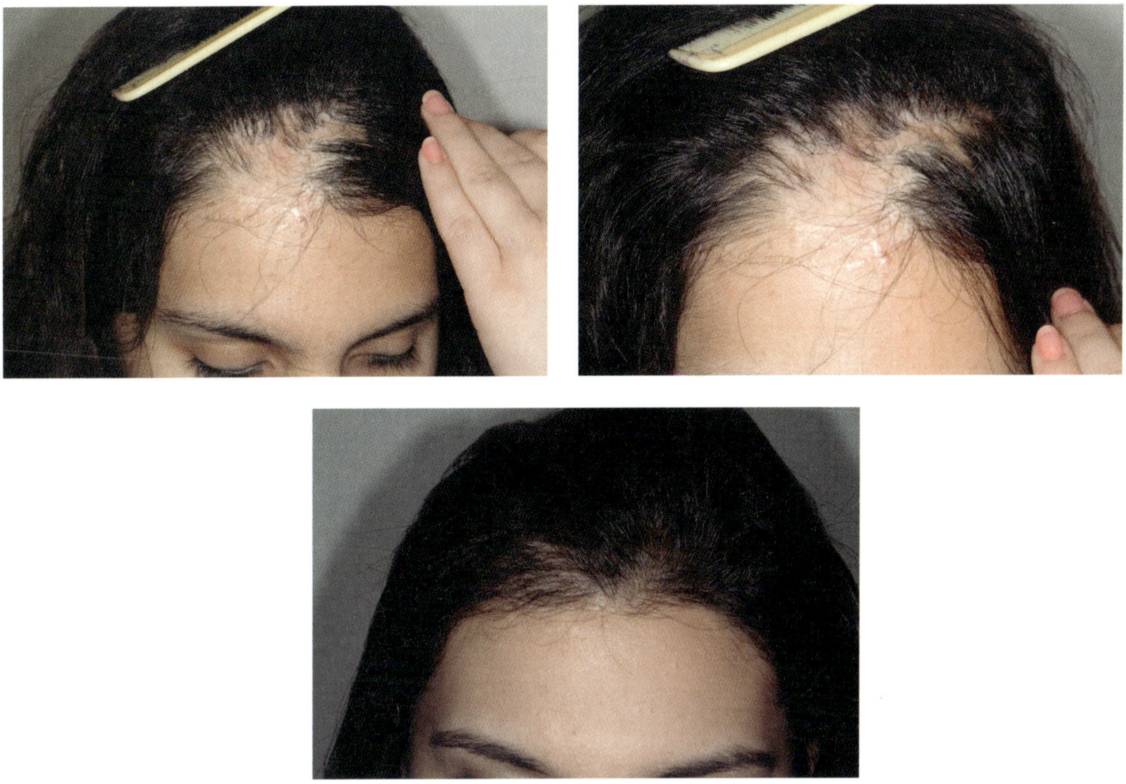

Figure 14.13 Young female with scarring alopecia of frontal scalp from an automobile accident. Shown before and a year postoperatively.

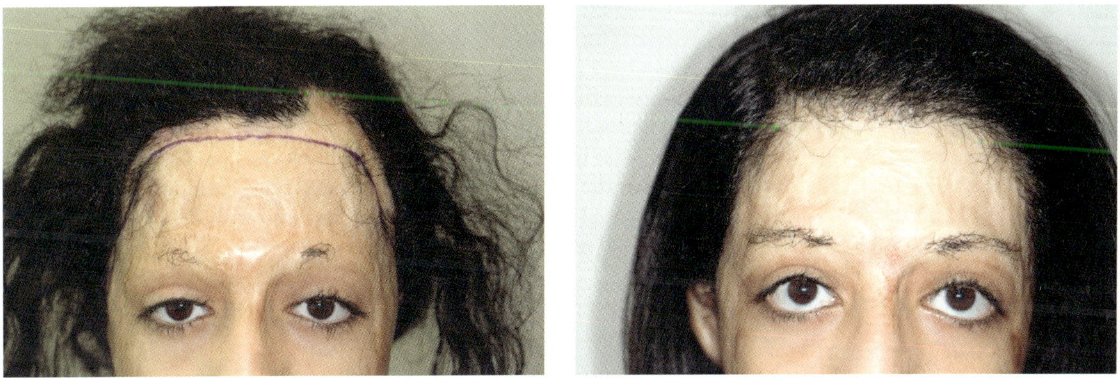

Figure 14.14 Young female with burn alopecia of the front scalp and eyebrows, shown before and a year postoperatively.

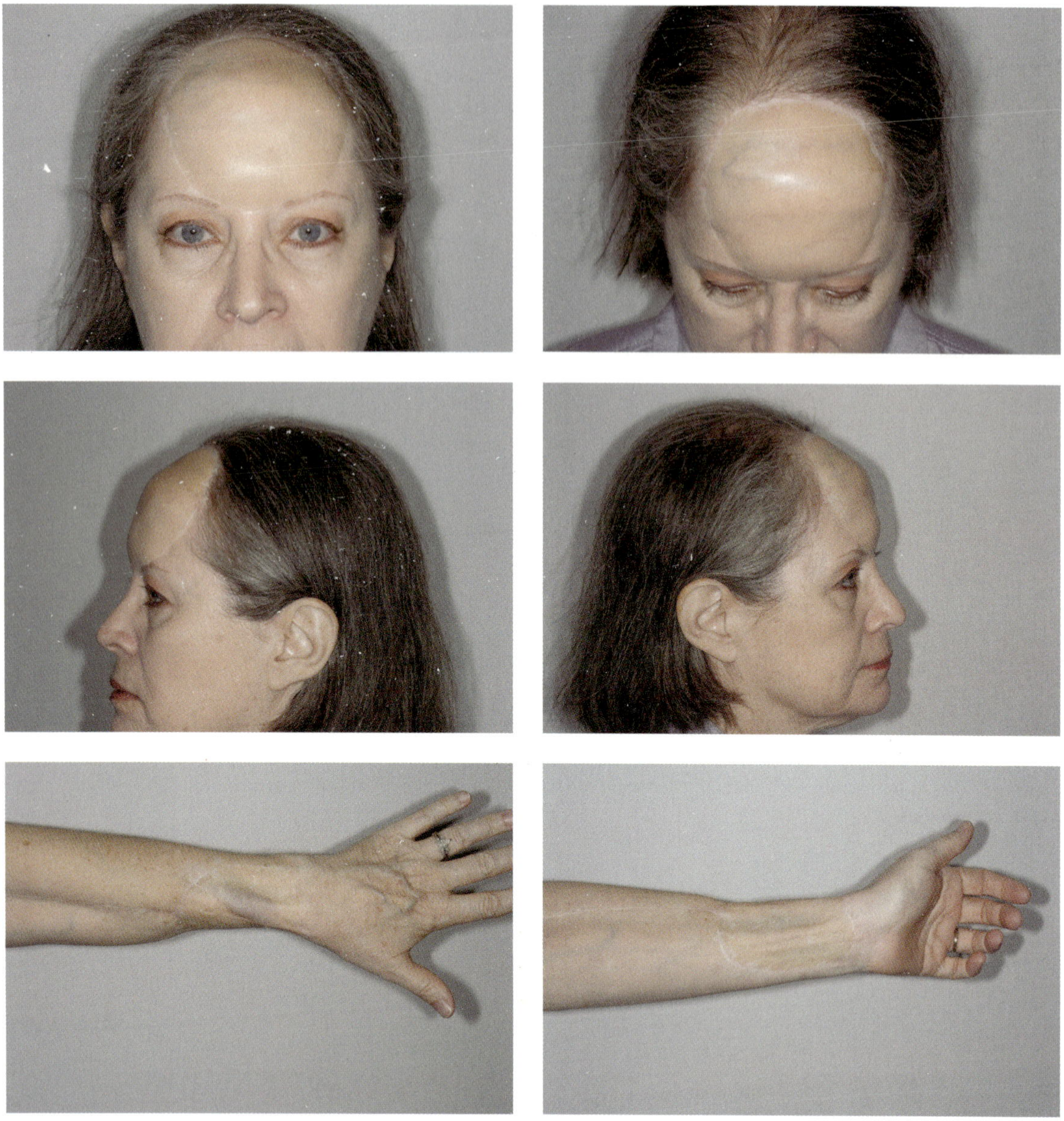

Figure 14.15 A 63-year-old female status post resection of malignant tumor of the scalp with bone involvement, underwent a craniectomy and methyl methacrylate reconstruction of the cranium and covered with a radial forearm flap reconstruction, one session of autologous fat injections was done to improve the conditions of the flap in preparation for hair transplantation, 6 months after the fat grafting she had the hair transplantation. Shown before and 6 months after the hair transplantation. Improved by simply framing her forehead with the new hairline, an additional session of grafting would enhance the final result by increasing the hair density. *(Continued)*

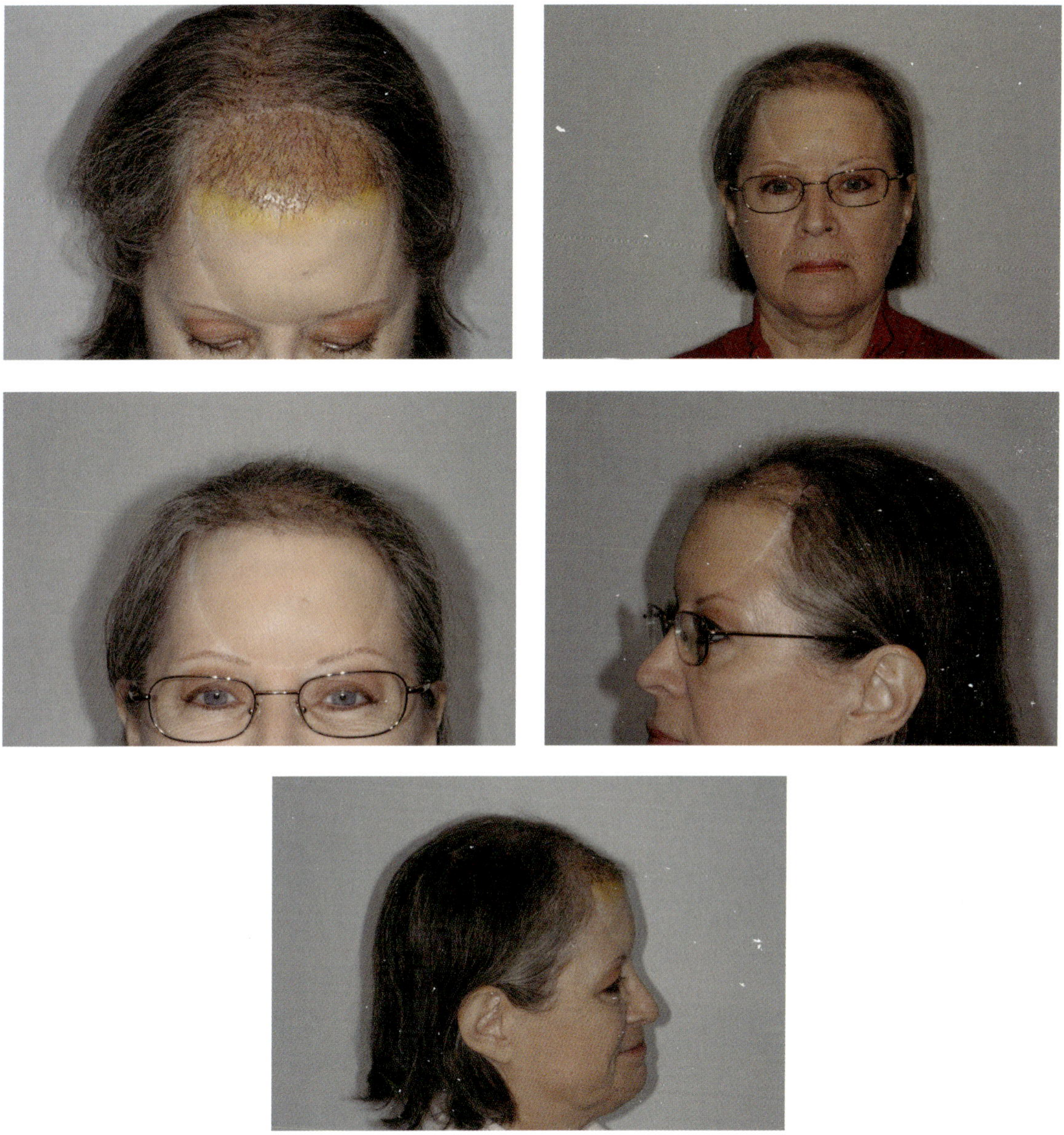

Figure 14.15 (*Continued*) A 63-year-old female status post resection of malignant tumor of the scalp with bone involvement, underwent a craniectomy and methyl methacrylate reconstruction of the cranium and covered with a radial forearm flap reconstruction. One session of autologous fat injections was done to improve the conditions of the flap in preparation for hair transplantation. Six months after the fat grafting she had the hair transplantation. Shown before and 6 months after the hair transplantation. Improved by simply framing her forehead with the new hairline, an additional session of grafting would enhance the final result by increasing the hair density.

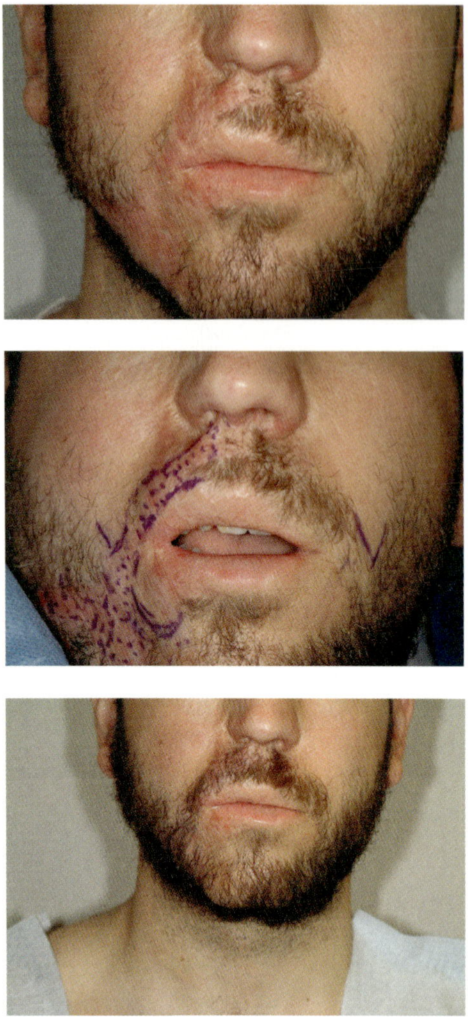

Figure 14.16 **Young man after third-degree burns around the mouth and chin on the right side due to accident in which his endotracheal tube caught on fire while having an electric procedure in a hospital. Shown before and a year after a single session of follicular unit hair grafting.**

DISCUSSION

It is much more difficult to work on some of these cases because of the severe degree of scarring and fibrosis. Obviously the graft take is less in those areas when compared to nonscarred areas.

In nonscarred areas the graft take may be up to 95%, of course, dissecting the grafts accurately and handling them atraumatically. On scarred areas this is a bit variable, generally around 60%, and we try not to densely pack the grafts as that in itself may reduce the graft take. Usually about 20–25/cm^2 per session will be transplanted.

It is very important to give realistic expectations to the patients and be certain they understand it will require several sessions for the most optimal result.

Hair grafts come with some fat cells and likely some stem cells; I have noticed that the grafted areas become healthier, softer, and thicker after hair transplantation.

CONCLUSIONS

In the patient with sufficient donor hair supply, follicular unit hair transplantation can safely and predictably enhance aesthetics in the reconstruction of the face and scalp.

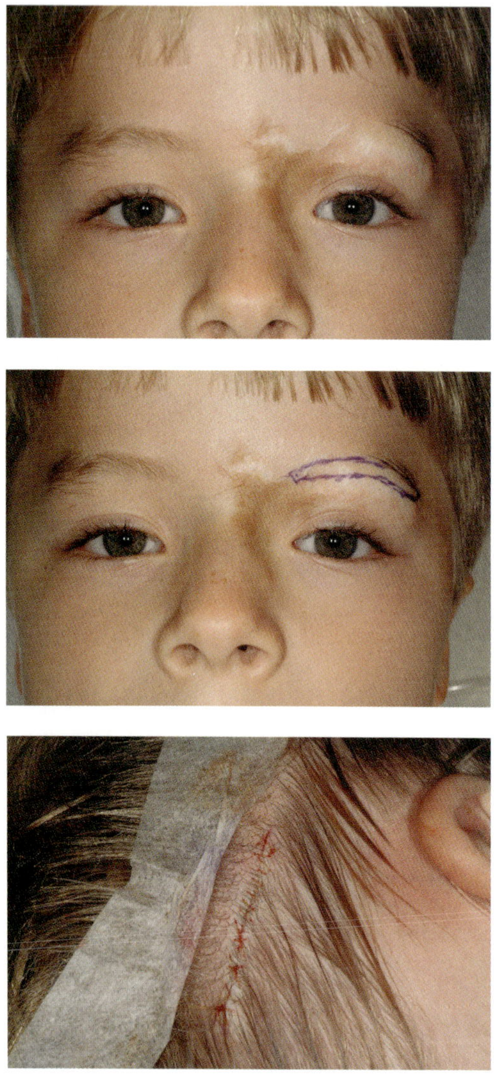

Figure 14.17 **An 11-year-old boy with scarring alopecia of the left eyebrow due to resection of a melanotic lesion. Shown before and after a single session of follicular unit grafting.** (*Continued*)

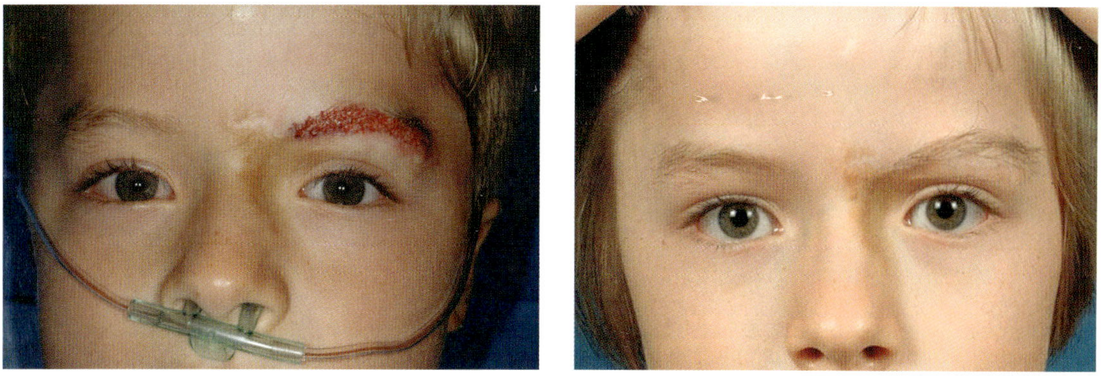

Figure 14.17 (*Continued*) An 11-year-old boy with scarring alopecia of the left eyebrow due to resection of a melanotic lesion. Shown before and after a single session of follicular unit grafting.

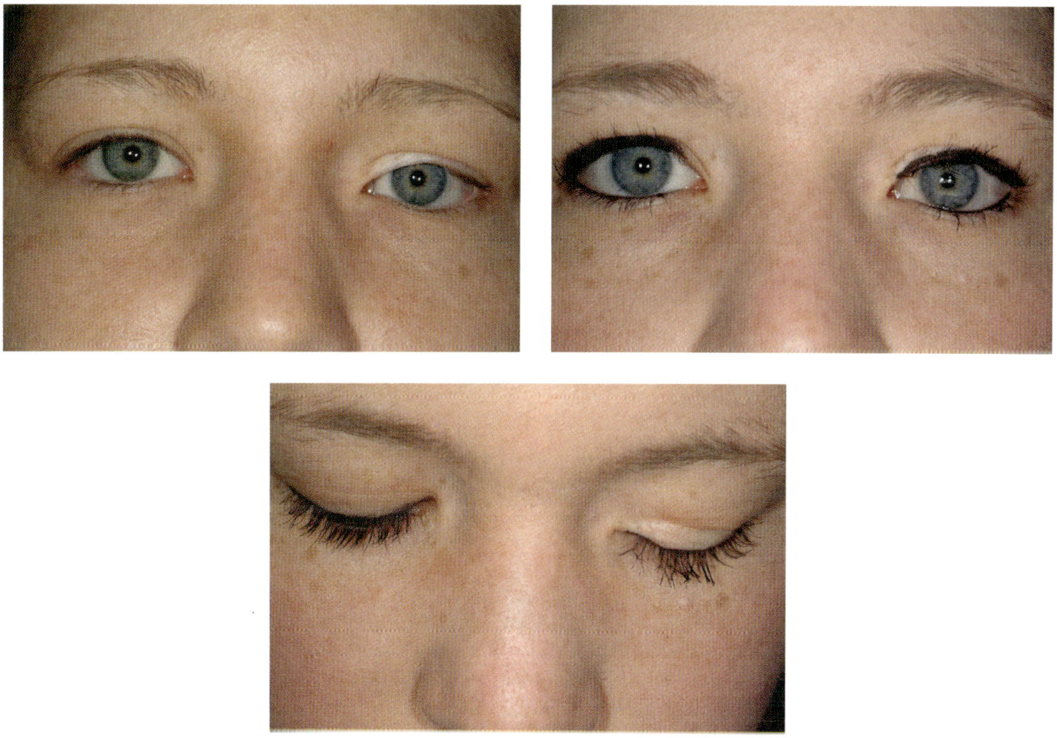

Figure 14.18 A 14-year-old girl after resection of a hemangioma of the left upper eyelid with loss of eyelashes. Shown before and a year after a composite strip scalp graft to the eyelash.

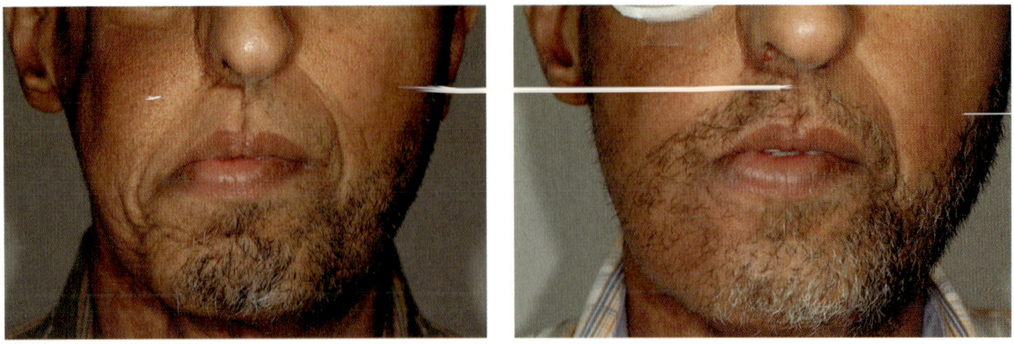

Figure 14.19 **A 43-year-old man after resection of a sarcoma of the maxilla and radiation therapy to the area and neck. Autologous fat grafting after 6 months follicular unit grafting, shown before and a year after the hair grafting.**

REFERENCES

1. Barrera A. The use of micrografts and minigrafts in the aesthetic reconstruction of the face and scalp. *Plast Reconstr Surg*. 2003;112(3):883–890.
2. Gandelman M. A technique for reconstruction of eyebrows and eyelashes. *Semin Plast Surg*. May, 2005;19(2):153–158.
3. Gandelman M. Eyelash and eyebrow reconstruction operative techniques in oculoplastic. *Oper Tech Orbit Reconstr Surg*. 2001;4(2):94–99.

15 Hair Transplantaion for aesthetic surgery of the scalp and body hair

Pierre Bouhanna and Eric Bouhanna

INTRODUCTION

In recent years, aesthetic surgery for male and female androgenetic alopecia or scarring alopecia has benefited from considerable progress. A diversity of techniques on the one hand, and a better assessment of their reliability on the other hand, allow surgeons to better focus their operations.

This surgery, which we limit here to hair transplant, obeys one overriding technical principle: the harvesting or preparation of autologous forms of micrografts or follicular units. Three techniques—mainly related to their sampling method—will be discussed here (follicular unit transplantation [FUT], follicular unit extraction [FUE], follicular units for long hair [FUL]). Automatic FUE transplanter or robotic FUE would be used for some indications.

Their indications are essentially guided by many parameters such as the area and the location of the alopecia; the sex, age, and ethnicity of the patient; characteristics of the scalp and hair; and the degree of alopecia evolution. A dynamic multifactorial classification combining all these parameters facilitates the choice of a suitable treatment for each case. A macrophotographic analysis or digitalized phototrichogram will implement this preliminary assessment.

FOLLICULAR UNIT TRANSPLANTATION

History

- In 1930, Sasagawa[1] reported the original hair transplantation method.
- In 1939, Okuda[2] mentioned for the first time the principle of autografts for the surgical correction of alopecia of the scalp, eyebrows, and mustaches.
- In 1943, Tamura[3] described pubic reconstruction in women with a one-hair transplantation.
- In 1953, Fujita[4] reported an eyebrow reconstruction puncture hair transplant among lepers.
- In 1959, N. Orentreich[5] published a method of harvesting cylindrical autografts with a cylindrical scalpel 4 mm in diameter (a "punch"). This process, which has prevailed for 25 years for the surgical treatment of male baldness, included some negative elements that led to its being neglected, such as an unsightly and unnatural appearance of tufts ("doll hair") and unsightly scars round "bees' nests" on the occipital donor area.
- In 1976 Bouhanna and Nataf[3,6,7] published a sampling technique for a graft strip procedure.
- Marritt[8] in 1980 proposed the use of micrografts for finishing earlier frontal hairline.
- Bradshaw and Limmer[9] in 1988 developed the anatomical concept of follicular units by cutting strips for micrografts (follicular unit transplantation [FUT]).
- In 1989 Bouhanna[10] published the technique of follicular units with long hair, by cutting strip under stereomicroscope without prior shaving (FUL).
- In 2002 Rassman and Bernstein[11] published the process of follicular unit extraction (FUE) with sampling with a microcylinder after prior shaving.

Principles

The main principle is to prepare micrografts or follicular units of one to four hairs:

- By follicular extraction[12] with a micropunch (by hand or motorized) of less than a millimeter (FUE).
- By follicular segmentation using a stereomicroscope of a strip of unshaved scalp (FUL)[10] or of shaved scalp (FUT).[9]

An essential point is that hairs harvested from the occipital region in men and the median occipital region in women keep their ability to grow definitively further once implanted on the bald or sparse area.

The goal

This process wishes to recreate the natural emergence of one to four hairs (the "follicular unit") through each pilosebaceous orifice (Figure 15.1):

- For the final transplant for bald areas of the scalp in a man, woman, or transgender in order to give the area an aesthetic and natural appearance.
- To blur some apparent scars (post-facelift, post-radiotherapy, after burns, stabilized pseudopelade, etc.).
- To make some hairy areas denser (eyebrows, eyelashes, beard, mustache, pubis).

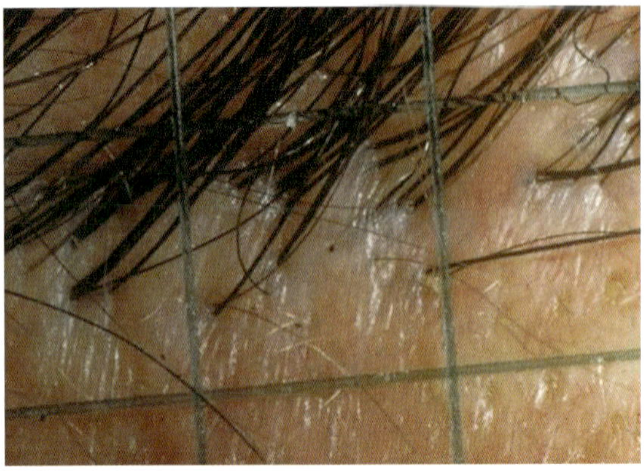

Figure 15.1 **One, two or three hairs (a "follicular unit") emerging through the same follicular orifice.**

Preoperative stage

A delay of 15 days between the consultation and intervention is required before any act of cosmetic surgery with complete information and the signed consent of the patient.

Medical photographs are always performed for the face—profile view, aerial view, and the surface to be implanted.

A digital phototrichogram is obtained of the donor area implementing the measurements of the multifactorial classification.

Preoperative blood tests and an electrocardiogram are routinely prescribed.

Drawing the anterior frontal hairline

A preliminary sketch with a dermographic marker delimits the area to be transplanted with the consent of the patient in front of a mirror (Figure 15.2).

In women, androgenetic alopecia usually allows a more or less hairy frontal line to persist.

In men, androgenetic alopecia determines a more or less complete recession from the frontal line.

The first stage of the design is one of the important aspects of reconstruction for frontal male alopecia. It takes into account several factors with a particularly harmonious equation between the aesthetic requirements, age, and ethnic peculiarities of the patient on the one hand and the hair capacity of the donor area, the characteristics of the hair, and aesthetic values on the other hand. ("Il disegno e una cosa mentale," "design is a process of the mind"—Leonardo da Vinci.) A previous photograph of the patient from a few years earlier may be helpful. The frontotemporal recession will need to be more or less deep and the frontal line more or less rounded and more or less symmetric, with some irregularities.

Local anesthesia

The preparation, disinfection, and anesthesia of the donor and recipient areas are similar to those used for the dermatologic surgery. Disinfectants based on flammable alcohol should be avoided on the scalp.[13,14]

Anesthesia of the scalp is obtained by

- A local anesthetic all around the bald or hairy surface to be treated by intradermal infiltration of 1% lidocaine with epinephrine. The addition of bicarbonates makes these injections painless.
- A nerve block infiltration of the frontal and occipital nerves. The prior application of EMLA® (lidocaïn-prilocaïn cream) cream could make these injections virtually painless.
- A premedication with Valium decreases the anxiety.

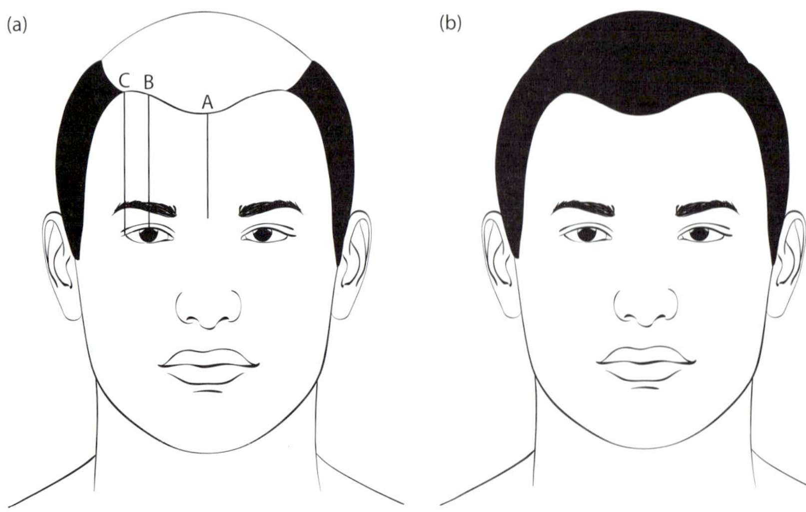

Figure 15.2 **(a,b) Schematic designs of the frontal hairline.**

- Sometimes the inhalation of a nitrous oxide gas (Kalinox–nitrous oxide) and a hypnosophrology session provide significant sedation in anxious patients.

Technique

Follicular unit transplantation (FUT)[18,20]

After a preshaving of the donor area, the conventional technical progress of removal of a strip and its segmentation into follicular units is then strictly similar to that of FUL described below.

Follicular units for long hair (FUL)

The hairs are not shaved and are therefore harvested with their stem length (Figure 15.3).[10,13,14,16]

The FUL technique we have described and refined since 1989[10] allows the removal and transplantation of grafts of varied shapes and sizes with long hair.

Without shaving the donor area, the strip will be segmented and taken under a stereomicroscope onto micrografts or follicular units with long hair.

The FUL process allows the patient immediately after surgery to mask scabs of the grafted area and thereby avoid a source of postoperative aesthetic embarrassment (Figure 15.4).

These long hairs will have two possible developments:

- The normal hair loss occurs for all or some of the transplanted hair in the third week, and regrowth occurs 3 months after surgery.
- All or part of the hair is still growing, eventually stimulated by medical prescriptions such as minoxidil lotion[17] or finasteride tablets[18] or platelet-rich plasma intradermal injection (PRP).[19]

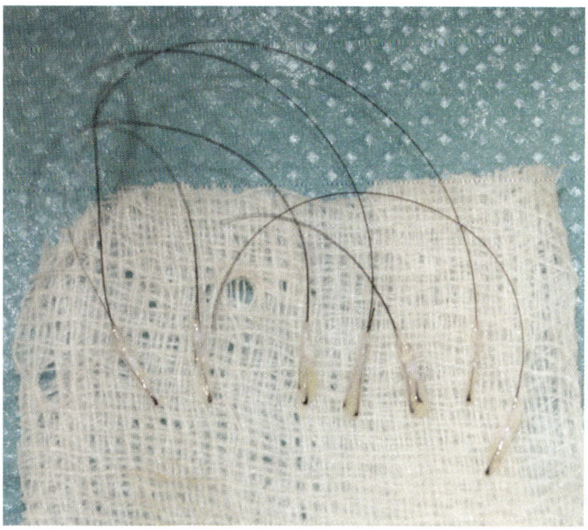

Figure 15.3 **Follicular units for long hair (FUL) after segmentation under a microscope.**

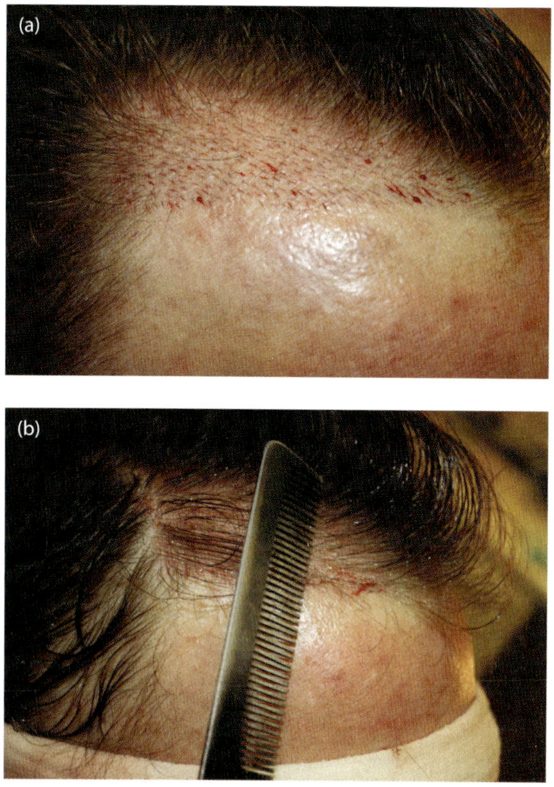

Figure 15.4 **(a) Frontal hairline with multiple microincisions. (b) Immediately after insertion of FUL, the new implanted hair is combed.**

Donor area: Preparation of follicular units. The strip removal of the unshaved occipital donor area previously infiltrated with saline is done by excision with a scalpel blade no. 11. The strip is about 10–30 cm long and 10–20 mm wide: the size depends on the desired number of follicular units[20,21] (Figure 15.5) and on the scalp laxity.

The closure of the edges of the donor area will be made with a resorbable suture with 3/0 thread or with skin staples (Figure 15.6).

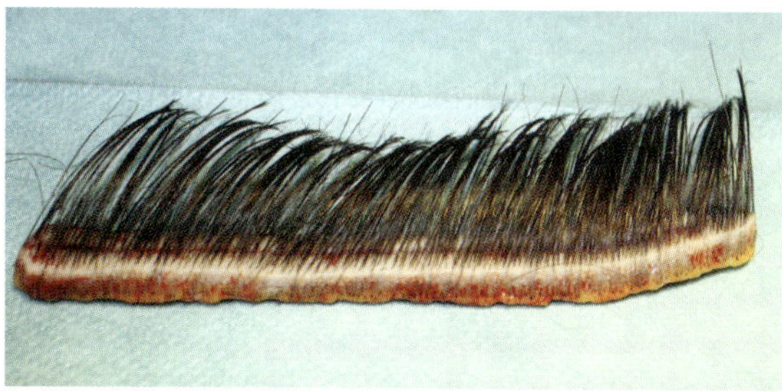

Figure 15.5 **Strip harvested with long hair.**

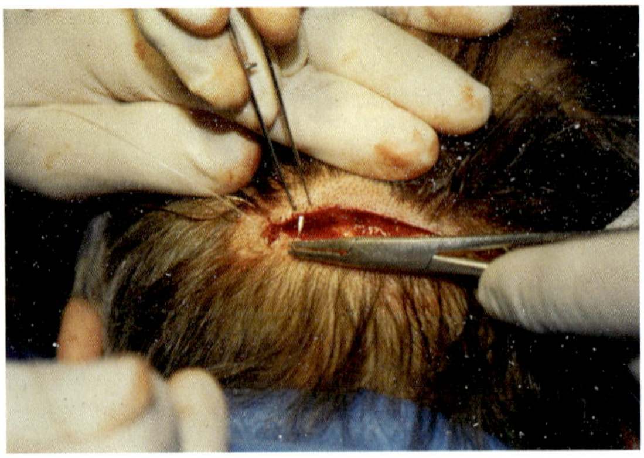

Figure 15.6 **Running absorbable suture for closure of the donor area.**

The strip graft is placed on a gauze in a Petri dish containing saline and then placed on a frozen container. The segmentation is performed by cutting the pieces on a wooden tongue depressor with a no. 11 blade or blades with large microtomes. One to four assistants cut the strip of scalp onto follicular units, under a good light and using magnifying glasses or stereomicroscopes (Figure 15.7). Cutting will be parallel to the bulb in the strip, held with fine forceps by the epidermis in variable portions according to the number, size, and shape of grafts required.

On average 500–1500 grafts (1000–4500 hairs) will be cut, and each element will be cleared of all hair shaft fragments or hypodermic debris before being placed in the receiving tray filled with chilled saline solution.

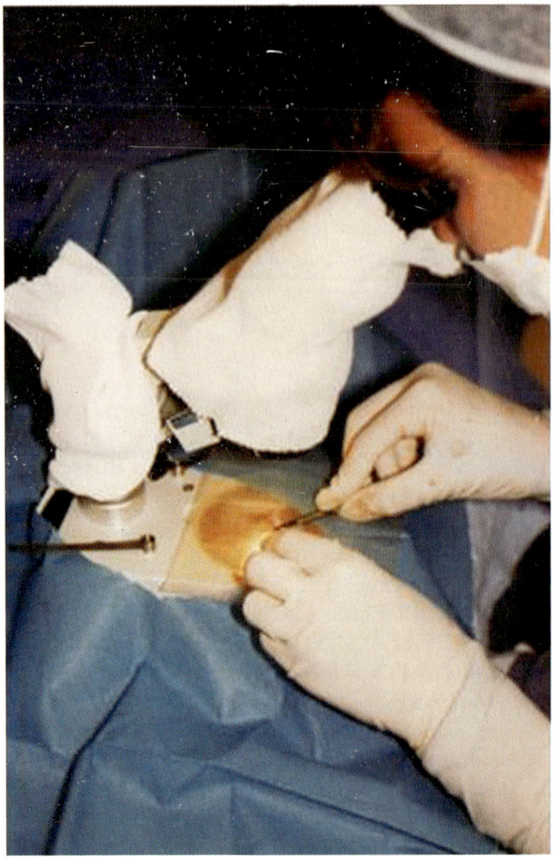

Figure 15.7 **Segmentation of FUL under a stereomicroscope.**

Preparation of the recipient area. During this cutting, the operator prepares the anesthetized recipient area with perforations and incisions.[8,16,21]

This step of perforation varies according to different physicians.

Most of them do a perforation of the skin surface with a Nokor needle of 16–18 gauge or ophthalmic microsurgical blades (spear point or chisel) (Figure 15.8).

Others use a drill with small punches of 1 mm in diameter, operated by hand or by a motor punch.

Implantation of the recipient area. Most authorities handle the skin fragments using unteeth forceps, very fine jeweler's forceps, or forceps with curved ends; others prefer straight tweezers (Figure 15.9).

Each follicular unit is delicately positioned to its full height in the clamp and threaded through the skin surface that has previously been perforated or incised.

Currently, it is possible during a session to transplant up to 1500 follicular units. When rebuilding a balding frontal region, the fragments selected to achieve the end of the line will be one hair (the puncture needle is a no. 18 gauge, intramuscular needle or microsurgical spear point) on the first row, then two or three hairs on the other rows (Nokor no. 18 gauge or chisel microblade).

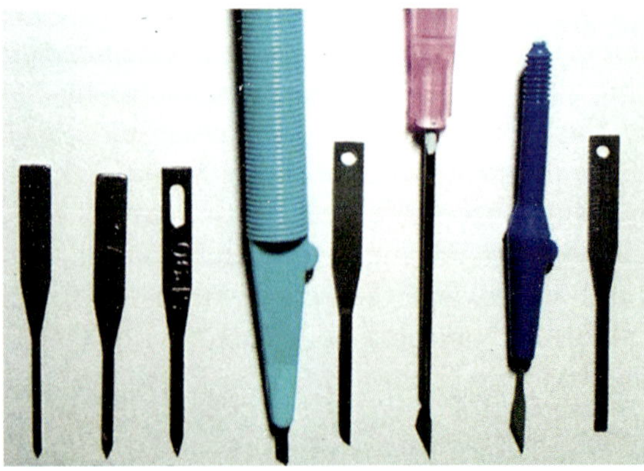

Figure 15.8 **Hardware needed for surgery: needles and microsurgery blades.**

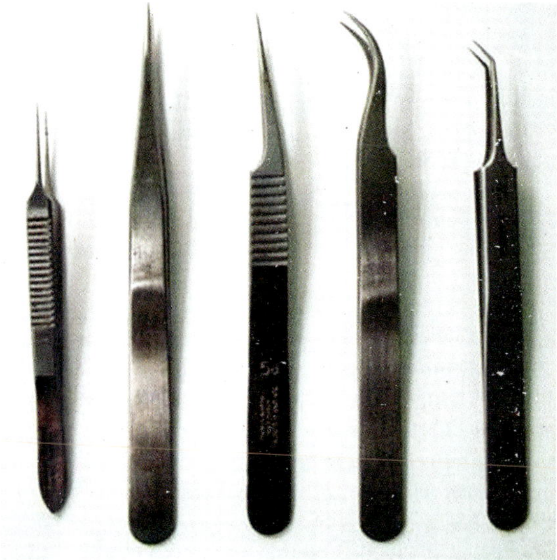

Figure 15.9 **Microsurgical forceps (straight or curved) for insertion of grafts.**

With a magnifying glass helmet, transplants are checked to control the correct insertion and proper orientation, or to swap some of them.

The patient should remain lying down for 1 to 2 hours. The advantages of FUL are

- For the patient:
  - The donor area of micrografts is unshaved. So the harvested donor area is immediately hidden by long hair.
  - The patient sees immediately the result, even though all or part of the hair can fall out in 2–3 weeks; the policy of "wait and see" has been replaced by one of "see and wait." Note the positive effect in the case of minoxidil and/or finasteride and/or PRP.
  - The scabs that persist for 10 to 12 days are hidden by long hair. Thus, the patient can quickly resume professional and social activities after 24–48 hours.
- For the physician:
  - A better assessment of the direction and angle of the hair (Figure 15.10).
  - A better choice, especially at the frontal hairline and whether hair is thick or thin, dark or light.
  - As for FUT a large amount of hair can be harvested with FUL at each session (4000 hairs per session).

The main drawback of the FUL technique, as for conventional strip harvesting (FUT), is be that it sometimes leaves a fine scar line. To avoid this it is possible to do a "trichophytic technique." This consists of removing about 1 mm of epidermis at the bottom edge of the excision of the strip. The hair will be able to grow through the epidermic and upper end to reduce the scar line edge. This method is borrowed from the "subepidermal technique" we described with Nataf for the front edge of the flaps for frontal reconstruction.[7,15]

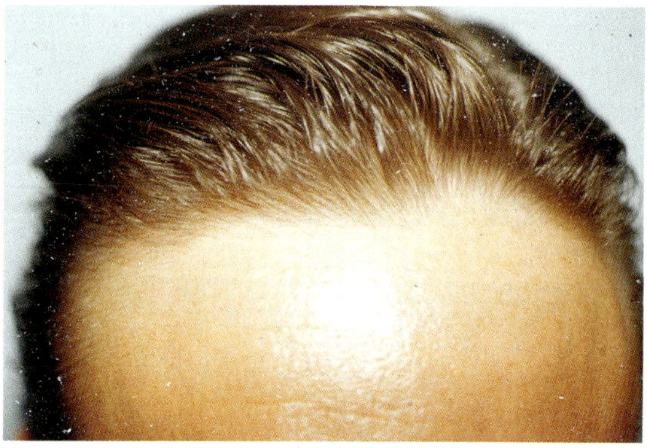

Figure 15.10 **A frontal region grafted with FUL allows a better choice of orientation, size, and color of hair.**

If the patient wants for personal reasons to shave his scalp and the fine scar line becomes visible, it is very easy to transplant in a second time a few follicular unit extraction (FUE) or to do an easy dermopigmentation (see Chapter 17).

Follicular unit extraction (FUE)

Follicular unit extraction (FUE) consists of a preliminary shaving of the donor area and then raising follicular units with the use of a punch (0.7–1 mm in diameter) at the occipital and temporal donor areas.[11,22,23]

Although the quality of the sample is directly dependent on the experience of the operator, improvements on the instrumentation have increased the speed of withdrawal and significantly reduced the loss of follicular units per transection.

Technique. The harvesting area region is shaved (Figure 15.11). On average an area of 100 cm² (20 × 5 cm) can provide usually 500–1500 follicular units.

The procedure is performed under local anesthesia.

The position of the patient during graft harvesting is the lateral or prone position. For the prone position a specific prone-pillow is used to ensure adequate comfort.

The basic principle of follicular unit extraction is to make, using a punch, a section around the follicular unit by a rotation across the dermal layer. Once after realizing a section of hair arrector muscle, the follicular unit can be extracted with forceps.

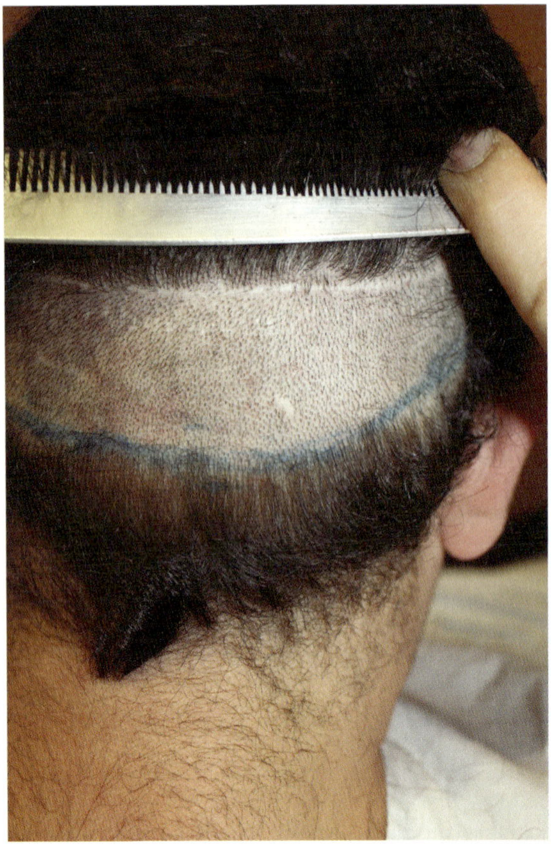

Figure 15.11 **The donor area is shaved for FUE harvesting.**

The instrumentation used for follicular extraction is relatively brief.

Special FUE punches with diameters ranging from 0.7 to 1 mm are used with a handle and microforceps.

There are two steps involved for the FUE procedure. In the first step, a sharp punch is placed over the follicular unit and aligned according to the direction of the hair shaft. The punch rotation must be realized without any axial pressure.

During the first step two parameters must be respected: depth and obliquity.

The rotation of the punch placed around the follicular unit allows the epidermis and dermis to be penetrated until the section of the arrector muscle insertion, which is 2–3 mm in depth.

It is important to measure the depth of insertion of the punch, which tends to vary from one person to another.

In the case of insufficient depth, the follicular unit cannot be extracted. In the case of a deep penetration, there is a risk of roots transection.

The second parameter is the respect of the obliquity. The emergence of the hair shaft varies according to the different axes of the follicles when performing a penetration of punch into the dermal layer; if the punch is oriented along the axis of the emergence of the hair, the follicle will be transected. In order to avoid this transection, the perfect angle must be found. This angle is estimated after viewing the first 10 harvested FUEs.

Usually the angle is verticalized from 5° to 10° relative to the angle of emergence of the hair.

In the second step, fine-toothed forceps are used to apply a gentle traction to the top of the follicular unit until it is extracted from the deeper dermal and subcutaneous connections.

Follicular units are extracted one by one using micropunches of 0.7–1 mm in diameter (Figure 15.12a–c). The instrument is rotated either manually or by a motor (Figure 15.13a). Each graft is extracted with jeweller forceps (Figure 15.13b).

The grafts are checked to control their quality and maintained in ice-cold saline before being inserted (Figure 15.14).

On average 1000 follicular units are removed in 2–3 hours.

Each follicular unit contains one to three hairs, so 1000 follicular units corresponds to approximately 1000–3000 hairs.

After harvesting all the follicular units, the patient is placed in a sitting position.

Local anesthesia is done on all the recipient areas.

The recipient area is perforated with ophthalmic microsurgical blades (spearpoint or chisel).

The insertion of follicular units is done with jeweler's forceps or using a Choi implanter[24] (Figure 15.18). The Choi implanter allows the assistant to store the graft in the microslot while it is inserted by the operator.

The procedure is done in about 3–4 hours, depending on the length of the session.

Sometimes the process is called "stick and place": one operator does the perforation and the other operator inserts immediately each FUE.

Indications for FUE

- Patients who have male or female androgenetic alopecia (Figure 15.15a–c).
- Patients who have a habit of shaving the hair (Figure 15.16a and b).
- Patients with limited laxity of the scalp (a limiting factor for strip harvesting).
- Patients with sufficient hair density in the donor area.
- Patients who do not want a scar line after harvesting a strip, since the latter, although very thin, can be blurred by some FUE in a second session.

Advantages of FUE

- The microscars in the donor area are, usually, almost imperceptible.
- The microperforations associated with harvesting follicular units in the occipital and temporal regions heal within a few days after surgery.

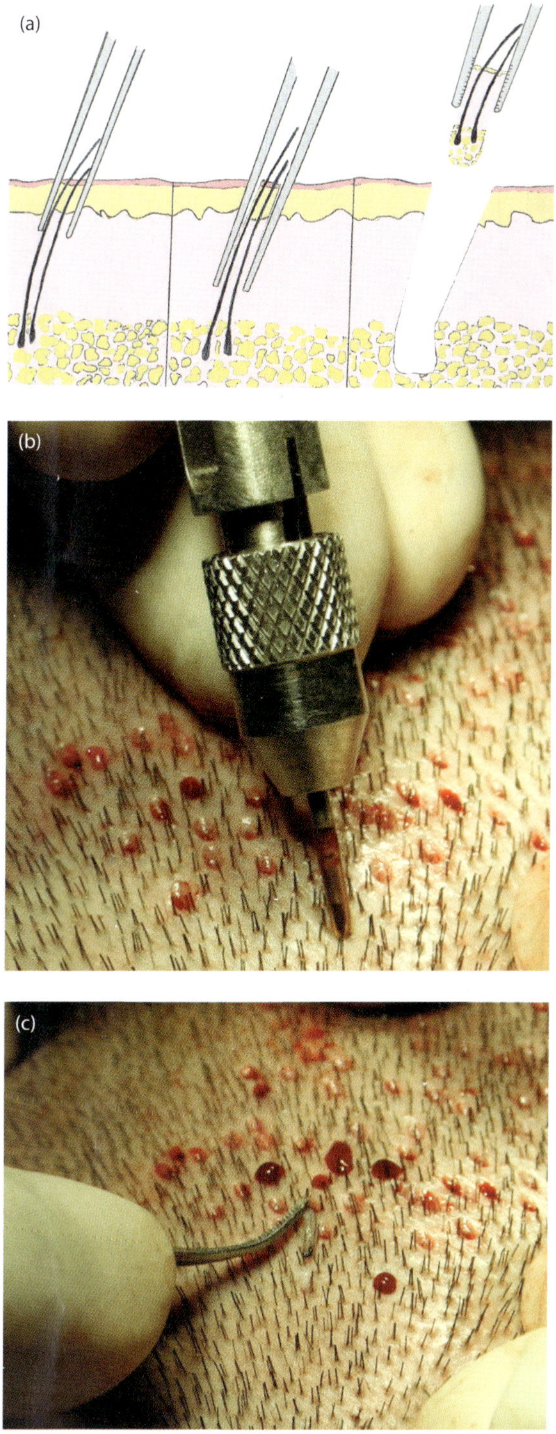

Figure 15.12 (a) Incision and extraction of FUE, (b) incision with the punch, and (c) follicular unit extraction with forceps.

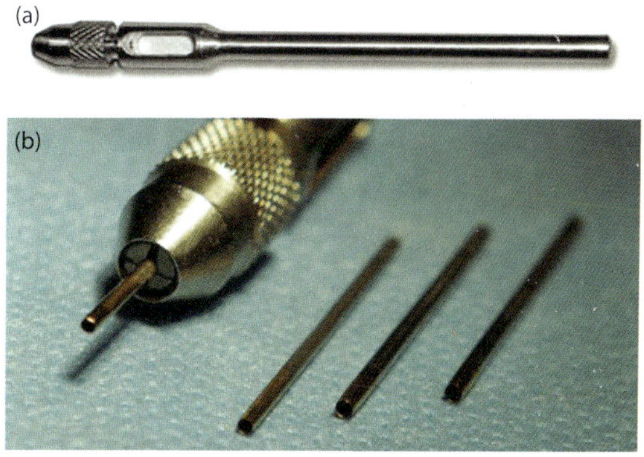

Figure 15.13 (a) Micropunch of 0.7–1 mm for FU extraction. (b) Handle for manual micropunch.

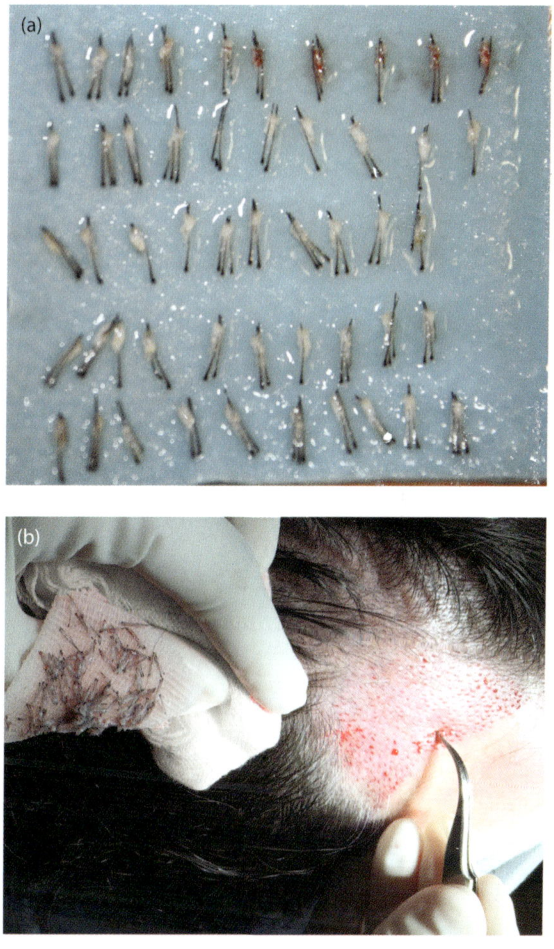

Figure 15.14 (a) Aspect of follicular units immediately after extraction. (b) Recipient area incisions and FUE implantation on male frontal recession.

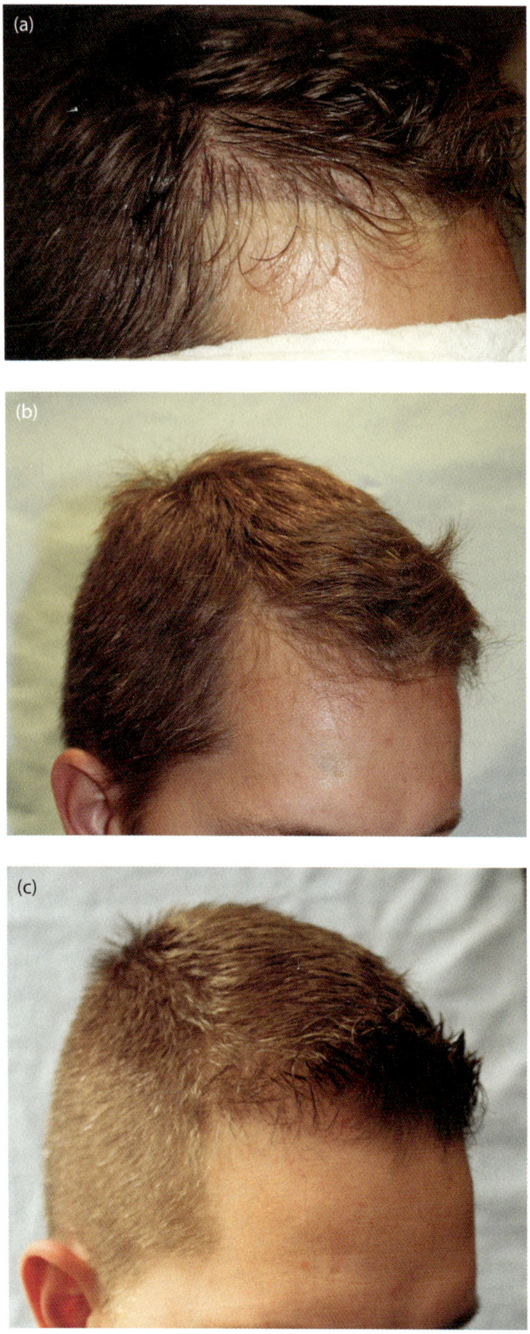

Figure 15.15 **(a) Aspect immediately after insertion of FUE on a frontal hairline. (b) Frontal recession before treatment. (c) Nine months after one FUE session.**

- There are no sutures and at most moderate postoperative pain.
- In some cases it is possible to harvest body hair, such as chest hair, for small FUE reconstruction.

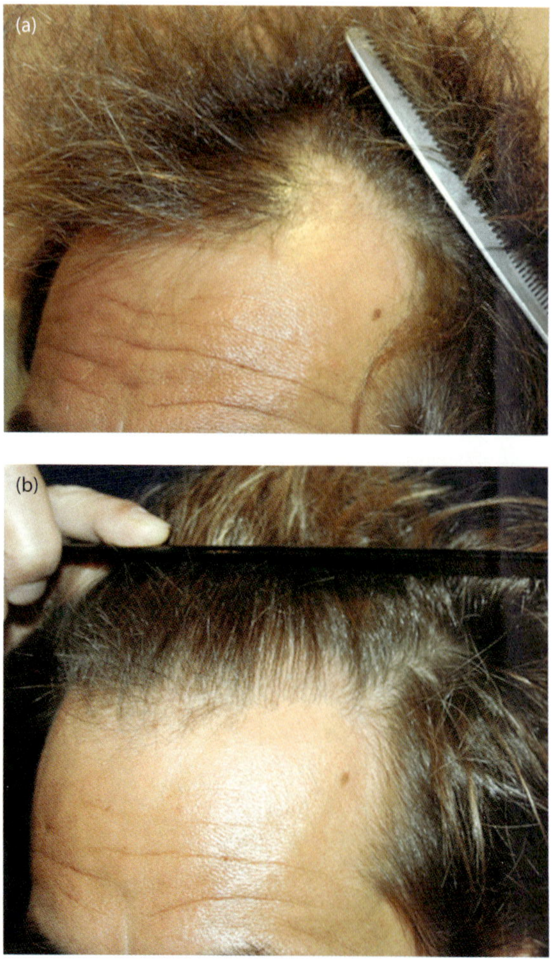

Figure 15.16 **A frontal hairline (a) before and (b) 9 months after one FUE session.**

Disadvantages of FUE. Usually, FUE is selected for small and medium baldness, especially in men.

In women, a sparse donor area often contraindicates FUE, especially since women rarely agree to have a preshave.

The FUE is more hazardous during any subsequent sessions according to the remaining donor hair capacity.

The FUE is worst for choosing the best angle and orientation during the implantation step.

In post-op FUE scabs are not hidden by the hair shaft.

The capacity of the donor area will be reduced if there is inexorable evolution of the alopecia process to greater baldness.

An essential point is that there is no regrowth of hair in the donor area for those which have been harvested.

It is possible now to do a FUE harvesting on a non-shaven scalp if a small session is indicated.

Postoperative course after follicular transplant

- A bandage is sometimes applied for one night in order to avoid bleeding after itching on the graft.
- A first cleaning with shampoo can be made the next day, and long implanted hairs can be dried with a mild air dryer.
- Swelling in the forehead may appear within 24–48 hours after surgery and will disappear 2–4 days later.
- Small crusts and implanted hair shafts will take approximately 7–10 days to fall out. Some long hair may remain implanted.
- Implanted follicles can have interrupted hair growth during the first 3 postoperative months.
- Regrowth of new hair is expected 3–4 months after surgery.
- Follicular units are extremely reliable, but we should still report the occurrence of secondary cysts due to the unfortunate inclusion of skin debris or a second hair transplant into the hole. This exceptional small complication should be treated as an outbreak of acne vulgaris with antibiotic, orally and locally, sometimes with an incision of the cyst.[22]
- Twelve months are necessary to evaluate the final outcome of the surgery.

Actions stimulating hair growth on transplants

Effect of minoxidil lotion

Usually 2–4 weeks after a hair transplant, the scabs over the transplants fall out, involving the bulbs of transplanted hair.[10,17,18] This fall-out, albeit transient with an average regrowth 3 months later, is sometimes aesthetically annoying.

An independent personal study[17] has shown that the application of minoxidil 2% lotion before and after transplantation allows persistent growth of part or all of the hair on more than two-thirds of the grafts, and causes fall-out in less than half of the transplanted hair on less than one-third of the grafts.

So it seems that the pre- and postoperative use of minoxidil 2% or 5% lotions, or taking orally finasteride 1 mg,[18] allows the continuation of the anagen process in a large amount of transplanted hair.

Effect of platelet growth factors (PRP)

Platelets contain "growth factors" (see Chapter 19; Figure 15.17).

The PRP process is a technique that involves isolating platelets from a blood sample, concentrating them by centrifugation, and injecting them back into the scalp.

Various evaluations show it is possible to observe an increase in the number of hairs per square centimeter due to an increase in hair diameter of vellus.

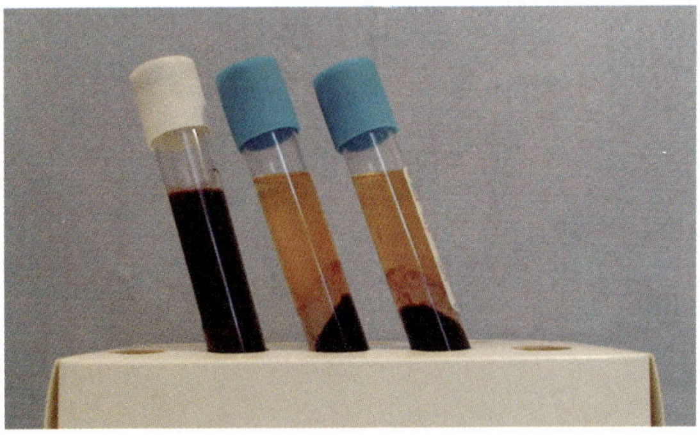

Figure 15.17 **Platelet growth factors (PRP) after centrifugation of a blood sample and before transdermal injection.**

The PRP injected in the recipient area may stimulate the regrowth of grafted hairs.[19,25]

New instruments for hair transplants

In recent years, various instruments or devices have been proposed and tested for their interest, reliability, and safety.

- *The Choi hair transplanter*[24] allows the introduction of follicular units (Figure 15.18). It may possibly be used for the reconstruction of the frontal hairline with hair implanted "one by one" in a more close-set manner and a better aesthetic refinement.

  It is a sterile device. The needle size must fit the hair follicle size and thickness (sizes of 0.8 or 1 mm).

  Each follicular unit (FUE, FUL, or FUT) is located in the needle with smooth forceps.

  The needle is then inserted deep into the scalp, and the cursor is pushed to implant the follicular unit.
- *The automatic FUE transplanter*[23] (Figure 15.19a) (SAFER/NeoGraft) may be recommended in the absence of contraindication to FUE. Compared to the conventional manual FUE technique, it avoids the need for additional assistance; however, for good results in practice, a long apprenticeship is essential.

  The SAFER/NeoGraft for hair transplantation is a patented medical device (Medicamat) used to both extract follicular units from the donor area and implant them in the recipient area via a suction-based system.

The extraction handpiece

It consists of an autoclavable hollow-shafted contra angle on which is fixed a motorized punch with a rotation system (five diameters: 0.8, 0.9, 1, 1.25, and 1.4 mm), and

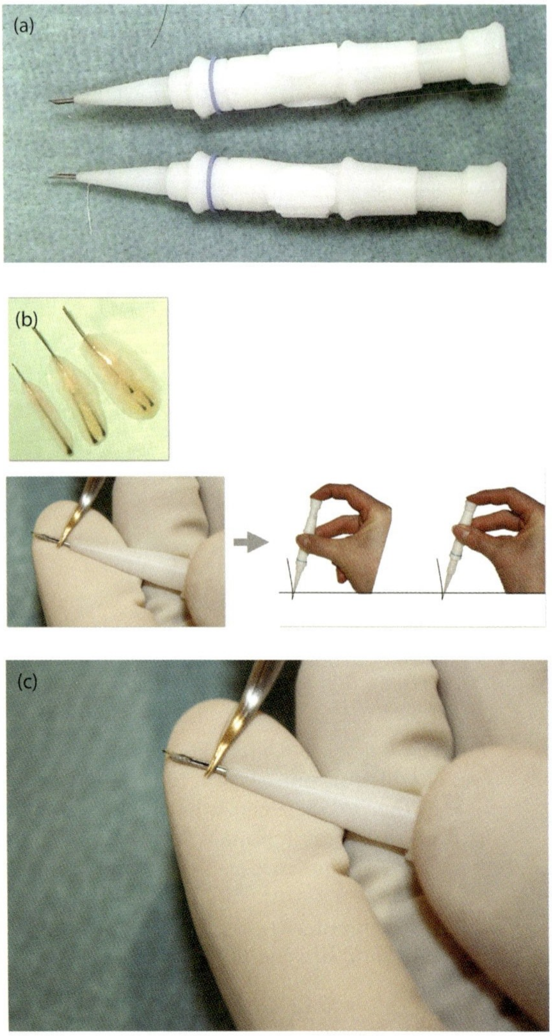

Figure 15.18 **(a,b,c) Choi implanter (Lion HT) for combining skin puncture and insertion of the micrograft.**

a controlled pneumatic negative pressure to smoothly extract every single graft from the donor area, into a micro flask fixed on the handpiece (Figure 15.19b).

The extraction handpiece superficially penetrates the patient's skin, until the arrector pili muscle is cut (≅2 mm deep). This superficial penetration avoids any risk of graft transection or trauma, allows a better quality graft (more cells around the graft), and reduces the time of surgery.

Once the graft is harvested from the tissue, it is sucked through a tube into the small flask.

When approximately 50 grafts are extracted from the scalp, the chamber, always wet with saline, is opened and the grafts are manually placed in a saline holding solution.

The recipient site incisions are done in the donor area using conventional instruments, such as 16- or 18-gauge needles or microblades.

The implantation handpiece

It consists of a hollow needle (diameter 0.8 mm and 1 mm) surmounted by a piston allowing the operator to gently implant the grafts into the premade incisions in the bald area with extreme precision and without any "popping" risk, using positive pneumatic pressure (Figure 15.19c). The two implantation handpieces connected to the device allow two operators to work simultaneously, substantially reducing the duration of surgery.

In this step the advantage of the SAFER/NeoGraft is that the grafts are inserted into the recipient site without forceps, thereby reducing potential injury from the forceps (Figure 15.19d).

Advantages of the SAFER/NeoGraft technique

- Productivity 500 grafts per hour
- Average hairs per graft of one to four
- A transection rate between 1% and 5%
- Donor area scarring that is nearly undetectable
- A technique that avoids the possible injury of forceps during implantation
- Gives eventually the possibility of working alone

The Robotic FUE (Artas)[26,27] (Figure 15.20a) is an interactive, computer-assisted, and physician-controlled robotic system used for the FUE harvest. A double concentric punch on a mechanical arm is guided by a video image. Its purpose is to minimize human error and fatigue while taking a greater number of transplants than the conventional extraction techniques allow (≈2000 grafts in 2 days). It also needs a long apprenticeship.

The system is composed of a cart with a six-axis articulated robotic arm.

The needle mechanism houses stereo cameras and force sensors that guide the dissection (Figure 15.20b). The dissection system uses a needle-in-needle (inner needle) configuration that is concentrically arranged within a blunt outer punch. A skin tensioner is maintained for the dissection process (Figure 15.20c). Sharp scoring incision, blunt punches (1.0 mm, 0.9 mm) dilate and dissect with automated depth control and angle adjustment.

The FU selection algorithms allow preferential treatment for multihair FU and adjusts minimum harvest spacing between incisions.

Stereo cameras precisely measure and calculate the angles and direction of each FU (Figure 15.20d). Each FU is then extracted manually with forceps. The surgeon makes slits in the recipient area and the extracted follicles

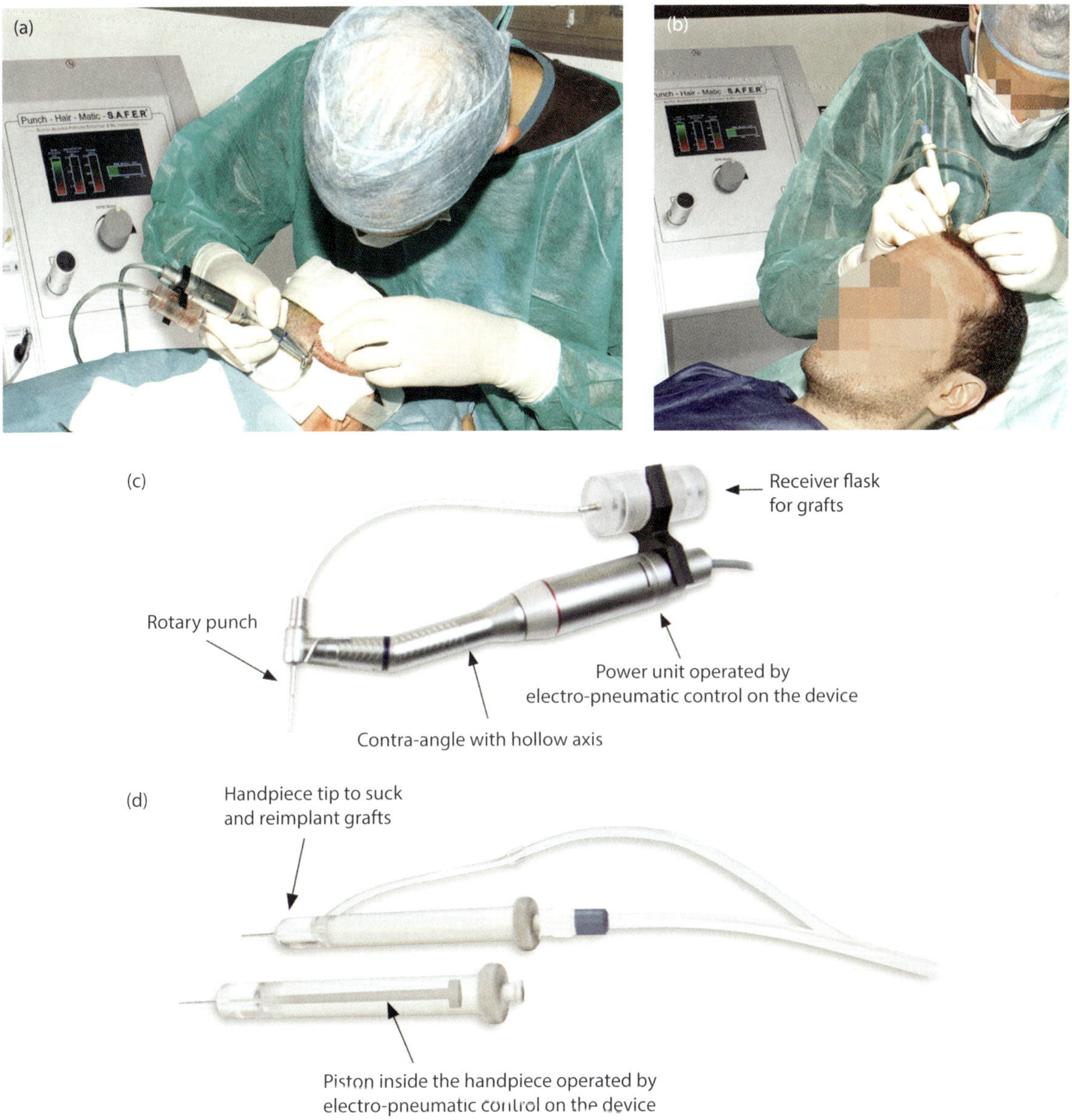

Figure 15.19 **(a) Extraction with the automatic system and transplantation of FUE (SAFER/NeoGraft). (b) Aspirating extraction of FUE collected in a chamber. (c) The implantation handpiece. (d) Implantation with the automatic system. (Courtesy of Medicamat.)**

are inserted manually with forceps in the slits after proper processing.

To detail the clinical performance, the transection rate is about 8% and the productivity is 500 grafts per hour with an average hairs per graft of 2,4 (evaluation done on 92.485 hair follicles). The donor area scarring is less detectable.

INDICATIONS FOR MICROGRAFTS

The goal is to obtain a harmonious balance between the aesthetic requirements (age, ethnicity, gender, and psychology), the evaluation of parameters for different classifications, the degree to which the alopecia has evolved, the capacity of the donor area, and the technical possibilities of the surgery.[28]

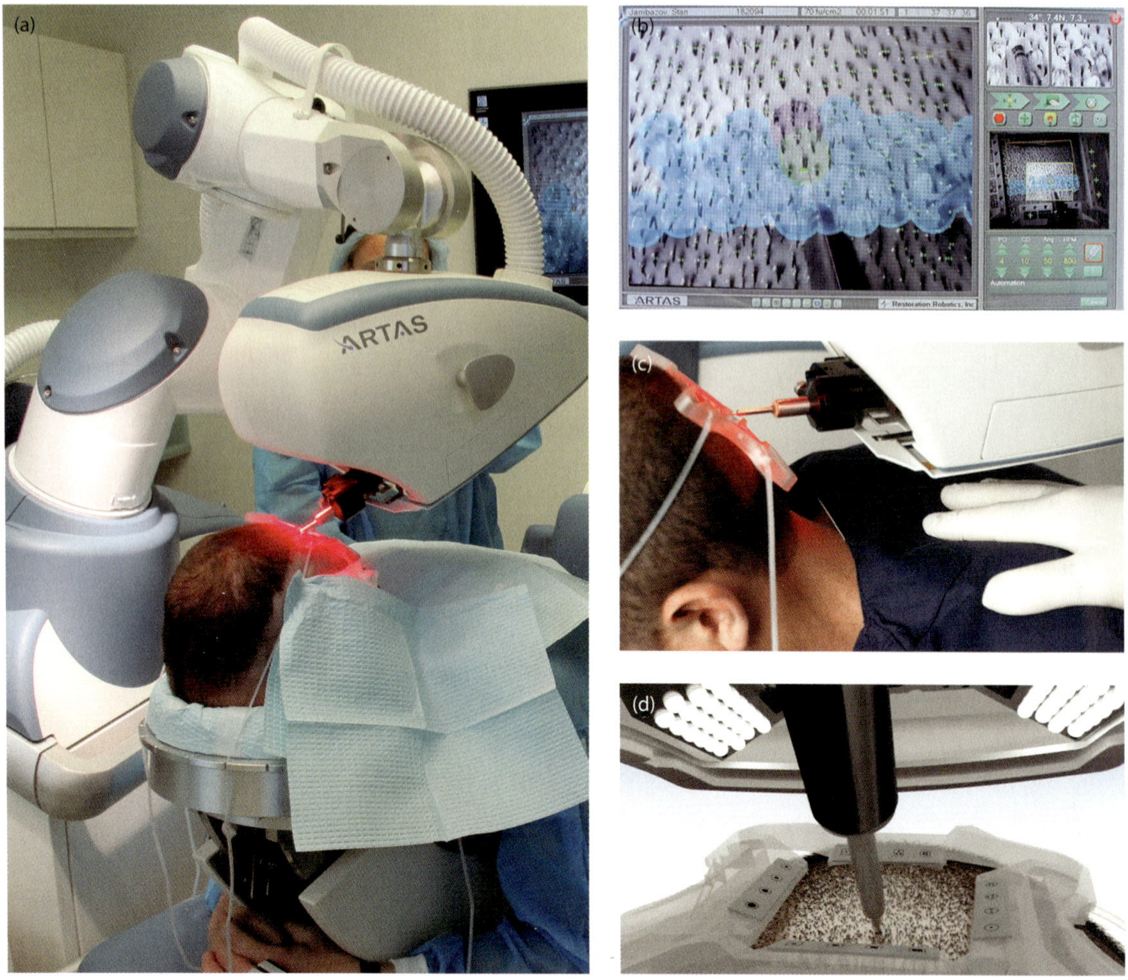

Figure 15.20 **(a) The ARTAS robotic system. (b) A stereocamera guides the dissection process. (c) A skin tensioner maintains the skin. (d) A stereocamera calculates the angle of each FU. (Courtesy of Dr. Bernstein and ARTAS.)**

Androgenetic alopecia

Various parameters of the Bouhanna multifactorial classification

Measurements are evaluated according to the Bouhanna multifactorial classification that takes into account multiple factors, such as the extent of the bald and hairy surfaces relative to some fixed points of the face, the laxity and thickness of the scalp, and the strength of the hair covering according to the density, size, shape, length, growth rate, and color (Figures 15.21a and b; see Chapter 5).[29,30]

Predictive evaluation is made of the residual medio-occipital hairy area in the stage of maximal baldness[29,30]: *superior axis*—eye external angle to earlobe apex; *inferior axis*—eye external angle to external auditory canal (Figure 15.21c).

The digital phototrichogram

The phototrichogram first described by Bouhanna in 1983[31] provides an objective scalp evaluation, using a digital camera, of the hairy surfaces, donor sites, and recipient sites for the transplant (Figures 15.22a and b).[31–33] The parameters of the hair growth—their density, size, number of miniaturized hairs, number of terminal hairs, and growth rate—will be measured and digitalized

Male androgenetic alopecia

The degree of baldness is graded to one of three schematic stages of the Bouhanna simplified classification[7] (Figure 15.23) or, more accurately, through the multifactorial classification[33] (Figures 15.21a–c).[30,34]

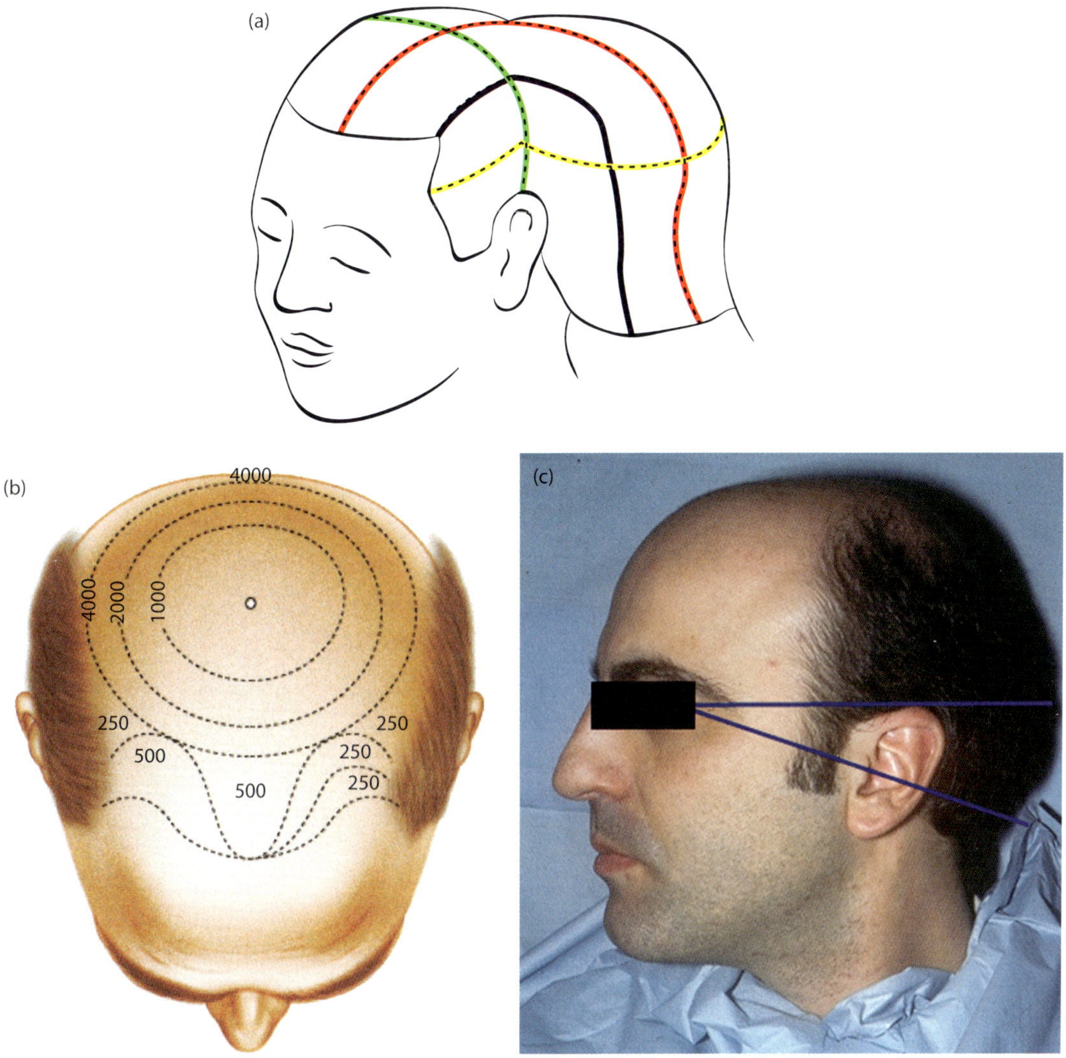

Figure 15.21 **(a) Patterns of multifactorial classification with the evaluation of the four axes. (b) Evaluation of the number of hairs required depending on the location and the transplanted area. (c) Predictive evaluation of maximal baldness according to superior and inferior axes. ([a] Adapted from Bouhanna P. *Dermatol Surg*, 2000;26: 555–561.)**

An essential point is that, in our opinion, to estimate the number of transplanted hair needed, the measurement unit is a hair and not a graft, as the graft may not always take.

Surgical correction involves transplantation of micrografts, as adapted schematically for one of these three stages described in 1976[7]:

- Stage I (frontotemporal recession, with possible crown alopecia at the vertex): Implantation of 1000 hairs in one session (Figure 15.24) (implantation of 2000–3000 hairs is sometimes required when there is associated crown alopecia) (Figure 15.25).
- Stage II (recession of all the frontal line to the vertex, with a possible crown alopecia): Implantation of 2000–3000 hairs in one to two sessions (up to 4000 hairs when there is associated crown alopecia) (Figures 15.26a and b).
- Stage III baldness (called "Hippocratic") where the hair remain only on the temporo-occipital region and up to 7000 hairs in one to three sessions are implanted (Figures 15.27a and b).

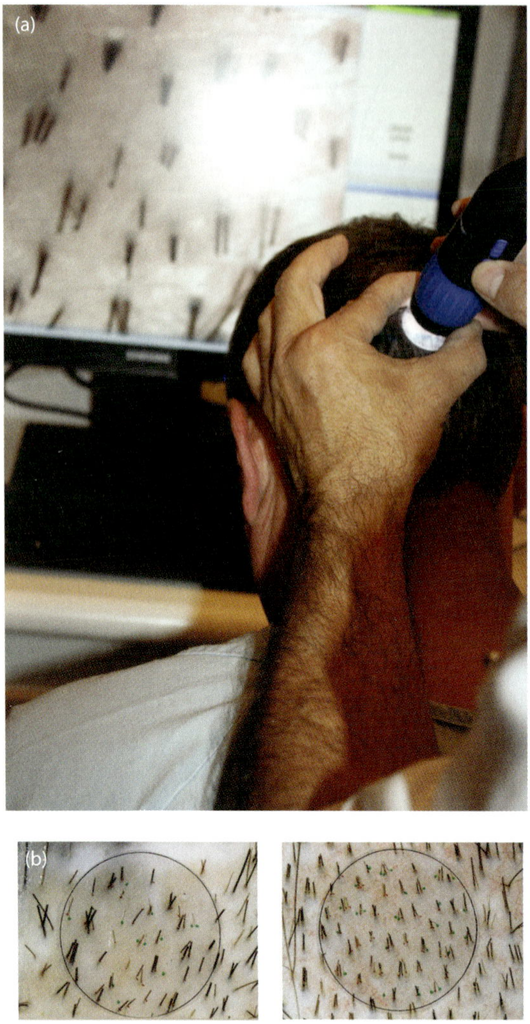

	1 cm²
Total hair count	94
Hair <40 μm	19
Hair >40 μm	75

	1 cm²
Total hair count	171
Hair <40 μm	44
Hair >40 μm	127

Figure 15.22 **Digital phototrichogram of the donor and the recipient area: (a) videocamera and (b) macroscopic views of the recipient and donor areas.**

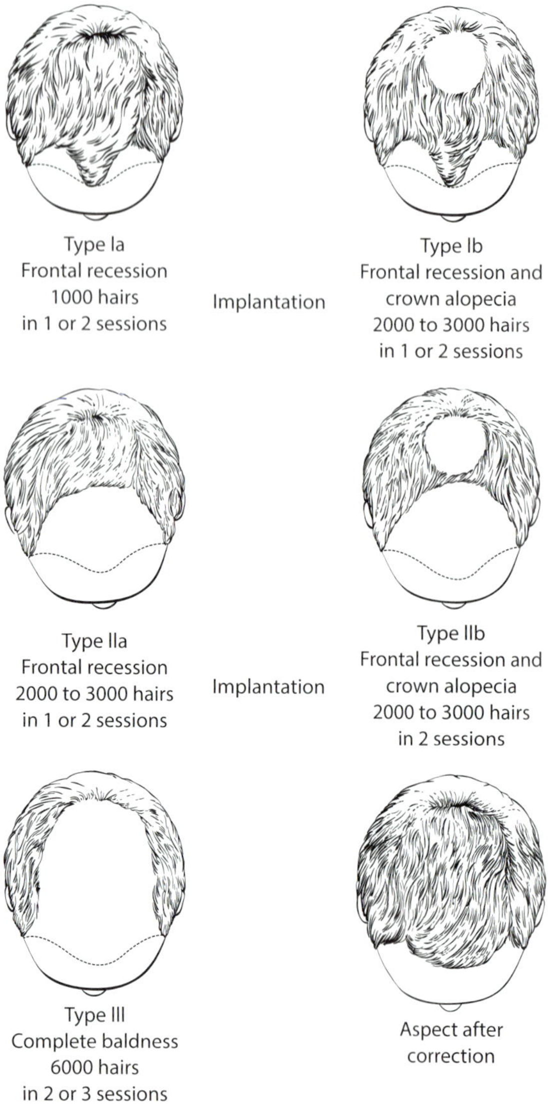

Figure 15.23 **The three stages of evolution of the classification of male androgenetic alopecia. (Adapted from Bouhanna P. Le cuir chevelu. Les alopécies définitives et leurs traitements. Thèse de doctorat en médecine, Université Paris XII, 1976.)**

The transplantation of micrografts may be combined with a local anti-hair loss treatment[17,18] (Figures 15.28a and b) (minoxidil 5%), intradermal injection of PRP (platelet-rich plasma), and/or general (finasteride 1 mg, orally), which aims to decrease the loss of residual hair between the grafts, to reduce the transient hair loss of grafted and nongrafted hair, and to accelerate the regrowth of grafted and nongrafted hair.

Female androgenetic alopecia

The degree of a female baldness androgenetic alopecia can be graded using the classification of Ludwig (1977)[35] or more precisely assessed through the multifactorial classification of Bouhanna.[13,14,21,29,30] Indications following the classification of Ludwig define three stages of evolution (Figure 15.29):

- Stage I: Moderate baldness on the vertex with respect of the frontal line: treated with implantation of 1000 hairs in one session (Figures 15.30a and b).

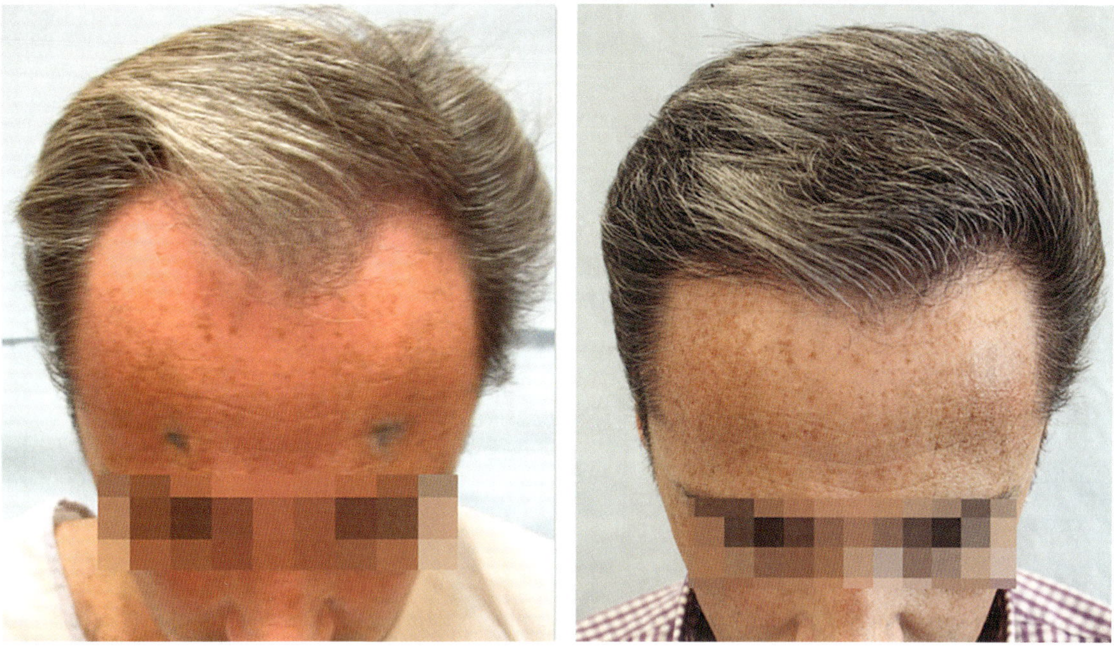

Figure 15.24 Male frontal alopecia (stage 1 or Hamilton IV) with FUL transplantation (1500 hairs) in one session.

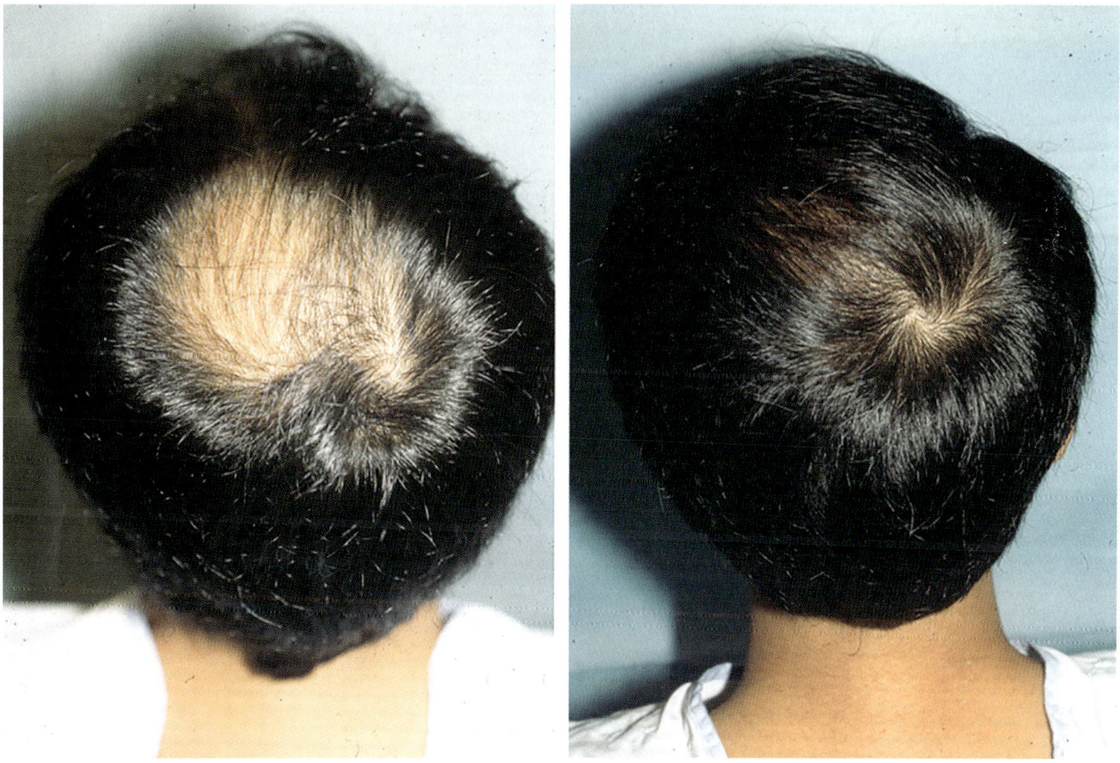

Figure 15.25 Male crown alopecia with FUL transplantation (1600 hairs) in one session.

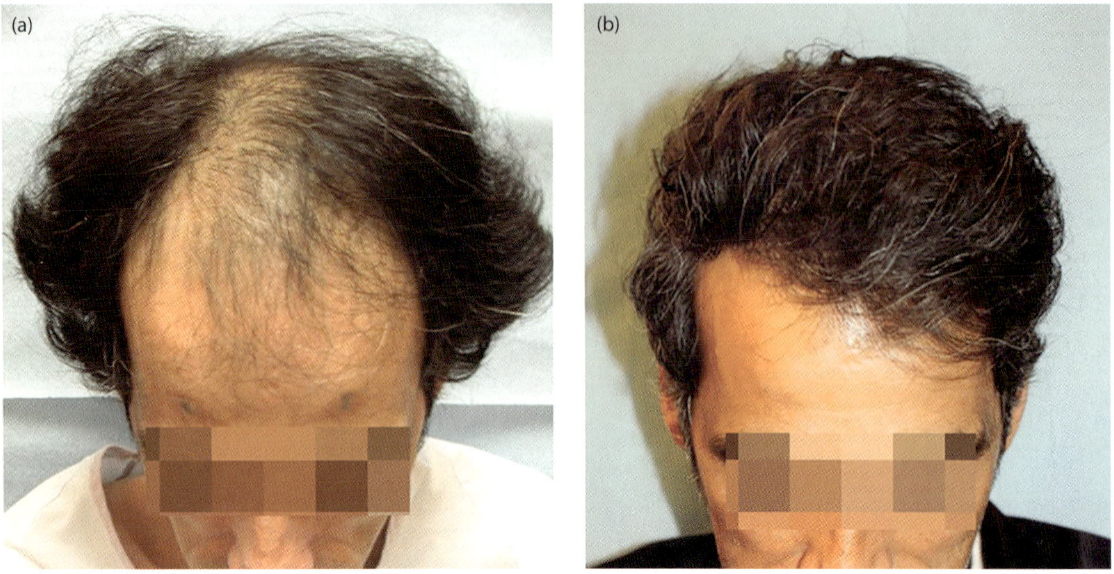

Figure 15.26 (a) Male androgenetic alopecia (stage 2 or Hamilton V), (b) with FUL transplantation (5100 hairs) in two sessions.

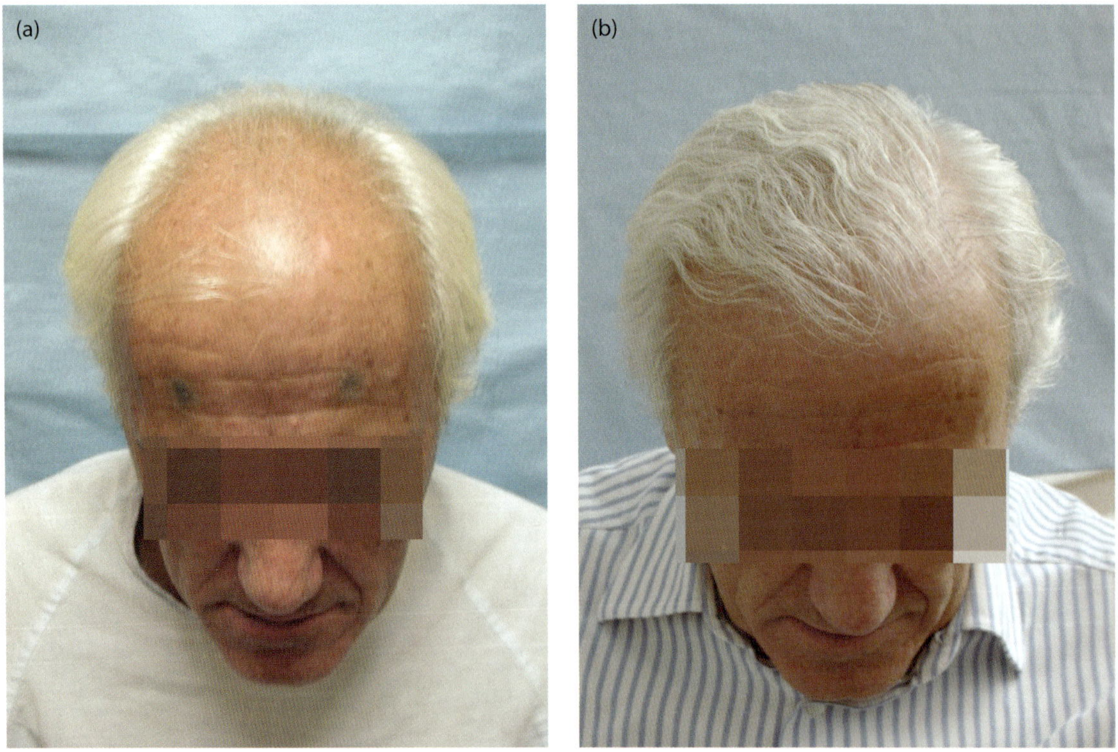

Figure 15.27 (a) Male androgenetic alopecia (stage 3 or Hamilton VI), (b) with FUL transplantation (2700 hairs) in one session.

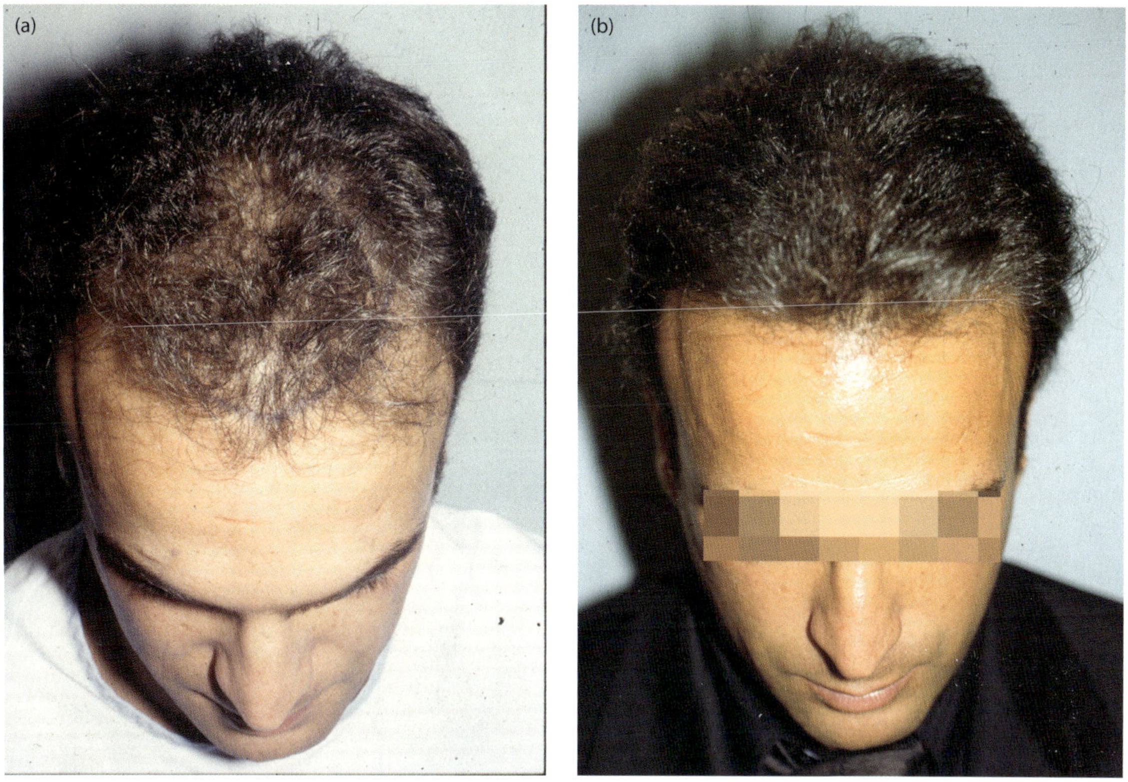

Figure 15.28 (a,b) **Male androgenetic alopecia with combining treatments: FUL transplantation in two sessions, minoxidil 5%, and finasteride.**

- Stage II: Alopecia with short hairs, located 1 cm behind the frontal line: treated with 1500–2000 hairs in one or two sessions (Figures 15.31a and b).
- Stage III: Almost important alopecia of the vertex, with preservation of a thin strip of remaining hair on the forehead): treated with 3000–4000 hairs in two sessions (Figures 15.32a and b).

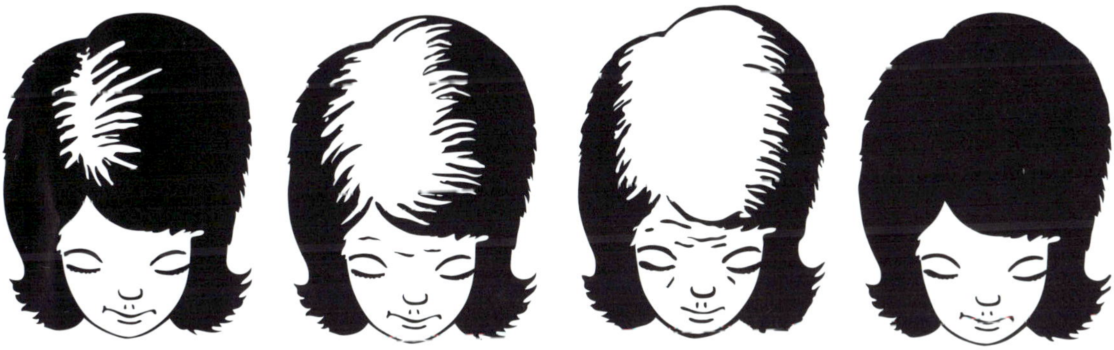

Figure 15.29 **The three stages of evolution of the classification of female androgenetic alopecia.** (Adapted from Ludwig E, *Br J Dermatol*. 1977;97:247–254.)

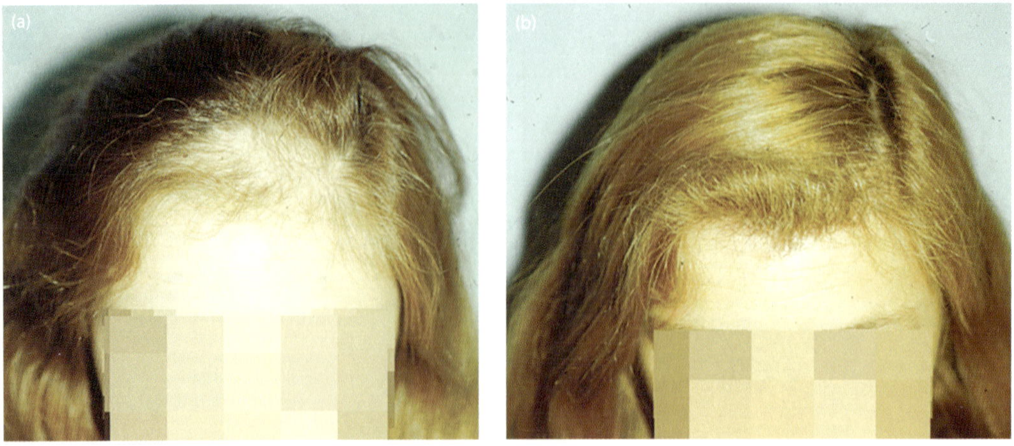

Figure 15.30 (a,b) Female androgenetic alopecia (stage 1) with FUL transplantation (1200 hairs) in one session.

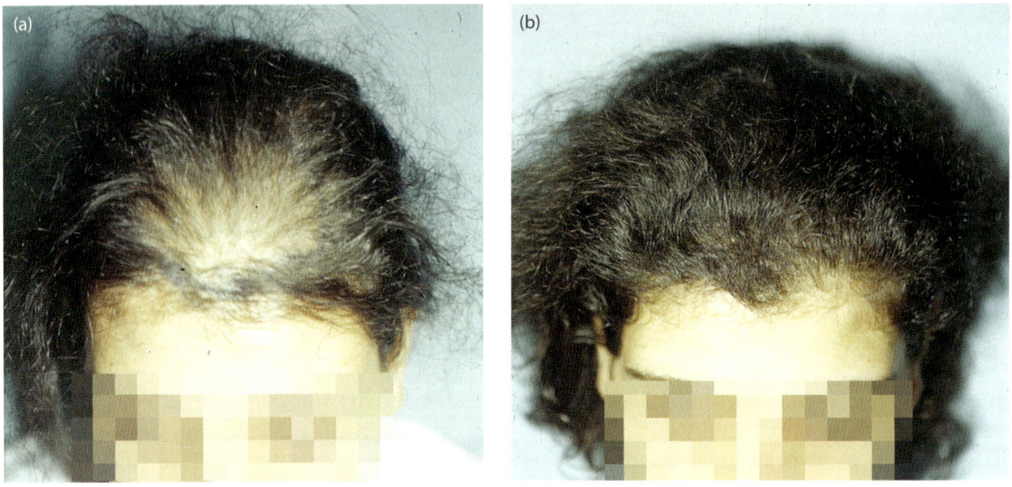

Figure 15.31 (a,b) Female androgenetic alopecia (stage 2) with FUL transplantation (1600 hairs) in one session.

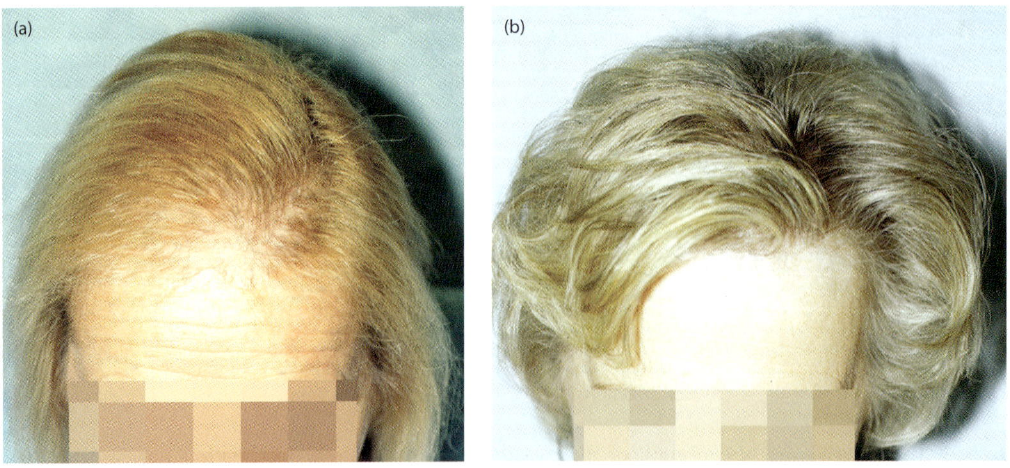

Figure 15.32 (a,b) Female androgenetic alopecia (stage 2) with FUL transplantation (1700 hairs) in two sessions.

The micrograft treatment may be combined with a local anti-hair-loss treatment (minoxidil 2%), intradermal injection of PRP, and/or oral anti-androgens such as cyproterone acetate or spironolacton.[28]

In transsexuals

We must fulfill the frontal recessions and give a fine frontal line of a feminine pattern.

OTHER ALOPECIA

- Traction alopecia[36]: Repeated traction (blow hair drying, straightening, braids, etc.), especially in African American patients (Figures 15.33a and b), can induce definitive alopecia of the frontotemporal region. Before considering implantation, one must control the absence of regrowth despite stopping traction for at least 6 months (see Chapter 12).
- Pseudopeladic alopecia, if stabilized and if the occipital donor area is not definitely spared.
- Alopecia and scars after facelift (Figures 15.34a and b).
- Scarring alopecia after burns, after radiotherapy, post-traumatic, etc. (Figures 15.35a and b).

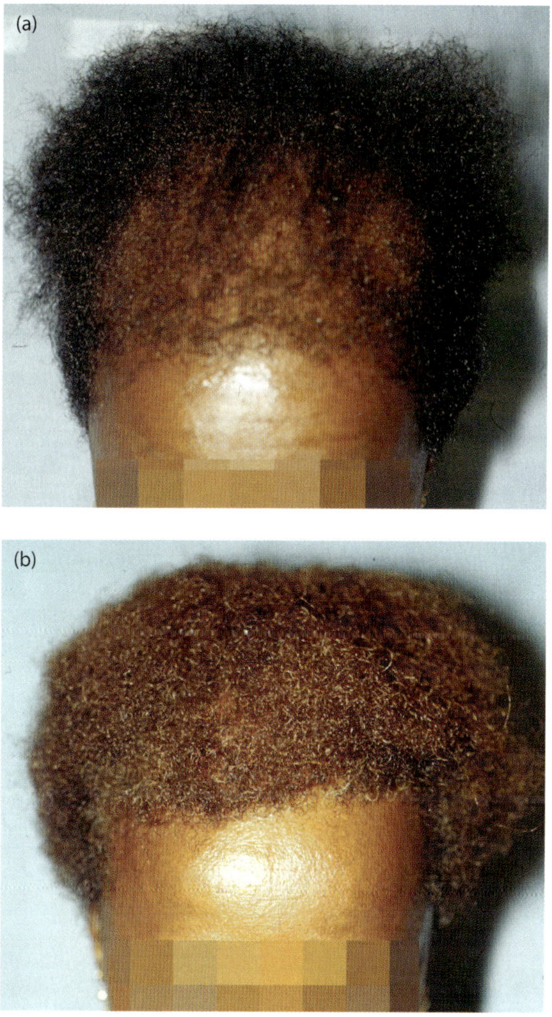

Figure 15.33 **(a,b) Definitive traction alopecia in an African American patient with FUL transplantation (1800 hairs) in two sessions.**

BODY HAIR ALOPECIA

Permanent alopecia of the eyebrows

Follicular transplantation is a simple surgical technique that corrects most of the definitive eyebrow alopecias.[37–39] It consists of implanting on the absent or sparse area of the eyebrow hair follicles harvested from the scalp or, more rarely, from a hairy area of the body.

Eyebrow alopecia causes

Alopecia of the eyebrow is relatively common in the population.[40] The most common causes are

- Eyebrow density loss related to aging. This usually starts at the tail of the eyebrow and then gradually affects the entire eyebrow. A few short and sparse hairs persist (Figure 15.36).
- Alopecia of the eyebrow tail linked to repeated aesthetic depilation (Figure 15.37).
- Post-traumatic alopecia or after removal of a lesion of the eyebrow.
- Alopecia areata is a common cause of alopecia of the eyebrow.
- Some eyebrow alopecias have been corrected with dermopigmentation (tattooing) (Figure 15.38).
- Except for alopecia areata, all the eyebrow alopecias can be corrected definitively with a single hair transplantation.

Eyebrow transplantation procedure

The design of the eyebrow is done according to three diagonals to locate the head, the body, and the tail of the eyebrow (Figure 15.39).[38,39,41,42]

The transplantation is performed under local anesthesia with previous oral sedation. A strip of scalp (6 cms × 1 cm) is harvested from the lower occipital area or the temporal region. The donor site is then sutured using absorbable running suture.

The strip is segmented under a microscope in order to get a group of micrografts containing one follicle and a group of micrografts containing two follicles (Figure 15.40).

Follicular units are combined and selected according to their shape (the goal is to get follicles with a large

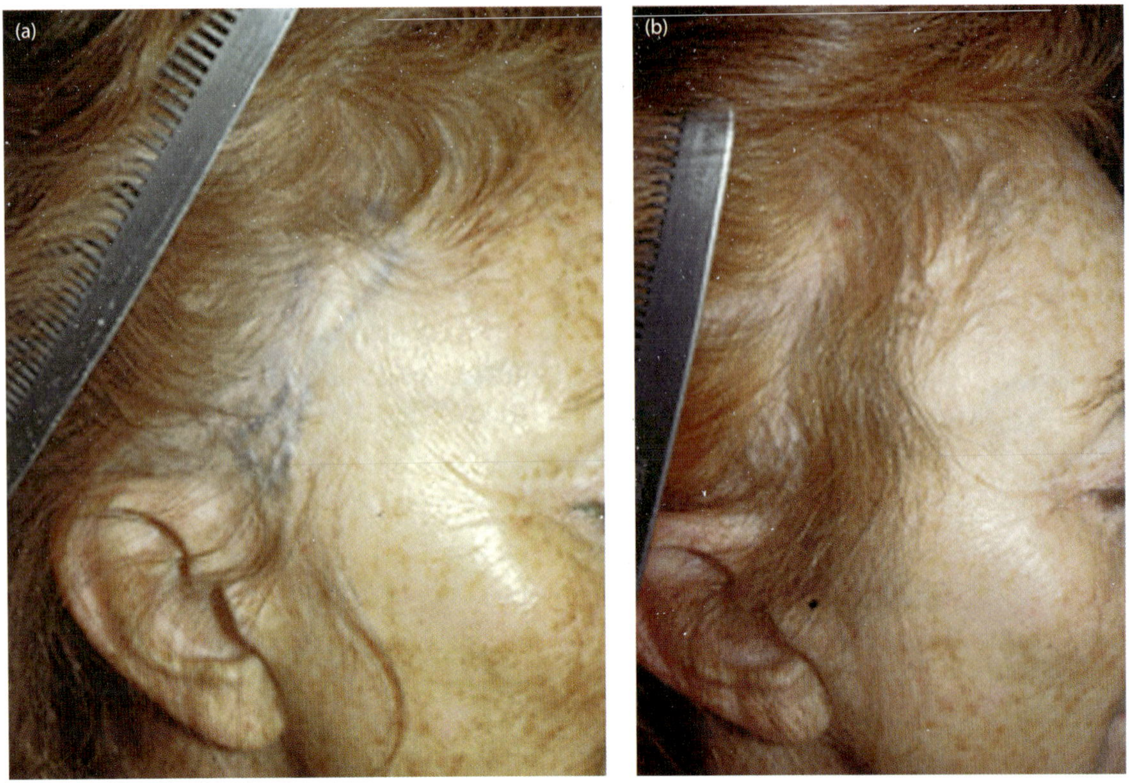

Figure 15.34 (a,b) Preauricular alopecia after a facelift with FUL transplantation (900 hairs) in one session.

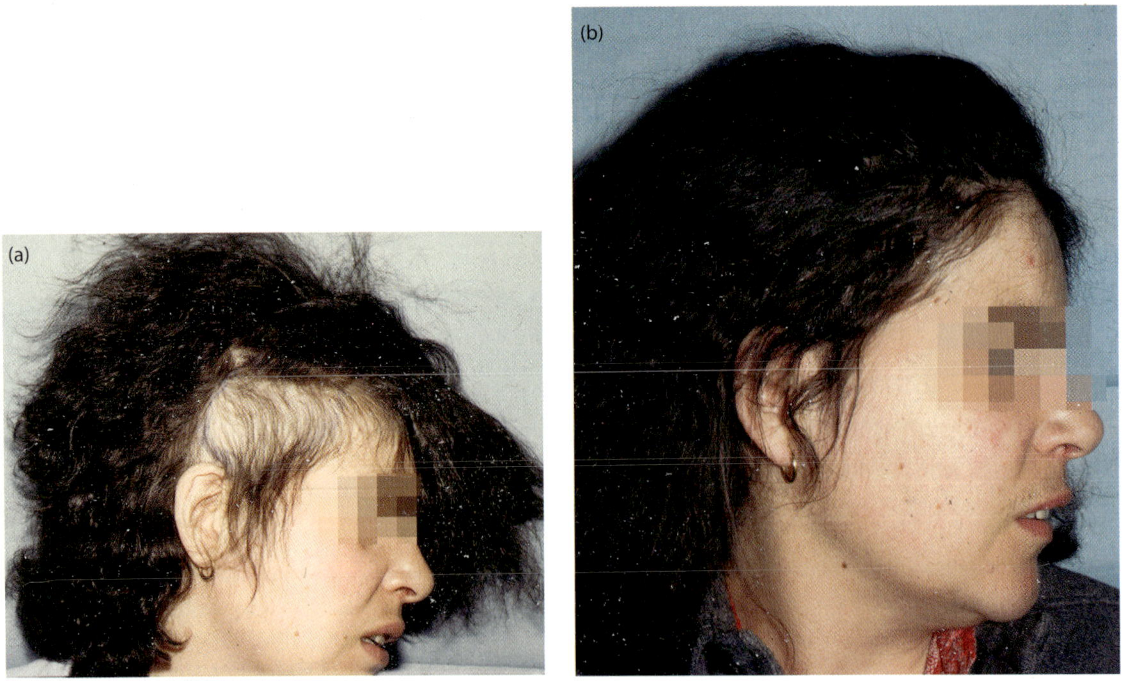

Figure 15.35 (a,b) Alopecia after radiotherapy for a malignant brain tumor with FUL transplantation (2200 hairs) in two sessions.

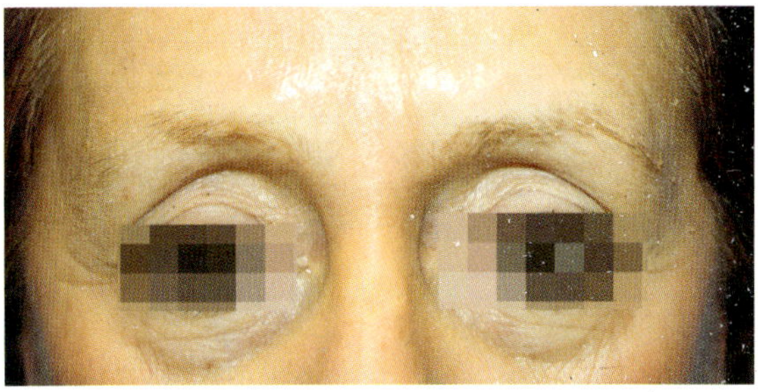

Figure 15.36 Eyebrows density loss due to aging.

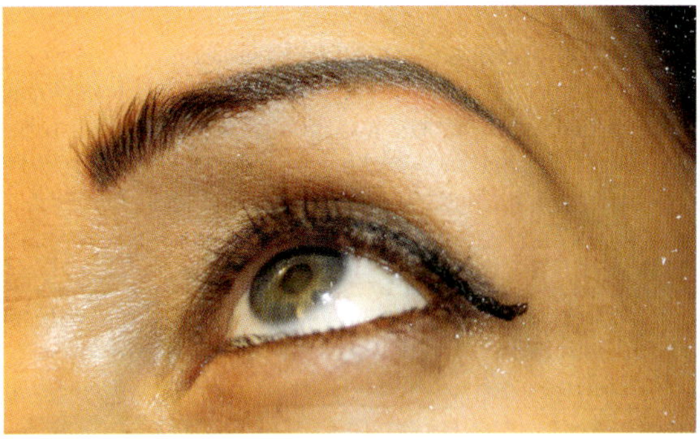

Figure 15.37 Eyebrow alopecia due to repeated depilation. (Courtesy of Dr. Eric Bouhanna.)

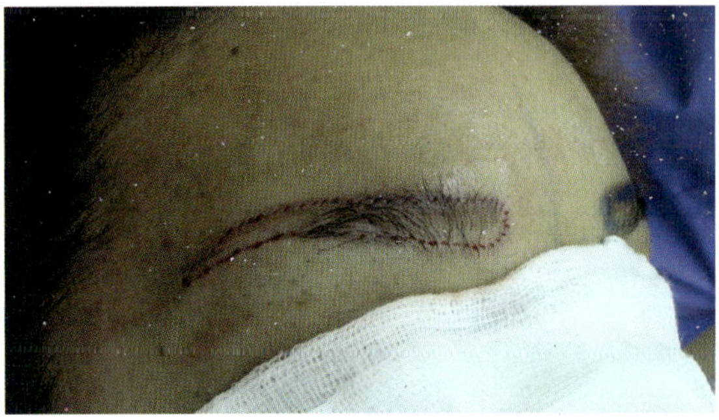

Figure 15.38 Eyebrow alopecia with a tattooing correction. (Courtesy of Dr. Eric Bouhanna.)

curvature) and thickness (selection of thick follicles and thin follicles).

The grafts are delicately placed on gauzes soaked in ice-cold saline to preserve them from dryness before implantation.

The eyebrow is anesthetized by infiltration of lidocaine with epinephrine 1%. The implantation is guided by the design done before surgery. The use of magnifying glasses is recommended to improve the precision of the graft insertion. Using a 18-gauge needle, twisted into "bayonet" fashion (Figure 15.41), microperforations on the recipient

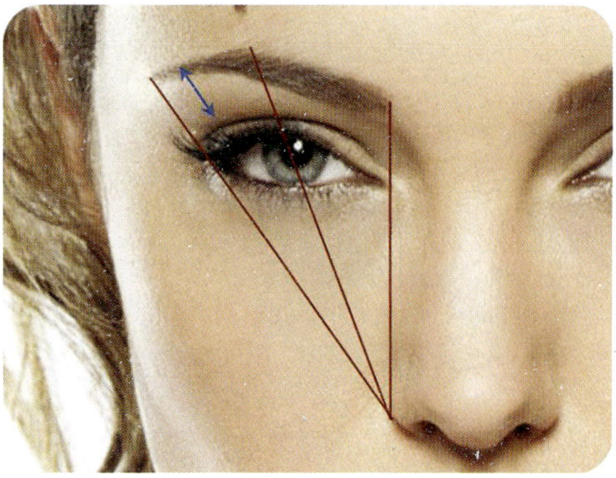

Figure 15.39 Eyebrow design according to the three diagonals. (Courtesy of Dr. Eric Bouhanna.)

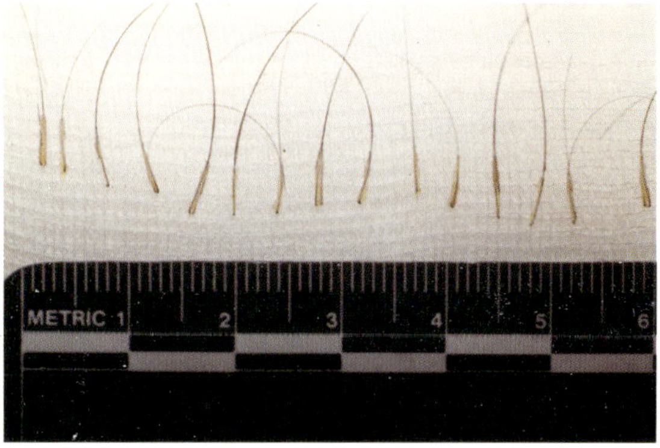

Figure 15.40 One and two follicular unit long hair (FUL) before the eyebrow transplantation.

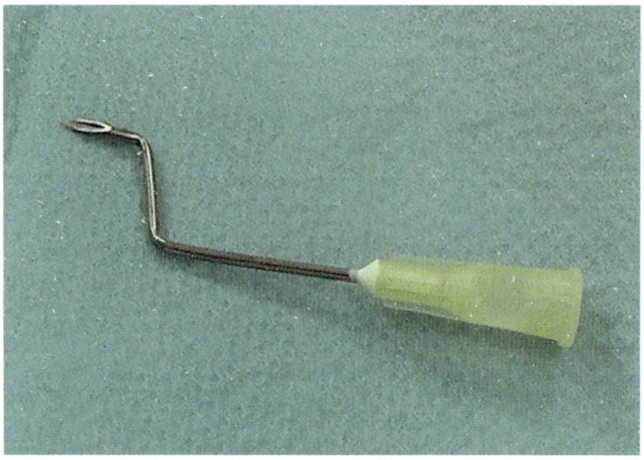

Figure 15.41 Microperforations with a 18-gauge needle modified in a "bayonet" fashion.

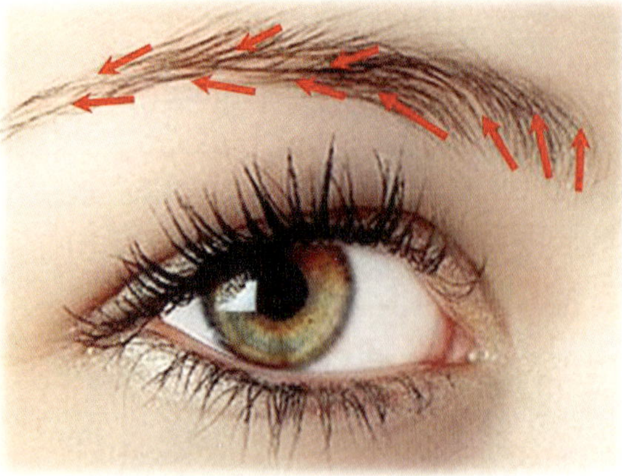

Figure 15.42 **Design of the eyebrow with the various hair orientations. (Courtesy of Dr. Eric Bouhanna.)**

area are carried out, taking care of the various orientations and remaining as tangentially nearly parallel to the skin (Figure 15.42).

After completing all the perforations on the recipient sites, micrografts are gently introduced with microsurgical forceps. The implantation must be done very gently to avoid any injury of the follicles. One-follicular implants with thinner shafts will be placed on the superior and inferior edges of the eyebrow, while thicker two-follicular implants are placed in the dense central body of the eyebrow. The oblique orientation of the hairs will be upwards to the head of the eyebrow, downwards to the tail of the eyebrow, and horizontally to the body of the eyebrow. These refinements are easier to do with the follicular unit long hair (FUL) (Figure 15.42).

Once all the follicles are implanted, meticulous control of the orientations of each graft is performed.

No dressing is necessary.

Eyebrow transplantation results

The preview result is immediate but sometimes transitory. Some of the implanted hair may fall during the postoperative weeks. A complete regrowth is expected 2 or 3 months later. To avoid any anxiety and feelings of failure, the patient needs to be well informed before and after surgery about this transient evolution.

The almost final result is observed 6–9 months later (Figures 15.43a and b).

Patients are informed about applying a modeling gel on the new implanted shafts, in order to guide smoothly all the hair of the eyebrow.

The eyebrows are trimmed according to the implanted hair growth about every 2 weeks.

Eyebrow transplantation is currently the best solution to seamlessly rebuild an eyebrow. The result depends on the quality of technical implantation and the careful selection of each implanted hair.

Ideally the hair with a highly curved or curly shaft is most suitable (Figures 15.44a and b and 15.45a and b).

Eyebrow grafting is satisfactory in most cases. It is, however, decreased in the case of smoking, or when the implantation is performed on fibrous scar tissue.

Sometimes the use of the extraction harvesting technique by FUE (follicular unit extraction) is possible for implantation of the eyebrows. However, with the prior scalp shaving, the natural curvature of the grafted hair shaft is not visible and this makes it difficult to get the correct positioning of implants. FUE is, however, indicated in some cases, especially for men who have workable hair on the chest or limbs.[43]

Alopecia of the eyelashes

The introduction of micrografts allows a definitive aesthetic reconstruction by implanting selected hairs "one by one."[43,44] The lashes will be cut to the desired length every 15–20 days.

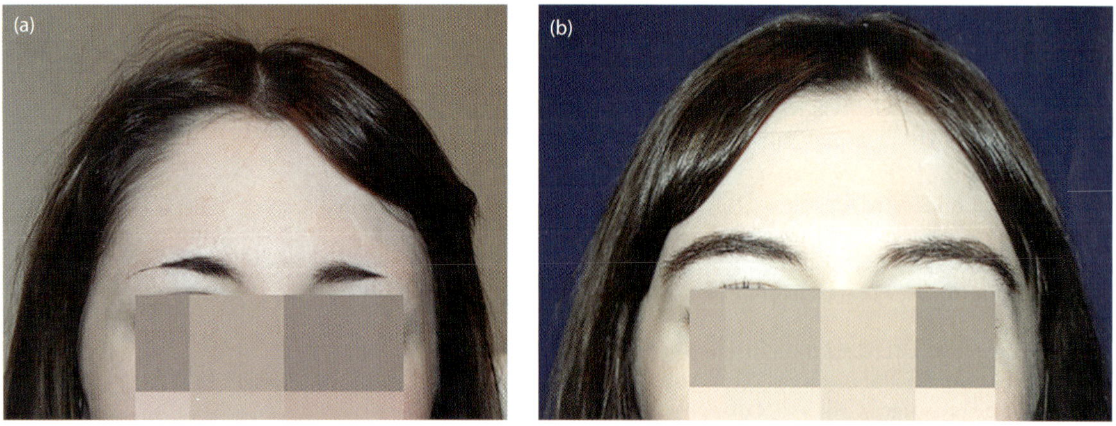

Figure 15.43 **(a) Tail eyebrow alopecia and (b) correction with one FUL transplantation session. (Courtesy of Dr. Eric Bouhanna.)**

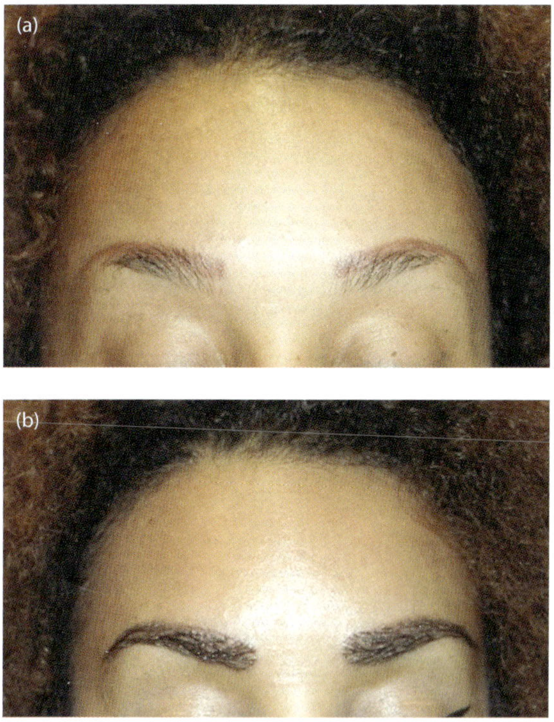

Figure 15.44 (a) Tattooed eyebrow and (b) correction with one FUL transplantation session. (Courtesy of Dr. Eric Bouhanna.)

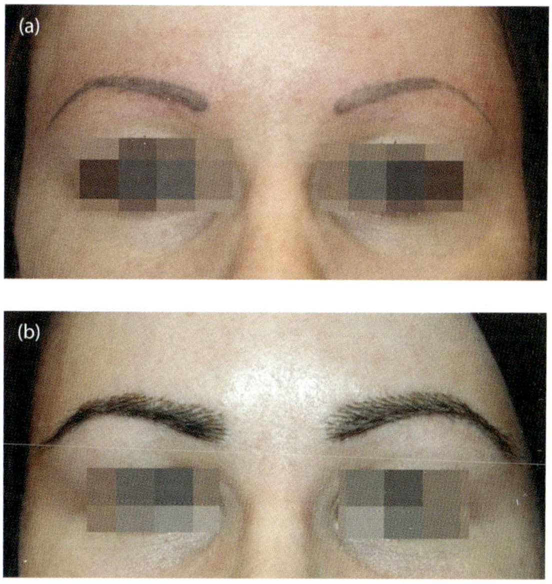

Figure 15.45 (a) Tattooed eyebrow alopecia and (b) correction with one FUL transplantation session. (Courtesy of Dr. Eric Bouhanna.)

Alopecia of the beard and mustache

Alopecia of the beard and the mustache is often of scar origin (harelip, acne scars) or a lack of beard due to ethnic origin (Asian male patients) (Figures 15.46a–c).[37,38] Increasingly, for ethnic and religious wishes (Middle East origin), a densification of the beard or mustache is

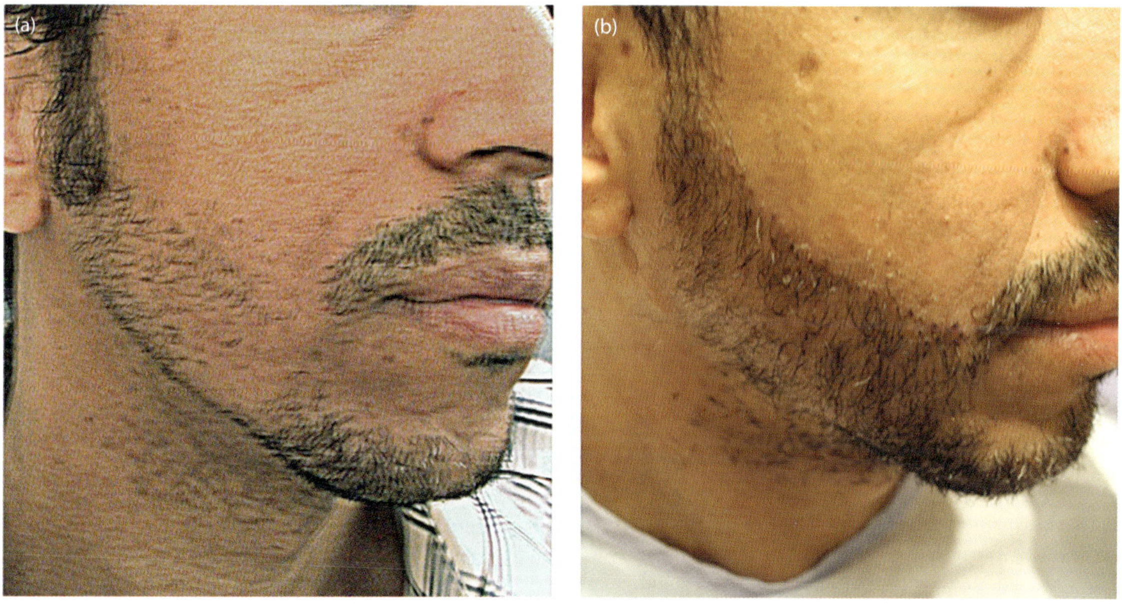

Figure 15.46 (a) Beard alopecia. (b) Four days after one FUL transplantation session.

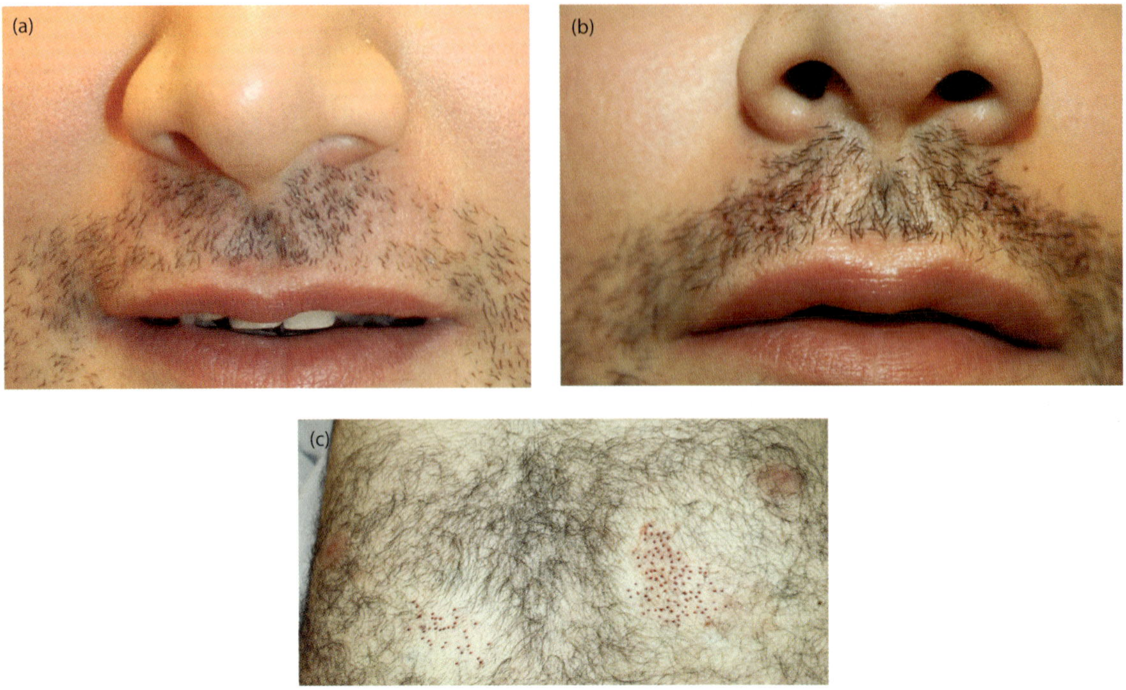

Figure 15.47 **(a) Male beard scars. (b) Four days after FUE transplantation. (c) Harvesting of FUE from chest body hair.**

requested. In these cases, it is very important to understand the psychological profile. The procedure is similar to that for the eyebrow and transplanted with one hair follicular unit, and in most cases with the follicular unit long hair (FUL) or sometimes with FUE. In a few cases, follicular unit extraction (FUE) is done by harvesting chest body hair (Figures 15.47a–c).

Alopecia of pubic hairs

This hair loss can be due to some gynecologic surgery procedures or postmenopausal hormonal effects.[37,38,43,45]

Reconstruction and densification of pubic hair are done according to many parameters.

An oblique centripetal orientation of the implants is of great importance to achieve a natural aspect.

Each one- to two-hair follicular unit long hair (FUL) are selected during segmentation and insertion.

The puncture perforations are done with 18-gauge needles with an obliquity nearly parallel to the skin. The needle is twisted into bayonet fashion to achieve a more acute angle incision.

No dressing is necessary.

CONCLUSION

Hair transplantation for male and/or female androgenetic alopecia can usefully be combined with the positive effect of various hair growth molecules (minoxidil, finasteride, intradermal injections of PRP, hormonal treatments, anti-androgens, etc.) densifying permanently bald areas. The aesthetic desire and the psychological profile are specific for each individual.

Follicular units of long hair (FUL), manual follicular extraction (FUE), automatic or robotic FUE, and conventional follicular unit transplant (FUT) can achieve most problems of hair thinning (scalp, beard, mustache, eyebrows, or pubis) for men and women and transgender. The methods also can treat most definitive alopecia of other etiology.

The follicular unit procedures are mostly selected according to ethnic origin (African American, Asian, etc.), the donor area density, and the extent of the baldness.[45,46]

Dermatological cosmetic surgery of the scalp requires, because of its specificity, a good knowledge of the anatomy of the scalp, the hair physiology and pathology, and a perfect handling of all the procedures of skin surgery. It is important to highlight seven key points:

- Establish an accurate analysis of the psychological profile of the patient (whether male or female).
- Present a precise planning of the immediate and future treatments, explaining the advantages and disadvantages of each procedure.
- According to the digital phototrichogram and the multifactorial classification, make an immediate and a prospective evaluation of the aesthetic result, taking into account the possible evolution of the alopecia process in the recipient area and in the donor area.

- Have a correct handling of all the procedures for selecting the best indications.
- Do not use any techniques that are unscientific, unreliable, or inadequately established.
- Be well aware of complications, the better to avoid or correct them.
- Examine the patient every year to control the evolution of the alopecia process and to determine if any additional refinements are required.

REFERENCES

1. Sasagawa M. Hair transplantation. *Jpn J Dermatol.* 1930;30:493 (in Japanese).
2. Okuda S. Clinical and experimental studies of transplantation of living hairs. *Jpn J Dermatol Urol.* 1939;46:135–138 (in Japanese).
3. Tamura H. Pubic hair transplantation. *Jpn J Dermatol.* 1943;53:76 (in Japanese).
4. Fujita K. Reconstruction of eyebrow. *La Lepro.* 1953;22:364 (in Japanese).
5. Orentreich N. Autografts in alopecias and other selected dermatological conditions. *Ann NY Acad Sci.* 1959;83:463–479.
6. Bouhanna P. Le cuir chevelu. Les alopécies définitives et leurs traitements. Thèse de doctorat en médecine, Université Paris XII, 1976.
7. Bouhanna P, Nataf J. A propos des transplantations de cuir chevelu. Critiques et propositions. *Rev Chir Esth.* 1976;7:17–23.
8. Marritt E. Single hair transplantation for hairline refinement: A practical solution. *J Dermatol Surg Oncol.* 1984;10:962–966.
9. Limmer BL. Elliptical donor stereoscopically assisted micrografting as an approach to further refinement in hair transplantation. *J Dermatol Surg Oncol.* 1994;20:789–793.
10. Bouhanna P. Greffes à cheveux longs immédiats. *Nouv Dermatol.* 1989;8(4):418–420.
11. Rassman WR et al. Follicular unit extraction: Minimally invasive surgery for hair transplantation. *Dermatol Surg.* 2002;28:720–728.
12. Bernstein RM et al. Standardizing the classification and description of follicular unit transplantation and mini-micrografting techniques. *Dermatol Surg.* 1998;24(9):957–963.
13. Bouhanna P, Dardour JC. Autogreffes. In: *Chirurgie de la calvitie.* Paris, France: Springer Verlag; 1994: 109–167.
14. Bouhanna P, Dardour JC. Autografts. In: *Hair Replacement Surgery.* Paris, France: Springer Verlag; 1996:70–114.
15. Bouhanna P. The post-auricular vertical hair bearing transposition flap. *J Dermatol Surg Oncol.* 1984;10(7):551–554.
16. Bouhanna P. Newer techniques in hair replacement. In: Roenigk RK, Roenigk H, eds. *Surgical Dermatology. Advances in Current Practice.* London, UK: Martin Dunitz;1993:527–553.
17. Bouhanna P. Topical minoxidil used before and after hair transplantation surgery. *J Dermatol Surg Oncol.* 1989;15:50–53.
18. Bouhanna P. Androgenetic alopecia: Combining medical and surgical treatments. *Dermatol Surg.* 2003;29:1130–1134.
19. Greco J., Brandt R. The effects of autologous platelet rich plasma and various growth factors on non-transplanted miniaturized hair. *Hair Transplant Forum Int.* 2009;19(2):49–50.
20. Limmer B. The density issue in hair transplantation. *Dermatol. Surg.* 1997;23:747–760.
21. Unger WP, Shapiro R, Unger R, Unger M. *Hair Transplantation*, 5th edn. Informa Healthcare; 2011.
22. Bouhanna P. Technique personnelle de minigreffes pour le traitement de l'alopécie de la femme ménopausée. *Actualités de Chirurgie Esthétique*, SOFCEP, Mole B. Paris, France: Masson; 1992;7: 46–59.
23. Bouhanna E. Greffe capillaire: Techniques actuelles. *Real Chir Plast FACE.* 2013;2:6–10.
24. Choi YC, Kim JC. Single hair transplanting using the Choi hair transplanter. *J Dermatol Surg Oncol.* 1992;18:945–948.
25. Bouhanna P., Amgar G. Platelet-rich plasma: A therapy for hair growth. *Prime.* 2013;3(4):20–31.
26. Bernstein RM. Integrating robotic FUE into a hair transplant practice. *Hair Transplant Forum Intl.* 2012;22(6):228–229.
27. Shin JW, Kwon SH, Kim SA et al. Characteristics of robotically harvested hair follicles in Koreans. *J Am Acad Derm.* 2014;72(1):146–150.
28. Bouhanna P. Hair research and the newest micrograft techniques. *Prime.* 2011;1(2):44–57.
29. Bouhanna P. Classification plurifactorielle des alopécies androgénétiques masculines et féminines. In: *Pathologie du cheveu et du cuir chevelu.* Paris, France: Masson; 1999.
30. Bouhanna P. Multifactorial classification of male and female androgenetic alopecia. *Dermatol Surg.* 2000;26:555–561.
31. Bouhanna P. The phototrichogram and a macrophotographic study of the scalp. *Bioeng Skin.* 1985;1(3): 265.
32. Bouhanna P. Le tractiophototrichogramme, méthode d'appréciation objective d'une chute de cheveux. *Ann Dermatol Vénéréol.* 1988;115:759–764.
33. Bouhanna P. The phototrichogram: An objective technique used in hair replacement surgery evaluation. In: Unger WP, Nordström REA, eds. *Hair Transplantation*, 3rd edn, revised and extended. New York, NY: Marcel Dekker; 1995: 61–68.
34. Bouhanna P. Traitements actuels des alopécies androgénétiques masculines et féminines. *Praxis.* 1997;86:996–999.

35. Ludwig E. Classification of the types of androgenetic alopecia (common baldness) arising in female sex. *Br J Dermatol.* 1977;97:247–254.
36. Bouhanna P. Les greffes de cheveux chez les patients afro-américains. *Dermatol Pratique.* 2010;344:12–13.
37. Bouhanna P. Microgreffes de cheveux et de poils: Leurs multiples indications. *Ann Dermatol Vénéréol.* 2002;129:837–840.
38. Bouhanna P. Microgreffes de cheveux et de poils: Les nouveautés. *Nouv Dermatol.* 2010;29:441–446.
39. Bouhanna E. Traitement de l'alopécie du sourcil par greffes folliculaires. *Nouv Dermatol.* 2011;30(2):97–100.
40. Velez N, Khera P, English JC III. Eyebrow loss: Clinical review. *Am J Clin Dermatol.* 2007;8:337–346.
41. Epstein SJ. Eyebrow transplantation. *Hair Transplant Forum.* 2006;16(4):121–123.
42. Laorwong K, Pathomvanish D, Bunagan K. Eyebrow transplantation in Asians. *Dermatol Surg.* 2009;35:496–503; discussion 503–504.
43. Pathomvanish D, Imagawa K. *Hair Restoration Surgery in Asians.* Tokyo, Berlin, Heidelberg, New York: Springer; 2010.
44. Sloan DF, Huang T, Larson DL et al. Reconstruction of eyelids and eyebrows in burned patients. *Plast Reconstr Surg.* 1976;58:340–346.
45. Bouhanna P. Unidades foliculares de pelos largos (FUL) y colgajos verticales en reconstrucciones pilosas immediatas. Otras terapéuticas: Plasma autologo rico en plaquetas. In: Camacho FM, Tosti A. *Montagna tercera Edicion -Tricologia Enfermedades del foliculo pilosabaceo.* Madrid, Spain: Biblioteca Aula Medica Editions; 2014.
46. Barrera A. Uebel C. *Hair Transplantation: The Art of Micrografting and Minigrafting,* 2nd edn. St-Louis, Missouri/Boca Raton, Florida, USA: CRC Press; 2013.

16 Follicular cell implantation: Research update on "hair cloning"

Jerry E. Cooley

Ten to fifteen years ago, most hair restoration physicians believed that "hair cloning," or cultured follicular cell implantation, would have become a practical reality by now. Several decades of basic animal research established the seeming inevitability that cell therapy would become a successful treatment for androgenetic alopecia, with the attendant hope for unlimited hair. Yet, the current situation suggests that cell-based treatments are no closer to successful realization than when the author last reviewed this topic 10 years ago.[1] The present review will cover published research over the past 10 years. The basic rationale and conceptual framework for using cell therapy to treat hair loss has been discussed in prior reviews.[2–4]

Although clinical trials are underway using cultured follicular cells, no published results in humans are available at the time of this writing. Furthermore, because of the inherent commercial potential of research findings, it can be assumed that much more is known than is publicly available. While knowledge of the cellular and molecular mechanisms underpinning hair growth has progressed substantially over the past 10 years, it appears that this has not yet translated into a clinically useful method to treat hair loss in humans using cell therapy.

The basis for cell therapy began in the fundamental research of normal mammalian hair growth. It has been established that hair growth occurs because of the dynamic interaction between epidermal and mesenchymal cell populations within the hair bulb. Using the rat whisker as a model, Oliver showed that the spherical aggregate of mesenchymal cells in the bulb known as the dermal papilla (DP) could induce new follicles when removed from the whisker and subsequently implanted into skin which normally lacks follicles.[5] Carrying this research further, Jahoda showed that rat whisker dermal papilla that had been cultured in vitro could induce new hair growth when implanted into incisions in the rat ear.[6] This research, published in the mid-1980s, initiated the race to develop cell-based treatments for hair loss. In the ensuing years, several commercial ventures were launched based on the work of Oliver and Jahoda.

Over the past 10 years, we have seen two major commercial ventures fail which were based on using implanted cultured autologous DP in humans. While some increased hair growth was claimed, it was largely agreed that simply implanting cultured DP in humans did not result in clinically meaningful hair induction (i.e., no follicular neogenesis occurred). What has become increasingly clear is that methods that routinely induce new hair follicles in mice and rats are largely unsuccessful in humans.

A third commercial venture is based on using not cultured dermal papilla, but the adjacent mesenchymal dermal sheath "cup" cells (DSC). This is based on the research of McElwee, who showed that implantation of cultured DSC cells from mouse whiskers could be injected into the ear, resulting in "colonization" of the dermal papilla of ear hair follicles with whisker cells programmed to produce thicker hair.[7] Early reports from clinical trials using cultured DSC in humans suggest it is safe and may produce some hair thickening. Rather than causing true follicular neogenesis, it appears that implantation of DSC cells may simply lead to the thickening of existing hair.

It is important to note here that no published reports exist of reproducible de novo hair follicle induction in humans (i.e., the formation of entirely new hair follicles in alopecic skin). What the current commercial ventures mentioned above do appear to show is that implantation of cultured follicular cells may result in clinically apparent thickening of native hair follicles. Whether these implanted cells incorporate into the structure of the native follicle and survive cycling or whether they merely secrete stimulatory factors that transiently promote thicker hair is an important distinction. If it is the former, then such a treatment may represent a true breakthrough in alopecia treatment with long-lasting or permanent effects. If it is the latter, then the expense of cell-based treatment may not justify the temporary benefits. Furthermore, the increasing popularity of injecting platelet-rich plasma (PRP) for hair loss,[8,9] as well as an injectable treatment under development containing growth factors secreted by cultured neonatal fibroblasts,[10] may produce similar gains at a fraction of the expense, without the burdensome regulatory requirements of cell therapy.

ANIMAL RESEARCH AND STUDY MODELS

These commercial ventures have their origin in basic research conducted on rats or mice. The seminal studies by Oliver and Jahoda were based on manipulating dissected rat vibrissa (whisker) which later proved cumbersome and limiting as research methods became more advanced. Over the years, more refined models have been developed which have allowed researchers to study the intricate inner workings of follicular neogenesis. Interestingly, the follicular neogenesis models that have been developed to study hair growth are now being retooled for cell therapy, with the goal of creating hair follicles in vitro first and then implanting these into areas of alopecia.

For many years, the silicon chamber model, pioneered by Ulrich and Yuspa[11] was the dominant model used by researchers in this area. Dermal and epidermal cells, either fresh or cultured, could be combined in full-thickness wounds on the backs of immunodeficient mice and covered with a bell-shaped silicon chamber that confines and protects the cells; after 1 week, the chamber is removed and new hair growth is apparent within 3 weeks. There are numerous variations on this technique, all of which can consistently and successfully produce hair growth via follicular neogenesis (Figure 16.1).

Qiao created a "flap graft" model that dispensed with the need for the chamber, allowing implantation of trichogenic dermal and epidermal cells below a flap of host skin.[12] This model still required the implantation, and subsequent removal, of a silicone sheet. Stenn developed a "patch assay" that consisted of injecting dermal and epidermal cells subcutaneously into immunodeficient mice. The resulting "hair ball" consists of hair bulbs located centrally with hair growth occurring radially outward.[13]

Almost all in vitro models have relied on mouse, usually embryonic, as the source of cells. It has been noted by researchers that successful hair follicle induction using mouse or rat cannot necessarily be translated into success using human cells. Although Stenn and colleagues reported success with their "patch assay" using adult human dermal cells, it is important to note that the epidermal cells were from human fetuses and the host was immunodeficient mice.[14]

One report stands alone in using only adult human cells and tissue. Krugluger described a human skin organ model in which injections of human DP and epithelial cells resulted in follicle induction and growth of vellus-type hair.[15] However, no follow-up studies from this group, or using this technique, have been reported in the many years since its original publication.

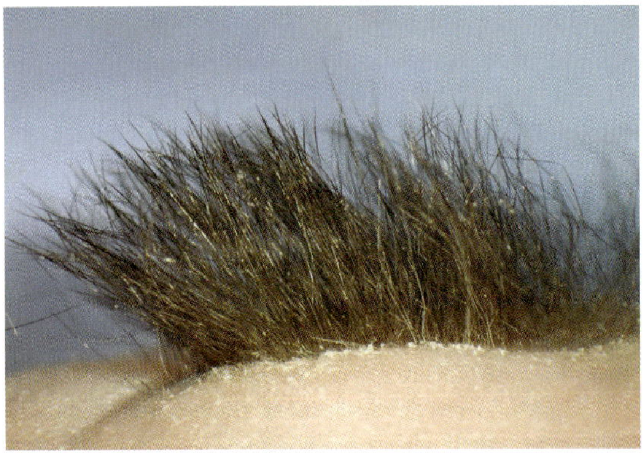

Figure 16.1 **Hair growth via follicular neogenesis can be consistently achieved in mice by a variety of methods using combinations of mesenchymal and epithelial cells. In this case, cultured dermal papilla and neonatal keratinocytes were combined in a protected chamber on the back of an immunodeficient mouse, followed several weeks later by abundant hair growth.**

CELL CULTURING CONDITIONS

Early experiments clearly showed that culturing conditions determined the success of dermal papilla-induced follicle morphogenesis. Cultured dermal papilla gradually lose their inductive ability as they are passaged and expanded in culture. Yoshizato showed that the presence of keratinocytes or keratinocyte conditioned media could keep cultured DP inductive through many passages.[16] Subsequent to this, it was found that the factors present in conditioned media were soluble WNT proteins excreted by keratinocytes[17] whose primary function appears to be keeping beta-catenin in the DP active, which is essential for maintaining inductive potential.[18]

In addition to the presence of soluble WNT factors to keep beta-catenin in cultured DP active, it has been found that three-dimensional culture conditions favor subsequent follicle induction over standard two-dimensional techniques.[19] Several reports have shown that cultured DP cells are more inductive when coaxed to aggregate into spheres rather than as the standard monolayers present in two-dimensional culture.[20–22] There is a growing consensus that these "3D" culture systems are superior to older "2D" methods.

CELL IMPLANTATION TECHNIQUE

While the techniques used by various researchers can be rather confusing, they can basically be divided into four distinct approaches (Figure 16.2). When the first reports of successful follicle induction in animals using cultured cells were released in the mid-1980s, it was assumed that not only would success in humans follow shortly, but that the envisioned treatment would consist of injections of dissociated cells directly into the scalp, where they would induce the formation of new follicles. Over the past 10 years, it has become increasingly clear that injection of dissociated dermal cells, with or without epidermal cells, is largely unsuccessful in inducing new follicle formation in humans.

Many reports using animal models have appeared focusing on modifying and augmenting the method of culture and implantation. The rationale is that by optimizing the culture and delivery of cells, follicle induction will be successful in humans. One report describes the comparative success of different implantation techniques on hair regeneration when using cultured DP alone (no epidermal cells). Cultured rat DP placed directly beneath the host epidermis using the "hemi-vascular sandwich" technique showed superior hair induction.[23] These researchers claimed that this technique allowed use of dissociated DP cells alone, and that success was due to

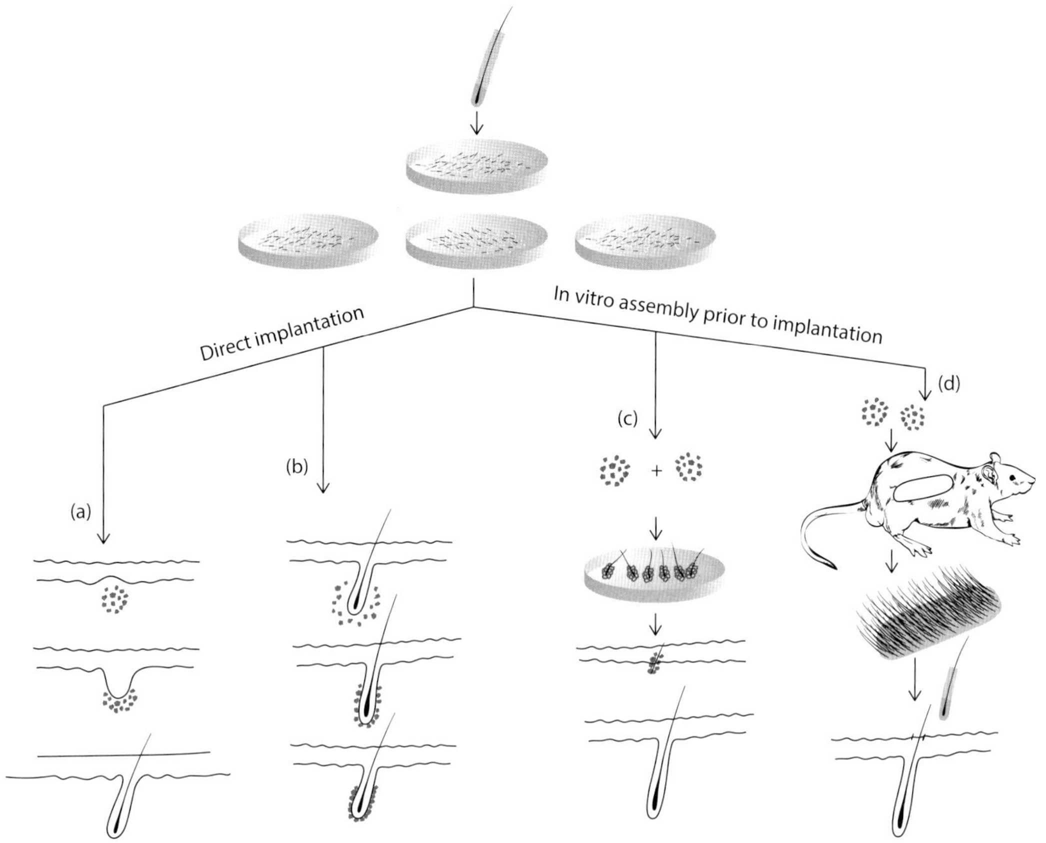

Figure 16.2 **Treating hair loss using follicular cell implantation may mean different approaches depending on the research team. Initially, the simplest approach that was tried involved injecting dissociated cultured dermal papilla (with or without keratinocytes) in an effort to stimulate follicular neogenesis (a). This approach has so far proved unsuccessful in humans. Animal evidence has suggested specific types of mesenchymal cells at the base of the follicle, called dermal sheath cup cells, can be injected into the skin and will attach to preexisting follicles, conferring the properties of the injected cells on the native follicles (b). This approach is currently in clinical trials. Another approach is to take cultured epithelial and mesenchymal cells and combine them using sophisticated in vitro incubation methods, spurring the creation of "proto-hairs," which can then be implanted (c). Perhaps the most promising technique to date involves taking cultured cells and implanting them into immunodeficient mice to serve as intermediate hosts. Once follicular neogenesis has occurred, mature hair follicles are harvested and implanted similar to modern-day hair transplantation techniques (d). See text for more detailed explanations of each approach.**

contact between DP cells and host epidermal cells as well as better oxygenation of the implanted cells.

TOWARD A NEW PARADIGM

Current research appears to be leading toward a treatment paradigm where dermal and epidermal cells are combined for a period of time *before* implantation. Since it is becoming clear that implantation of cultured cells does not lead to follicle neogenesis in vivo, researchers are attempting to create the follicles in vitro and then transplant these. In a method reported by Qiao, mouse dermal and epidermal cells were cocultured prior to implantation, resulting in the formation of primitive "proto-hairs" which could be subsequently transplanted, resulting in growth of mature, cycling hair.[24] It bears repeating that this involved animal cells, not human.

Along these lines, Lindner described the creation of "neo-papilla" using cultured human DP and components of extracellular matrix, followed by coculture with human keratinocytes and melanocytes. This resulted in the formation of in vitro follicles with vellus-like hair shaft growth.[25]

Similarly, Tsuji and colleagues reported that cultured DP and epidermal cells could be combined in a collagen gel to create a "bioengineered follicle germ," which could then be transplanted along with a fine suture which serves as a guide for follicle directionality and connection to the outside epidermis, thus preventing cyst formation.[26] When transplanted into the hairless skin of mice, these bioengineered "hair germ" grafts took root and produced hair, and analysis of these hair follicles showed all correct layers of normal follicles and accessory structures including connection with surrounding host tissue (i.e., arrector pili muscles and nerve fibers).[27] Normal hair cycling occurred, confirming the presence of necessary stem cell populations within the new hair follicles.

Furthermore, these researchers reported similar success using adult human follicle stem cells (DP and bulge region-derived epithelial cells), which may represent an important breakthrough. In a variation of their method, they implanted the bioengineered hair germ into the subrenal capsule of mice, providing a protected, vascularized space for induction to occur. After 2 weeks, mature hair follicles were seen in clusters and could be harvested for subsequent transplantation as one- and two-hair follicular units.[28] They suggested that these bioengineered hair grafts could be used in a manner similar to follicular unit transplantation (FUT). One might envision a treatment where the patient's follicles are shipped to the lab, where the cells are dissected out and multiplied in cell culture using the latest techniques in 3D culture, then combined in surrogate mice where follicular neogenesis occurs, after which the follicles are harvested and shipped back to the surgeon where they can be implanted via the FUT technique.

Finally, mention should be made of the latest developments in stem cell research which may affect follicular cell implantation for hair loss. Research models, as mentioned, frequently use neonatal keratinocytes which are rich in stem cells. In an autologous cell therapy for hair loss, adult keratinocytes will be needed, and in particular those with "bulge" stem cell properties. Xu recently reported the ability to generate these bulge stem cells from induced pluripotent stem cells using specified cellular signaling factors.[29] And Vacanti recently reported the ability to create pluripotent stem cells from somatic cells using acidic culture conditions.[30] This breakthrough suggests that nonstem somatic cells have the potential to convert into stem cells if given the right cues. Together, these research findings suggest that the requisite population of stem cells can be created through exogenous signals and culturing conditions prior to combining them for in vitro follicular neogenesis. While exciting, it should also be noted that, if successful, such maneuvers will greatly increase the complexity of a follicular cell implantation procedure, meaning many more years of testing and development. One major concern is that these implanted stem cells are not tumorigenic.

CONCLUSION

Follicular cell implantation for hair loss remains an exciting possibility, but true hair multiplication is a long way off from practical reality in the clinic. Cell-based treatments may come online first as "hair thickening" treatments, where periodic scalp injections produce modest clinical gains similar to finasteride and minoxidil. True hair follicle neogenesis in humans has proven far more complex than that which has been routinely carried out in rats and mice, but intricate models are now being developed which keep alive the dream of unlimited hair.

REFERENCES

1. Cooley J. Follicular cell implantation: An update on "hair follicle cloning." *Facial Plast Surg Clin N Am.* 2004;12:219–224.
2. Teumer J, Cooley J. Follicular cell implantation: An emerging cell therapy for hair loss. *Sem Plast Surg.* 2005:19(2):189–196.
3. Stenn K, Parimoo S, Zheng Y et al. Bioengineering the hair follicle. *Organogenesis.* 2007:3(1):6–13.
4. Higgins CA, Christiano AM. Regenerative medicine and hair loss: How hair follicle culture has advanced our understanding of treatment options for androgenetic alopecia. *Regen Med.* 2014:9:101–111.
5. Oliver RF. The experimental induction of whisker growth in the hooded rat by implantation of dermal papillae. *J Embryol Exp Morphol.* 1967;18:43–51.
6. Jahoda CA, Horne KA, Oliver RF. Induction of hair growth by implantation of cultured dermal papilla cells. *Nature.* 1984;311:560–562.
7. McElwee KJ, Kissling S, Wenzel E, Huth A, Hoffmann R. Cultured peribulbar dermal sheath cells can induce hair follicle development and contribute to the dermal sheath and dermal papilla. *J Invest Dermatol.* 2003;121:1267–1275.
8. Greco J, Brandt RJ. Preliminary experience and extended applications for the use of autologous platelet rich plasma in hair transplantation surgery. *Hair Transplant Forum Int.* 2007;17(4):131.
9 Park KY, Kim HK, Kim BJ, Kim MN. Platelet-rich plasma for treating male pattern baldness (letter). *Dermatol Surg.* 2012;38(12):2042–2044.
10. Zimber MP, Ziering C, Zeigler F et al. Hair regrowth following a Wnt- and follistatin containing treatment: Safety and efficacy in a first-in-man phase 1 clinical trial. *J Drugs Dermatol.* 2011;10(11):1308–1312.
11. Weinberg WC, Goodman LV, Morgan GC, Ledbetter S, Yuspa SH, Lichti U. Reconstitution of hair follicle development in vivo: Determination of follicle formation, hair growth and hair quality by dermal cells. *J Invest Dermatol.* 1993;100:229–236.
12. Qiao J, Philips E, Teumer J. A graft model for hair development. *Exp Dermatol.* 2008;17:512–518.
13. Zheng Y, Du X, Wang W, Boucher M, Parimoo S, Stenn K. Organogenesis from dissociated cells: Generation of mature cycling hair follicles from skin-derived cells. *J Invest Dermatol.* 2005;124:867–876.
14. Zheng Y, Nace A, Chen W et al. Mature hair follicles generated from dissociated cells: A

universal mechanism of folliculoneogenesis. *Dev Dyn*. 2010;239(10):2619–2626.
15. Krugluger W, Rohrbacher W, Laciak K, Moser K, Moser C, Hugeneck J. Reorganization of hair follicles in human skin organ culture induced by cultured human follicle-derived cells. *Exp Dermatol*. 2005;14:580–585.
16. Inamatsu M, Matsuzaki T, Iwanari H, Yoshizato K. Establishment of rat dermal papilla cell lines that sustain the potency to induce hair follicles from afollicular skin. *J Invest Dermatol*. 1998;111(5):767–775.
17. Kishimoto J, Burgeson RE, Morgan BA. Wnt signaling maintains the hair-inducing activity of the dermal papilla. *Genes Dev*. 2000;14:1181–1185.
18. Soma T, Fujiwara S, Shirakata Y, Hashimoto K, Kishimoto J. Hair-inducing ability of human dermal papilla cells cultured under Wnt/β-catenin signalling activation. *Exp Dermatol*. 2012;21(4):307–309.
19. Higgins CA, Richardson GD, Ferdinando D, Westgate GE, Jahoda CA Modelling the hair follicle dermal papilla using spheroid cell cultures. *Exp Dermatol*. 2010;19(6):546–548.
20. Osada A, Iwabuchi T, Kishimoto J, Hamazaki TS, Okochi H. Long-term culture of mouse vibrissal dermal papilla cells and *de novo* hair follicle induction. *Tissue Eng*. 2007;13(5):975–982.
21. Young TH, Lee CY, Chiu HC, Hsu CJ, Lin SJ. Self-assembly of dermal papilla cells into inductive spheroidal microtissues on poly(ethylene-co-vinyl alcohol) membranes for hair follicle regeneration. *Biomaterials*. 2008;29(26):3521–3530.
22. Huang YC, Chan CC, Lin WT et al. Scalable production of controllable dermal papilla spheroids on PVA surfaces and the effects of spheroid size on hair follicle regeneration. *Biomaterials*. 2013;34(2):442–451.
23. Aoi N, Inoue K, Kato H et al. Clinically applicable transplantation procedure of dermal papilla cells for hair follicle regeneration. *Tissue Eng Regen Med*. 2012;6(2):85–95.
24. Qiao J, Turetsky A, Kemp P, Teumer J. Hair morphogenesis in vitro: Formation of hair structures suitable for implantation. *Regen Med*. 2008;3(5):683–692.
25. Lindner G, Horland R, Wagner I et al. *De novo* formation and ultra-structural characterization of a fiber-producing human hair follicle equivalent in vitro. *J Biotechnol*. 2011;152(3):108–112.
26. Nakao K, Morita R, Saji Y et al. The development of a bioengineered organ germ method. *Nat Methods*. 2007;4(3):227–230.
27. Toyoshima KE, Asakawa K, Ishibashi N et al. Fully functional hair follicle regeneration through the rearrangement of stem cells and their niches. *Nat Commun*. 2012;3:784.
28. Asakawa K, Toyoshima KE, Ishibashi N et al. Hair organ regeneration via the bioengineered hair follicular unit transplantation. *Sci Rep*. 2012;2:424.
29. Yang R, Zheng Y, Burrows M et al. Generation of folliculogenic human epithelial stem cells from induced pluripotent stem cells. *Nat Commun*. 2014;5:3071.
30. Obokata H, Wakayama T, Sasai Y et al. Stimulus-triggered fate conversion of somatic cells into pluripotency. *Nature*. 2014;505(7485):641–647.

17 Platelet-rich plasma and stem cells

Gilbert Amgar, Joseph Greco, and Fabio Rinaldi

INTRODUCTION

Autologous cellular therapy is a medical paradigm that allows the safe use of our own cells to enhance surgical and nonsurgical procedures in the treatment of hair loss diseases.

Regenerative growth factors and stem cells in our body modulate the rate of repair that other healing cells perform. Think of them as the maestro leading the orchestra into a beautiful musical piece, first directing the horns to play, then calling the strings to join in, all the time, regulating the flow, depth, and tempo.

PLATELET-RICH PLASMA (PRP)

Currently, autologous platelet-rich plasma (PRP) has been used in diverse indications for more than 30 years with effective results. The first publication on this subject goes back to 1975[1] and deals with the use of platelets as physiological adhesives in corneal surgery. Since then, the literature has widely supported and covered their functions and effects. Most specialties were interested in PRP when a repairing process was necessary: Osseous regeneration in dental surgery,[2] healing of ulcers in diabetic patients,[3] large-scale burns,[4] in orthopedics,[5] in rheumatology, in sports medicine,[6,7] and in plastic surgery (cosmetology). There have been numerous reviews of published literature regarding autologous cellular therapy use in wound care, and Carter et al. published a 10-year systemic review and meta-analysis that included strict protocol inclusion of 24 peer-reviewed published papers from 8577 citations on acute and chronic wounds.[8] In 1996, biology showed a positive effect of growth factor on the hair follicle.[9] Since that time, this process has increasingly been used by physicians.

Definition: Physiology

Platelets are small particles without nucleus, coming from the fragmentation of the megacaryocytes. Their life span is about 10 days. They contain granulations. The morphology of the platelets changes when they become activated: They became round, with pseudopods, and they release alpha granules, within which those growth factors are stored. More than 60 factors have been identified.[10] The secretion begins 10 minutes after activation, and 95% of the factors are secreted in the first hour.

The most important growth factors for hair applications are (Table 17.1):

Table 17.1 Most Important Growth Factors for Hair Applications

Growth Factors	Area	Effect
PDGF	Epithelial cells and sebaceous glands of hair follicles	Hair canal formation
VEGF	Vascular plexus in dermal papilla	Improve follicle vascularization
EGF	Epithelial cells and fibroblast	Improve the ratio of anagen High doses of EGF can induce regression of the follicle
IGF 1	Keratinocytes	Slow down apoptosis
FGF	Keratinocytes and endothelial cells	Promote the anagen phase
NGF	Perifollicular neurogenic	Modulating effect on the hair depending on the receptor with which it interacts

- PDGF (platelet-derived growth factor) stimulates the growth of dermal mesenchyme.[9]
- VEGF (vascular endothelial growth factor) increases vascular permeability. The hair follicle is an avascular structure. The growth of hair depends on the vessel capillaries that form the vascular plexus in dermal papilla.[11]
- EGF (epidermal growth factor) stimulates mitosis on epithelial cells and fibroblasts, and improves the ratio of anagen. EGF inhibits the entry in the catagen phase, promoting the anagen phase.[12]
- IGF-1 (insulin-like growth factor) regulates at the cellular level the expression of a powerful messenger anti-apoptotic capable of preventing cell death.[13]
- FGF (fibroblast growth factor) stimulates the proliferation and differentiation of keratinocytes and endothelial cells.[14]
- NGF (nerve growth factor) stimulates hair growth and slows apoptosis. NGF has a modulating effect on the hair depending on the receptor with which it

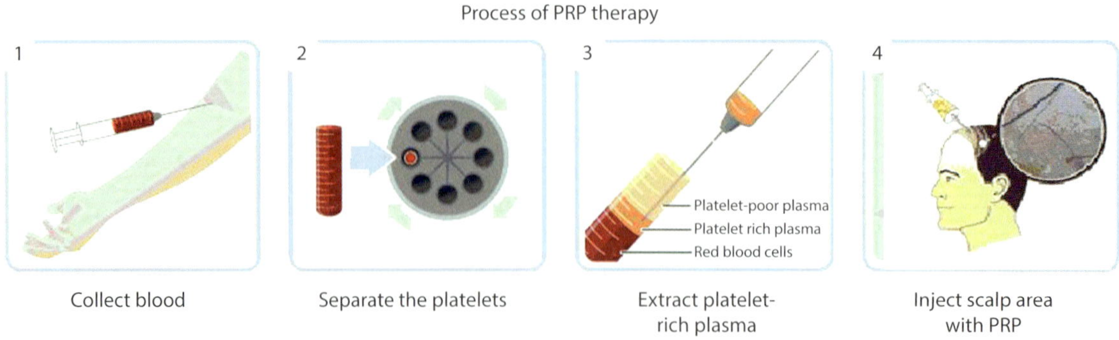

Figure 17.1 **General process for PRP extraction.**

interacts.[13] NGF acts also as a stress mediator. This is certainly a good way to explain the stress and hair loss correlation.[15]

Preparing procedure

The procedure to obtain PRP begins by doing a blood sample on an anticoagulated tube (Figure 17.1). Then tubes are centrifuged for about 5 to 10 minutes at 600–1200 G. (Speed and time depend on the kit protocol.) According to their density, the red cells go down in the tube (Figure 17.2). On the upper part, we find the plasma and the platelets. We usually talk about PRP when we have a concentration three to seven times normal standards.

The patient must sign an informed consent describing the procedure, the contraindications, the expected benefits, and the possible side effects.

The contraindications are cervicofacial cancer history, hematologic diseases, pregnancy, active local infection, and anticoagulant treatment. We have to pay attention to history of allergies because activated platelets also release histamine.

Application fields

In 2012, an in vivo animal study conducted by Li showed that the injection of activated PRP into the skin of mice once every 3 days for 3 weeks greatly stimulated hair growth. According to the results, PRP increased hair growth and hair follicle survival due to its promotion of cell proliferation and its anti-apoptotic properties. Thus, PRP can potentially prolong the anagen phase of the hair growth cycle.[16]

For humans, the three principal applications fields are androgenic alopecia (AGA), alopecia areata, and surgical procedures.

ANDROGENIC ALOPECIA

The prevalence of progressive AGA approaches 50% of Caucasian men and women beyond the age of 40; whereas in Asian, Native American, and African American men the prevalence is lower and AGA is less severe.[17]

Four studies bring us interesting results concerning PRP and androgenic alopecia.

The first from Rinaldi and Co[18] is an in vitro study realized on 50 patients. Twelve follicles were taken from each patient, four follicles were divided in PRP, four in Ringer solution, and four in standard solution. Then, the mitotic activity was measured. The result shows a significant increase of mitotic activity and reduction of apoptotic process in the PRP group.

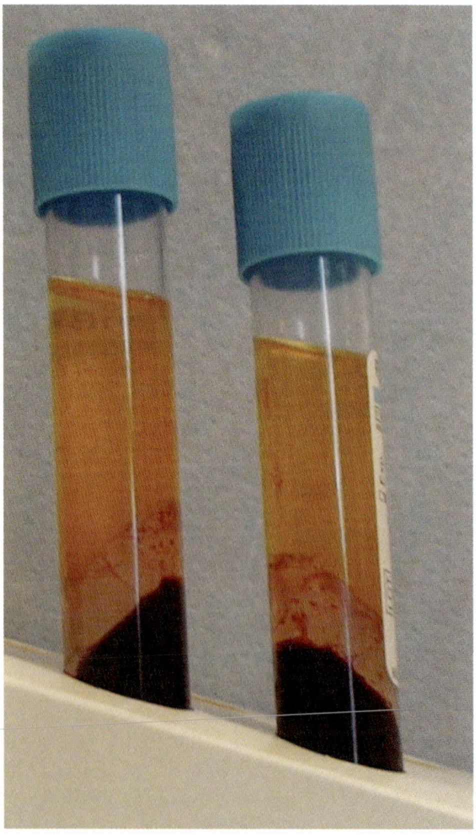

Figure 17.2 **Once centrifuged.**

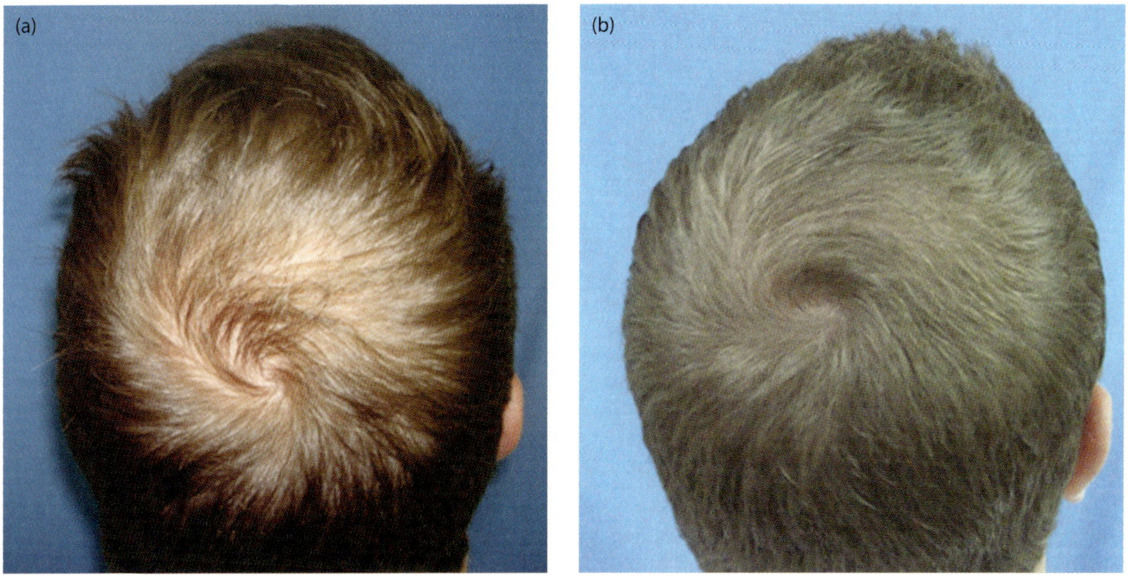

Figure 17.3 **Male androgenic alopecia. (a) Before and (b) 8 months after PRP session. (Courtesy of Dr. Greco.)**

The study by Kiyosawa and Co[19] was conducted on 26 volunteers with thin hair who received five local treatments. They were evaluated for 12 weeks. Areas were photographed and digitally measured. The result shows that PRP improves the density 16% at 12 weeks.

In another study, Greco and Brandt[20] show that traumatizing and infusing growth factors into the scalp reversed miniaturization over an 8-month period when compared to control. Ten hair samples were taken from each patient, five patients in the control group (CG) and five patients from the treatment group (TG). Hair diameter was measured with a Starrett micrometer.

The CG demonstrated a 2.8% average decrease in hair shaft diameter at 4 months and 3.5% decrease at 8 months. (This is the classical evolution of androgenic alopecia.) An increase of 9.7% in average hair shaft diameter at 4 months and then 6.1% at 8 months was observed in the TG (Figure 17.3).

A recent evaluation conducted by Amgar and Bouhanna brings objective parameters for the human scalp[21] (Figures 17.4 through 17.6). Seventy patients (male and female) were included. They all got digital measurement (Figure 17.7) (tattoo mark, hair density, caliber, and terminal/vellus ratio) and standard photographs. Blood, 60 cc, was drawn, and 10 cc of PRP was processed without any activation. The scalp was first traumatized with a 1.5 mm micro needling roller. Patients got two sessions with 3 months between them. At 3 months, they observed a density variation of 19.7%. That means [(third-month density–initial density)/initial density]. At 6 months,

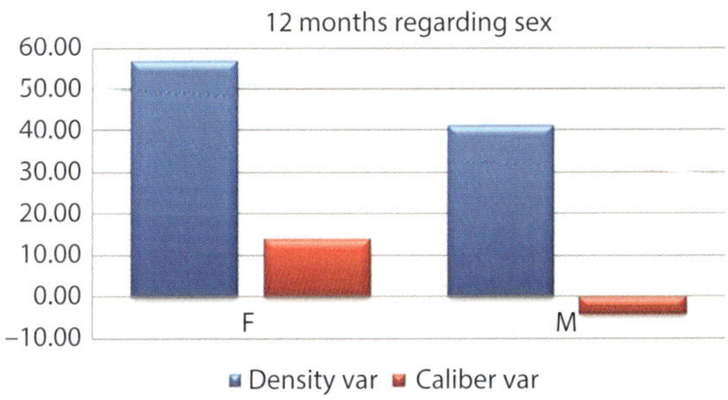

Figure 17.4 **Twelve months density and caliber variation in male and female study—two PRP sessions with 3 months between them.**

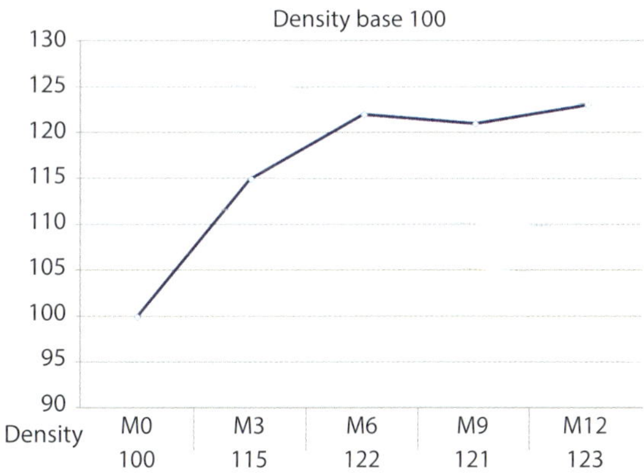

Figure 17.5 **Twelve months density variation in base 100.**

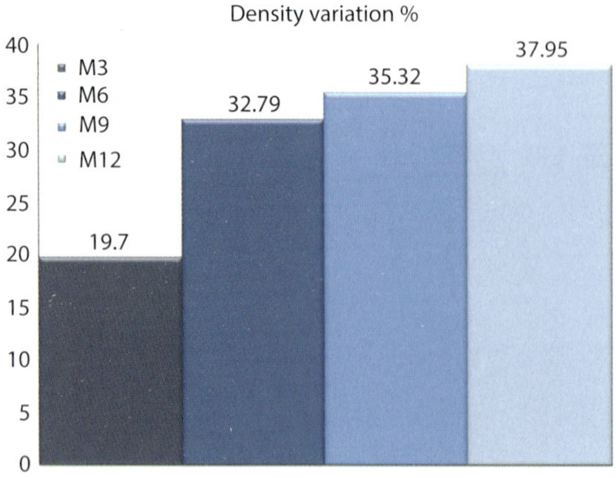

Figure 17.6 **Twelve months density variation.**

density variation reached 32.79%, and it was 38% at 12 months. The other way to evaluate the yield of this method is to report the result to a base 100 (as if every patient had 100 hairs/cm^2 at day 0). The yield is 23%.The mean caliber did not show variation, but if we separate the male and female population we observe an improvement for women. We can also observe that this curve is not linear but logarithmic. That caused the authors to think that they did not create new follicles but just saved from apoptosis some follicles that were unable to provide a hair. Once the capability is recovered, an annual session can maintain it.

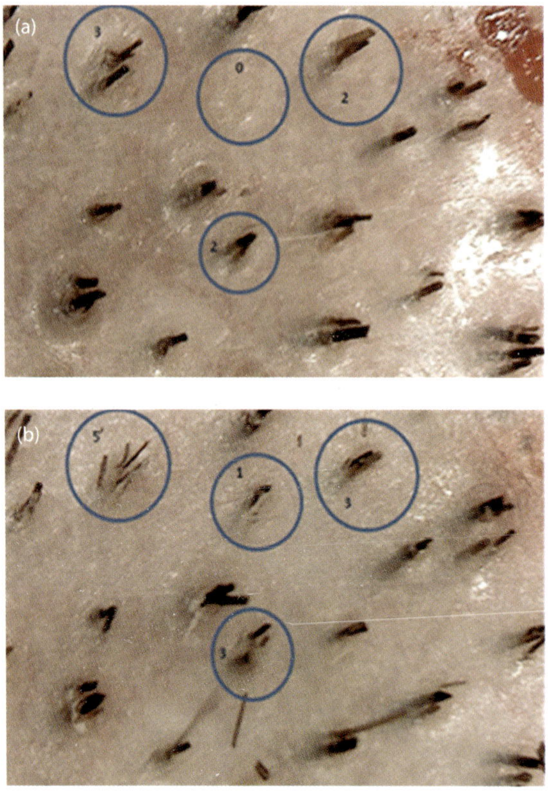

Figure 17.7 **(a) Before and (b) 3 months after PRP session. (Courtesy of Dr. Amgar and Dr. Bouhanna.)**

ALOPECIA AREATA

Alopecia areata (AA) is the most common condition to cause inflammation-induced hair loss, having a calculated lifetime risk of 2% (Figures 17.8 and 17.9).[22] It is characterized by well-demarcated patches of hair loss, which can progress to complete loss of hair from the scalp (alopecia totalis) or from the whole body in severe cases (alopecia universalis).[23] Most patients are relatively young, and the disease burden is commonly substantial, leading to overwhelming effects on the patient's quality

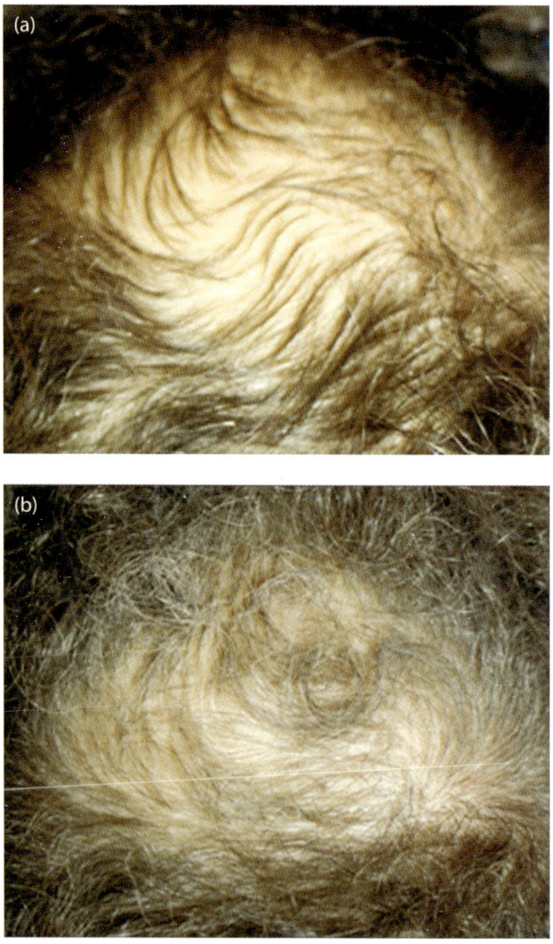

Figure 17.8 **Male androgenic alopecia. (a) Before and (b) 9 months after two PRP sessions. (Courtesy of Dr. Amgar and Dr. Bouhanna.)**

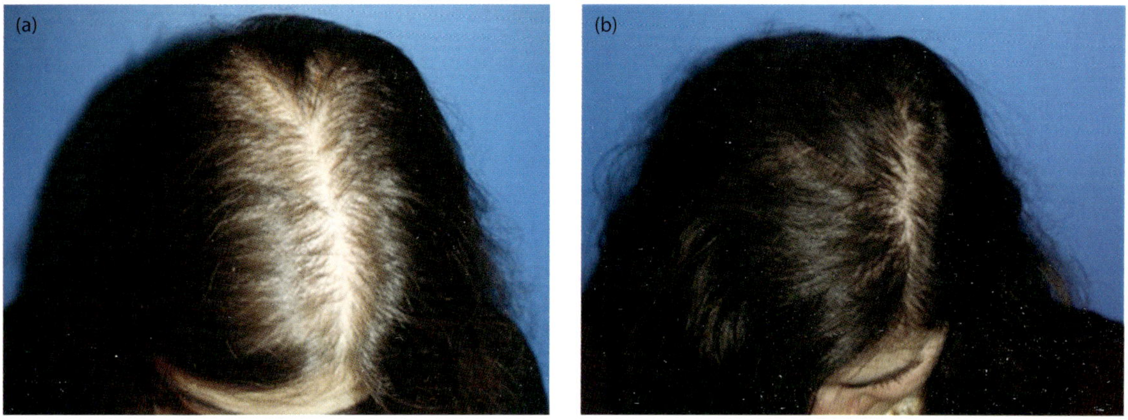

Figure 17.9 **Female androgenic alopecia. (a) Before and (b) 9 months after two PRP sessions. (Courtesy of Dr. Amgar and Dr. Bouhanna.)**

of life and self-esteem. It is considered an organ-specific autoimmune disease, stemming from loss of the hair follicle's (HF) immune privilege; therefore, therapies are mostly immunosuppressive. Nevertheless, treatment is still a challenge in AA, and no treatment is either curative or preventive.[24] Finding new therapies for this condition, and improving effectiveness of existing therapies, are therefore of utmost importance.

Platelet rich plasma (PRP) is an autologous preparation of platelets in concentrated plasma.[16] It has been investigated in several disciplines in medicine for its role in wound healing, especially orthopedics and dentistry.[25] Recently, it has also been found to be beneficial in dermatology, for example in acne scarring, wound healing, and fat transplantation. It has also been shown to promote hair survival and growth, both in vitro and in vivo.[16,26]

Rinaldi et al. conducted a randomized, double-blinded, placebo and active-controlled, half-head, parallel group study to evaluate the effects of PRP on AA in vivo and showed that PRP administration leads to major improvements in AA lesions (Table 17.2), with 60% of patients achieving complete remission at study termination. Currently, triamcinolone acetonide[27] is considered as the treatment of choice for patch-stage AA.[28]

The PRP is known to contain more than 20 different growth factors, which are important in promoting cell proliferation and differentiationn.[19] These properties are thought to lead to its beneficial effects on acne scarring[29] and wound healing.[30] More recently, the role of PRP in promoting hair growth has also been investigated. Uebel et al. have shown that storing hair grafts in PRP can enhance graft survival, improve hair density, and stimulate growth of transplanted follicular units.[26] Still, the mechanisms by which PRP exerts its effects on HFs are still obscure. A recent study has shown in vitro that PRP increases the proliferation of dermal papillae cells and activates the signaling pathways' extracellular signal-regulated-kinase and Akt.[25] Additionally, fibroblast growth factor-7 and beta catenin, which are both stimulators of HF growth, were stimulated after PRP administration. Our study gives further support to the growth-promoting effect of PRP in hair, by providing evidence that levels of Ki-67, a marker for cell proliferation, are increased after PRP administration in humans.

In addition to its proliferation-inducing effects, PRP is a potent anti-inflammatory agent, which can suppress cytokine release and thereby limit local tissue inflammation.[31] Since AA is characterized by an extensive inflammatory infiltrate, responsible for secretion of a variety of inflammatory cytokines, it is probable that the anti-inflammatory effects of PRP may be of great benefit in this condition.

Taken together, this study suggests PRP as a new treatment modality for AA, being a safe and a more efficient alternative for TrA, the current treatment of choice for AA. However, further controlled and randomized studies are needed to validate our findings in a larger cohort of patients.

TRANSPLANTATION SURGERY

The primary use for PRP in hair restoration surgery demonstrated an increased follicular yield when utilized as a graft storage medium by Uebel, and similar studies in hair transplant surgery by Perez-Meza demonstrated the positive use of autologous growth factors for wound healing and hair growth.[32–34] In 2007, Greco and Brandt suggested expanding the use of PRP in all aspects of hair restoration surgery.[35]

THE ROLE OF GROWTH FACTORS AND HAIR

Growth factors are present in the bulge area, where stem cells are found, and they interact with cells of the matrix, thus activating the proliferative phase of the hair. Stem

Table 17.2 Evaluation Parameters of AA Patches after Treatment with Placebo, TrA or PRP

	Placebo		TrA		PRP	
	Untreated	Treated	Untreated	Treated	Untreated	Treated
SALT score						
T1	4.87	4.93	3.27	13.2***###	4.33	25.6***###†††
T2	6.2	5.33	5.8	18.8***###	5.73	27.6***###†††
T3	5.93	7.27	5.07	23.8***###	6.13	40.73***###†††
Dermoscopic evaluation						
T0	2.67	2.67	2.6	2.6	2.67	2.6
T1	2.67	2.73	2.53	1.53***###	2.8	1.4***###†††
T2	2.13	2.6	2.67	1.27***###	2.6	0.8***###†††
T3	2.6	2.47	2.07	1.2***##	2.4	0.53***###†††
Burning/itching sensation						
T0	2.6	2.6	2.67	2.8	2.73	2.73
T1	2.33	2.67	2.47	1.07***###	2.47	0.53***###†††
T2	2.33	2.53	2.53	0.4***###	2.6	0.07***###†††
T3	2.4	2.6	2.67	0.2***###	2.27	0.07***###†††
Ki-67 levels						
T0	13.15	13.55	13.65	13.72	13.21	12.75
T1	15.53	19.84	13.72	32.37##	12.94	50.06***###
T2	17.61	19.81	13.81	35.59##	12.75	55.79***###†
T3	20.68	21.83	12.23	37.39##	12.88	69.09***###†

Note: Evaluation scores at four time points: T0 = beginning of study, T1 = 2 months, T2 = 6 months, T3 = 1 year. N = 15 for each treatment modality.
Student t test, $^{***}p < 0.001$ when compared to placebo; $^{\#\#}p < 0.01$, $^{\#\#\#}p < 0.001$ when compared to untreated side of the scalp; $^{\dagger}p < 0.05$, $^{\dagger\dagger\dagger}p < 0.001$ when compared to TrA treatment.

cells are more primitive and of ectodermal origin; they give origin to the epidermal cells and the sebaceous glands. Cells of the dermal papilla, which are found at the capillary base, are of mesenchymal origin. Both cells need each other, and when they interact through the action of various growth factors, they will give rise to the future follicular unit.

The main function of platelet-derived growth factor is to stimulate cell replication (mitogenesis) of healing-capable stem cells. It also stimulates cell replication of endothelial cells. This will cause budding of new capillaries into the wound (angiogenesis), a fundamental part of all wound healing. In addition, PDGF seems to promote the migration of perivascular healing-capable cells into a wound and to modulate the effects of other growth factors.

Numerous studies and practical applications have demonstrated how growth factors are essential for regulating the cellular events involved in wound healing by attracting cells to the wound, stimulating proliferation, and significantly influencing matrix deposition.[36]

The TGF-beta is extremely important because it affects most aspects of tissue wound repair, namely, initiation and termination, and promotes differentiation and proliferation.[37] The PDGF improves dermal regeneration, acts locally to promote protein and collagen synthesis, causes endothelial migration or angiogenesis,[38] and induces the expression of TGF-beta.[39]

METHOD OF USE IN HAIR RESTORATION SURGERY

Phase I: Harvesting

PRP in donor site strip harvesting and follicular unit transplantation FUT

After the subcuticular layer is closed with 3 Monocryl, PRP gel is injected into the wound edges from end to end. The second layer is approximated with a running 3 Prolene suture, and PRP is then injected back into the wound (Figure 17.10).

PRP in follicular unit extraction follicular unit transplantation FUE

Since individual follicular units are extracted in the FUE procedure, PRP is injected into the donor site before extraction to promote hemostasis. After all follicular units are extracted a platelet gel is then covered over the extraction sites and a Sylon dressing is applied for 24

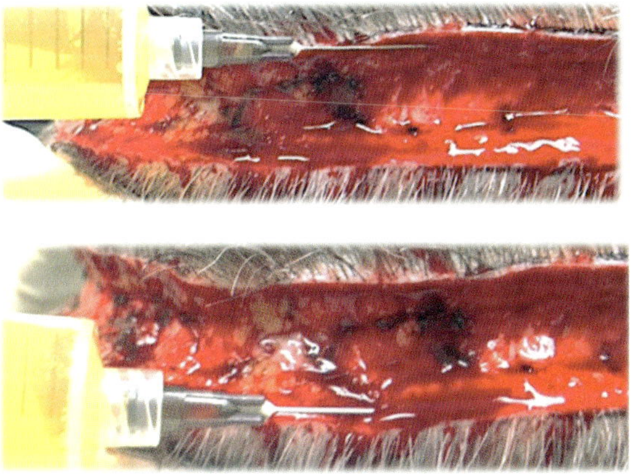

Figure 17.10 **Injections of PRP at both skin edges.**

hours with a bandage to promote more rapid healing of the extraction sites (Figures 17.11 and 17.12).

Phase II: Grafts cultured in PRP

After the follicular units are dissected, they are cultured and bathed in PRP prior to implantation so the growth factors can attach to the stem cells in the bulge region of the dissected follicular units[33] (Figure 17.13).

While dissection is ongoing and the graft design pattern is completed, the PRP is then injected into the recipient scalp area to maximize the effects of the growth factors on hair (Figure 17.14).

The growth factors in PRP provide an enriched environment to promote angiogenesis. In 2001, Yano identified VEGF as a major mediator of hair follicle growth and cycling, providing the first direct evidence that the improved follicle vascularization promotes hair growth and increases follicle and hair size[11] (Figure 17.15).

The latest studies conclude that autologous growth factors demonstrate a considerable effect on the time of hair follicle formation and the yield of hair follicle reconstitution, and higher levels of growth factors were more effective at 15% versus lower levels at 2% or control at 0%.[40]

Injecting PRP into the recipient area (Figure 17.16), may have other advantages for the nontransplanted hairs. This patient had hair transplantation in the frontal half of his head and his crown was injected with 10 mL of 15% PRP and no hair transplantation was done. Notice the miniaturized hair in the crown at 9 months after PRP injections.

In the final analysis, this author's experience utilizing PRP in all phases of hair restoration surgery the past 7 years has been positive. Autologous growth factors in PRP enhance the procedure by (1) decreasing scaring and promote preservation of the donor site, (2) increase the yield of grafts, (3) and promote hair follicle reconstitution.[40]

STEM CELLS

In recent years, adult human hair follicle neogenesis has been an important target in regenerative medicine, both for biological research and clinical interest (Table 17.3). Starting from the studies of the inductive capacity of the intact dermal papilla to produce new follicle formation in recipient human skin, much research has been developed to find other biological sources for hair follicle neogenesis.[41,42]

For this reason, stem cells have been studied for their therapeutic potential in many medical fields, and in hair treatment. Stem cells and regenerative medicine applications evolved rapidly during the last years, especially thanks to the use of adipose tissue-derived stromal cells (SVF and ADSC).

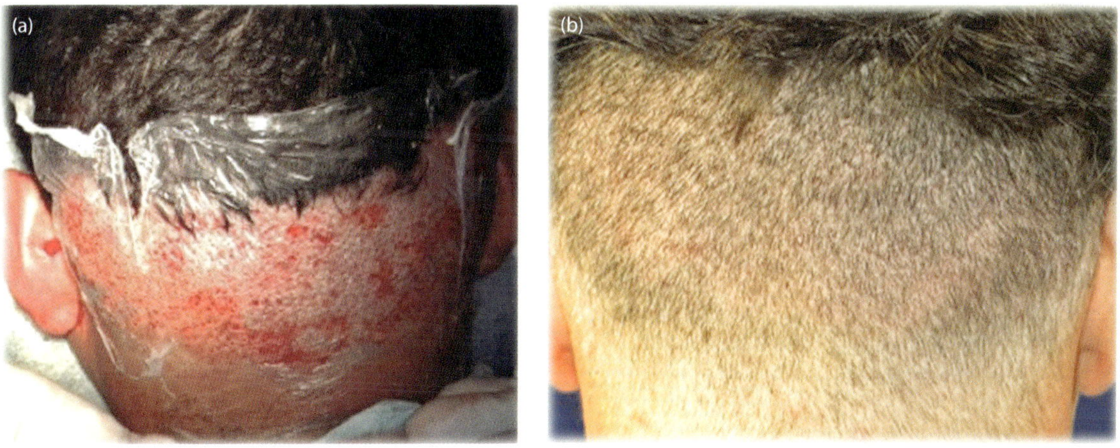

Figure 17.11 **PRP/Sylon dressing applied (a) post-op and at (b) day 7.**

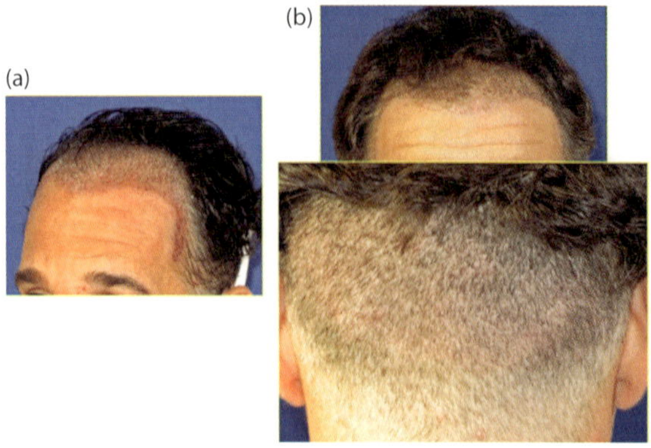

Figure 17.12 **PRP-FUE patient at 1 week. (a) Recipient area and (b) donor area.**

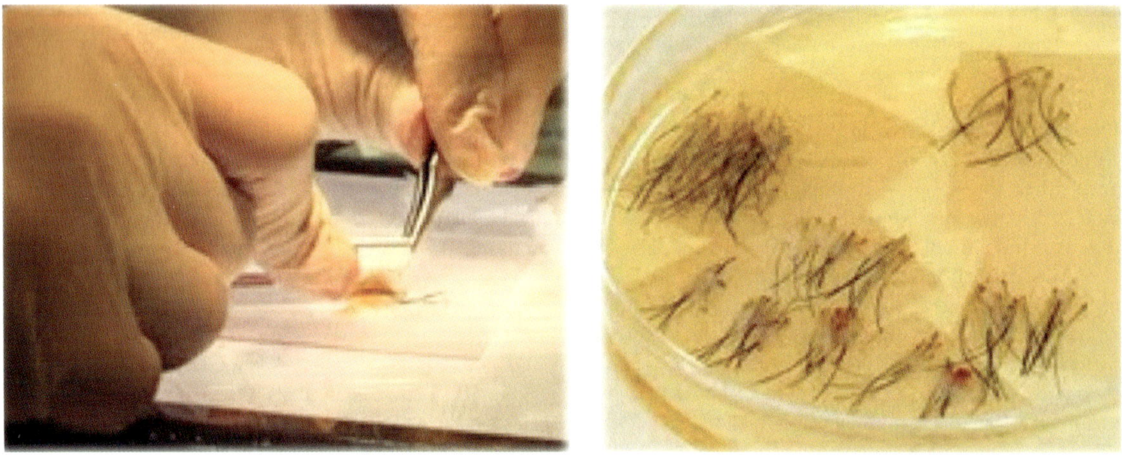

Figure 17.13 **Follicular units cultured in PRP.**

Stem cells are undifferentiated biological cells that can differentiate into specialized cells that can undergo mitosis to produce more stem cells. Stem cells can be divided into two main groups[43]:

- Embryonic stem cells, derived from the epiblast tissue of the inner cell mass of blastocyst (early stage embryo, 4–5 days old in humans, consisting of 50–150 cells).[44]
- Adult stem cells, derived from various tissues of child as well as adult organisms.

Embryonic stem cells are pluripotent and give rise during development to all cell types of the three primary germ layers: ectoderm (nervous system and skin), endoderm, and mesoderm.

At the moment there are no approved medical treatments using embryonic stem cells.

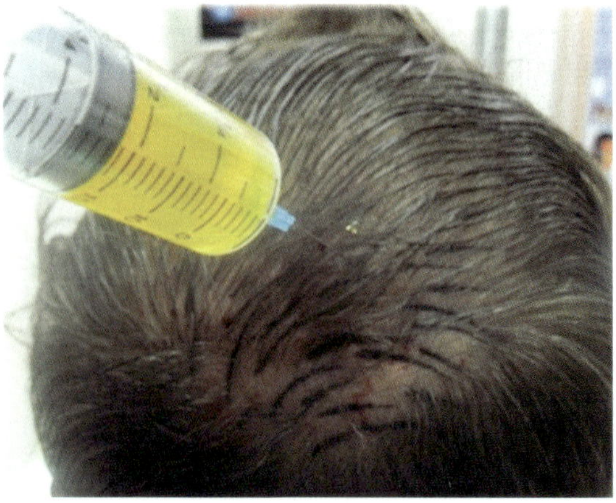

Figure 17.14 **PRP injected into the recipient's scalp.**

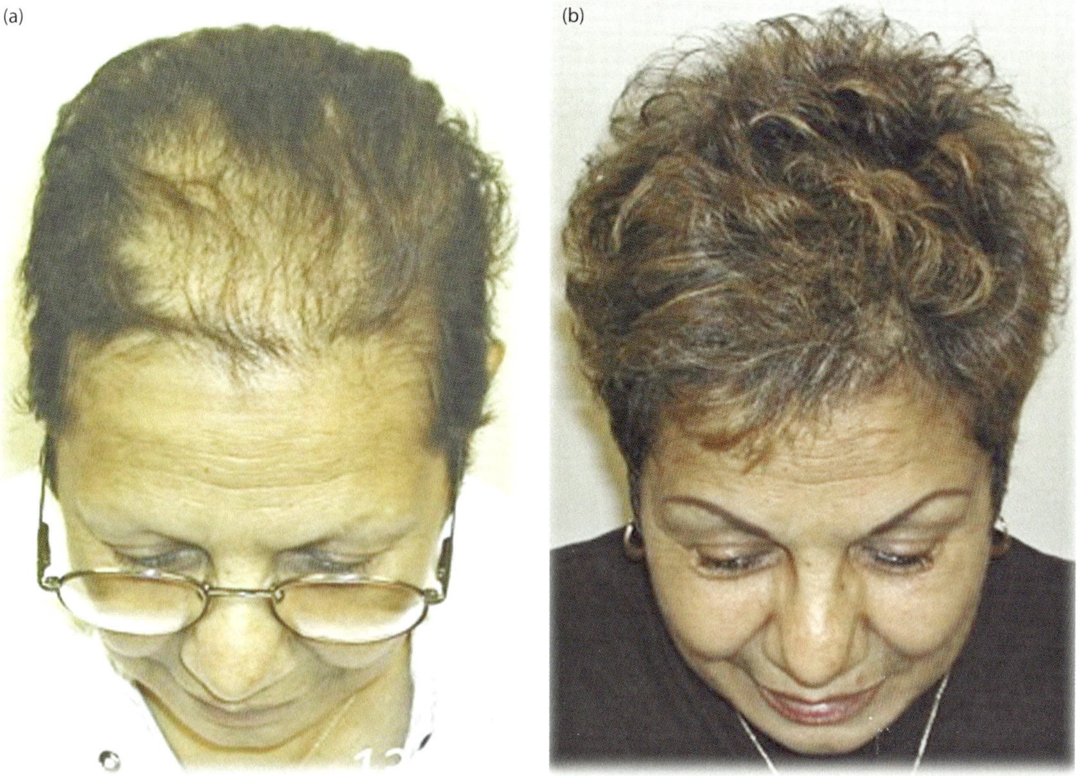

Figure 17.15 PRP-Surgical combination. Result of PRP hair transplantation at 9 months. This Ludwig III female patient did not have a dense hair character and this is her result at 9 months. (a) Before and (b) after.

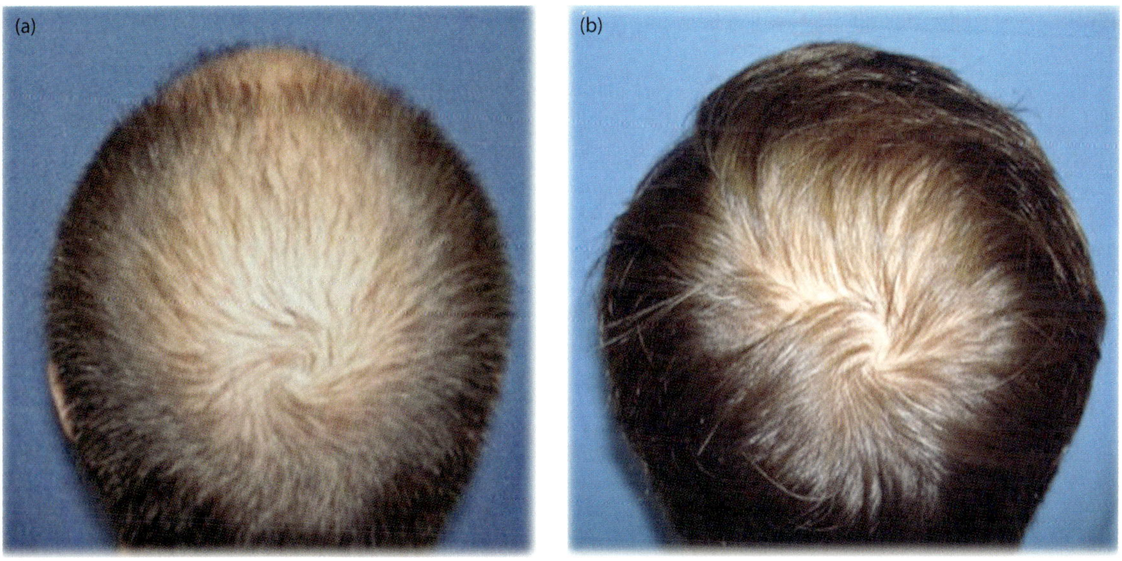

Figure 17.16 Male androgenic alopecia. (a) Before and (b) after 9 months PRP injections in posterior crown.

Table 17.3 Stem Cells Properties

Self-Renew: Several Cell Mitosis, Maintaining the Undifferentiated State	Asymmetric Replication
Potency: capacity to differentiate into specialized cell types	Stochastic differentiation Totipotent SC Pluripotent SC Multipotent SC Oligopotent SC Unipotent SC

Source: Adapted from Pittenger MF et al. *Science*. 1999;284 (5411):143–147.

Fetal stem cells located in the organs of the fetus are referred to as fetal stem cells.

Adult stem cells can be found in children and adults and can be pluripotent and multipotent stem cells[45,46]:

- Pluripotent stem cells in humans are small in number and can be found in umbilical cord blood, amniotic fluid, and bone marrow.
- The typical adult stem cells, present in many tissues, are multipotent (lineage restricted), and they only can originate the same differentiated cell types from the tissue of origin. Many adult stem cells have been identified:
  - Hematopoietic stem cells, differentiate into all mature blood cells.
  - Neural stem cells, differentiate into neurons, astrocytes, and oligodendrocytes.
  - Mesenchymal stem cells differentiate into fibroblasts, adipocytes, osteoblasts, chondrocytes, and skeletal muscle cells.[47]

Many other stem cells have been identified, although they are not yet well characterized.

Adult stem cells in research and therapy have been used for many years, especially in the treatment of leukemia and related bone cancers and blood cancers through bone marrow transplants.[48]

Recently, autologous stem cell transplantation has been proven to be effective and to have broad prospects in regenerative medicine.[49]

Many studies have shown that adipose-derived stem cells (ADSCs) have surface markers and gene profiling similar to bone marrow-derived mesenchymal stem cells (BMSCs) (the most effective mesenchymal stem cells). ADSCs have their own capacities of multidirectional differentiation, weak immunogenicity, lack of morbidity at the donor site, contrary to BMSCs.[49]

It has been proven that ADSCs can enhance wound healing by promoting collagen synthesis and the migration of dermal fibroblasts.[50,51] ADSC transplantation induces neovascularization in the ischemic myocardium, and the skin flaps by paracrine vasculogenesis promoting growth factors.[52] Histologic examination of skin in animals has shown that ADSCs transplantation increased the number of blood vessels to support sufficient oxygen and nutriments to the newly formed tissue.[53]

Because of its abundance and its easy sampling, performing a small liposuction from the lower abdomen or thighs, adipose tissue is a rich source of ADSC. It represents a significant alternative to bone marrow mesenchymal stem cells, even though the frequency of ADSC is higher in adipose tissue than that of mesenchymal stem cells in bone marrow.

Therefore, ADSCs have great potential for accelerating skin growth. In adipose tissue, ADSCs are localized in the periendothelial layer of the blood vessel. After collagenase digestion, 1×10^5, ADSCs could be harvested from a human lipoaspiration of 20 mL of fat.[54]

Then, via plastic adhesion, the cells could be expanded to purification. By the later stages of culture, 90% of the adherent cells assume a more homogeneous profile with consistently high levels of stromal markers. It has been shown that ADSCs secrete VEGF, FGFb, EGF, hepatocyte growth factor, transforming growth factor, and KGF. Among these factors, VEGF and FGFb are the most important factors in angiogenesis. After FGFb stimulates angiogenesis, VEGF regulates the proliferation and inhibits the apoptosis of endothelial cells.[55–57]

From these data, it has been rational to try to use ADSCs and SVF in hair treatment.

Adipose-derived stem cells (ADSCs), or sometimes adipose-derived stromal cells, must be distinguished from the crude stromal vascular fraction (SVF). After the extraction of adipose tissue by lipoaspiration from the body, fat must be treated by collagenase digestion to obtain crude SVF.[49]

The SVF is highly heterogenous and contains many cell types, including mature adipocytes, a mixture of endothelial cells, smooth muscle cells, fibroblasts, mast cells, pericytes, a reservoir of immature stromal cells, and hematopoietic cells (up to 20% of total fraction). The SVF is a complex fraction that contains ADSCs (5%–10% more or less) but cannot be defined as a stem cell or mesenchymal stem cell fraction. The ADSCs should be named only the fraction containing the isolated and expanded ADSCs.[49]

Once collected, fat tissue is processed to isolate the SVF using different medical devices able to separate ADSCs from adipose tissue particles (via enzymatic digestion or via mechanical separation). The SVF must be immediately injected in the recipient area[58] (Figure 17.17).

An adipose tissue sample obtained by liposuction is processed to obtain purified ADSCs, and then banked for subsequent cellular expansions in order to obtain a large number of cells stored for further treatments.[59]

Today ADSC can be applied in treatments for which fat transplantations already occur, giving results 10 times

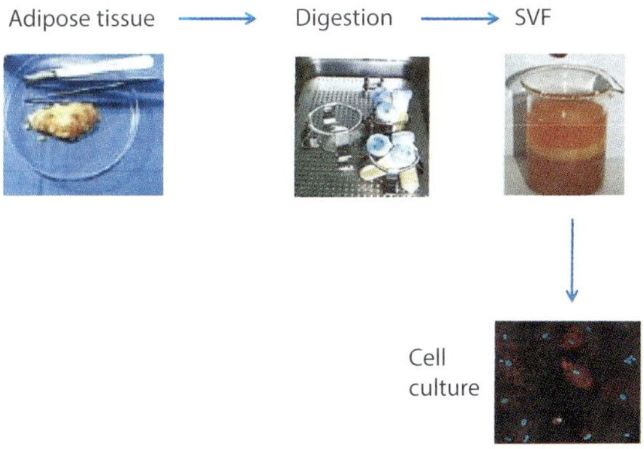

Figure 17.17 **Schema: fat tissue is processed to isolate the SVF.**

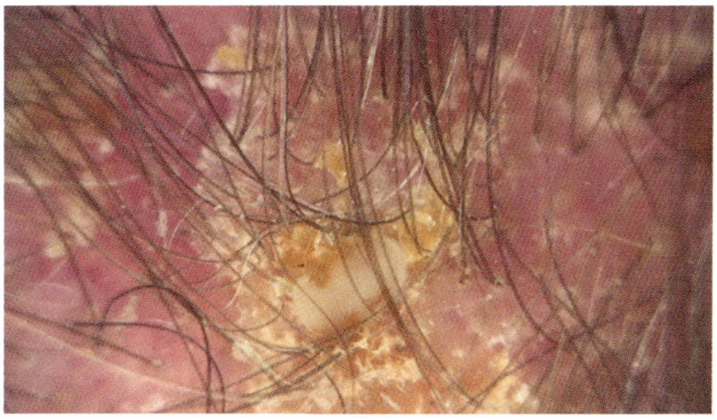

Figure 17.18 **Infectious and necrotic reaction.**

higher in aging, burns, scars, breast augmentation, wound healing, wrinkle correction, and breast reconstruction.[60]

The ADSC demonstrated strong angiogenic features in ischemic hind limb, myocardial infarction, and wound healing. In this field they seem to be more efficient than their bone marrow counterpart; they also have the ability to modulate immune and inflammatory functions, probably mediated via paracrine activity.

Research on Crohn disease reported that expanded ADSC are more efficient than the freshly prepared in controlling inflammation and improving healing processes, and the strong immunosuppressive effects of ADSC lead to a planned trial in multiple sclerosis.[49]

There is quite a rich literature on the use of ADSC for soft tissue augmentation in plastic and reconstructive surgery, but no reported experience in the treatment of hair diseases, to our knowledge.

Our personal data (not yet published) include different clinical trials on patients suffering from androgenic alopecia (Table 17.4) and alopecia areata.

In our experience in androgenic alopecia, using SVF we had three very good/good results (improvement of hair shaft diameter, improvement of anagen/telogen ratio, new hair growth) on 15 patients and 12 poor or no results. With this technique we had two patients with important side effects: in one case (Figure 17.18) we had an infectious and necrotic reaction with temporary loss of hair in the area. Infection resolved after antibiotic therapy in 14 days, and original hair regrowth occurred after 3 months.

In the other case, the patient had an unexpected patch of alopecia areata (Figure 17.19) after 22 days from the treatment. We treated this patch with topic corticosteroids, and we had resolution of AA after 2 months. This patient never suffered from AA.

Cultured ADSCs gave us a significant result with seven patients with very good/good results (same score, 46.6% improvement) with no side effects reported, after 12 months from the treatment. The hair follicle neogenesis and neangiogenesis could be the rationale of the efficacy of ADSCs in androgenic alopecia (Figure 17.20, Table 17.5).

Table 17.4 Androgenic Alopecia

	SVF	ADSCs
# Patients, men, II–IV Hamilton	15	15
Score efficacy (average)	Very good: 1 patient Good: 2 patients Poor : 3 patients No result: 9 patients	Very good: 4 patients Good: 3 patients Poor : 3 patients No result: 5 patients
Side effects	1 patient: infection 1 patient: onset of one patch of alopecia areata in the side of injection	No side effects in all patients

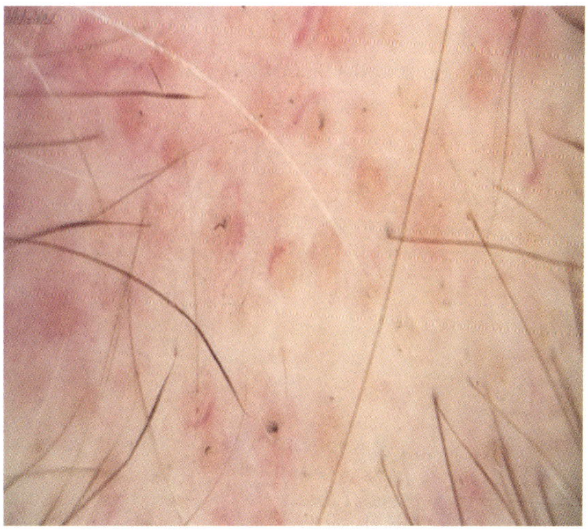

Figure 17.19 **Unexpected patch of alopecia areata.**

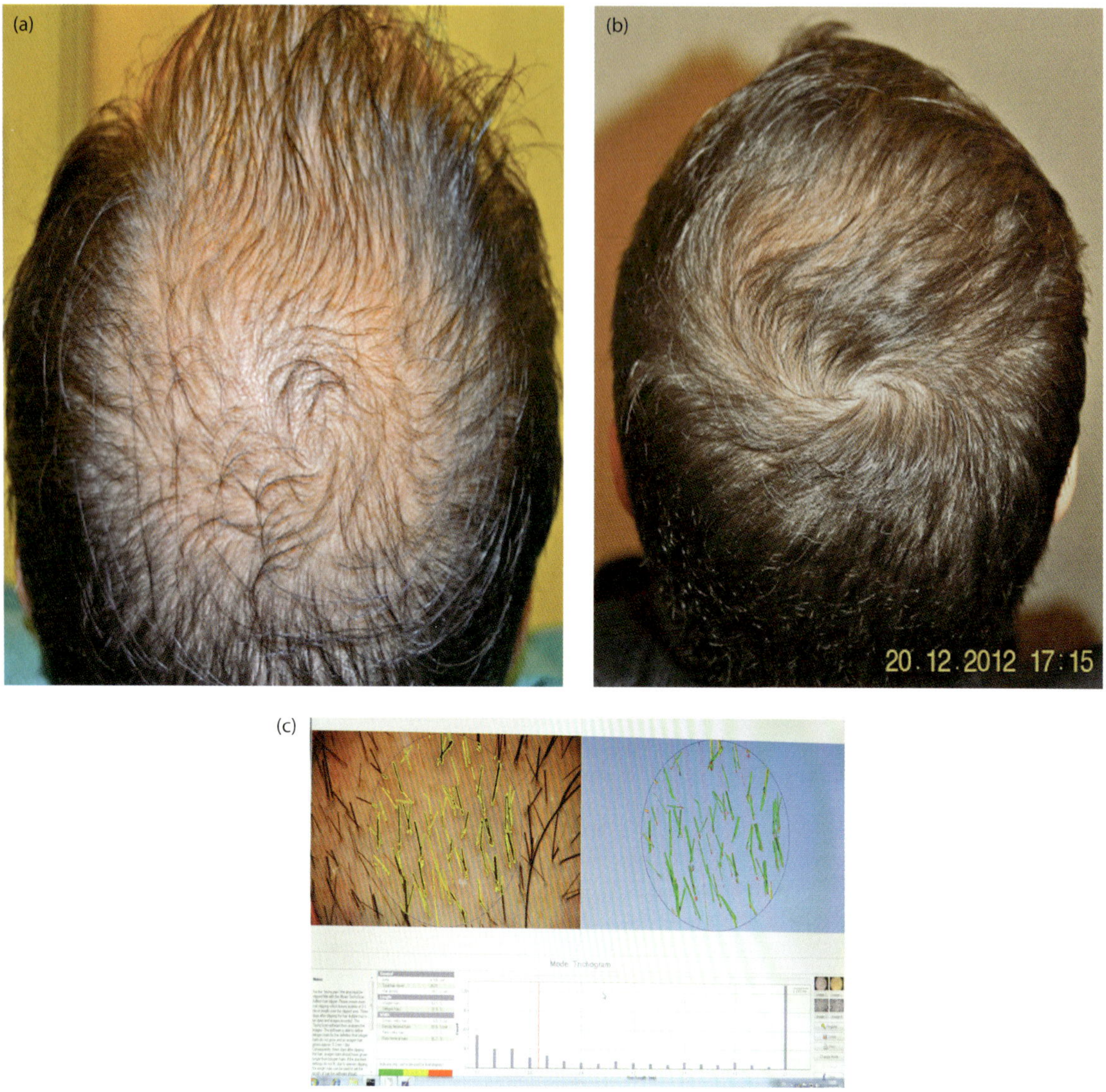

Figure 17.20 **Male androgenic alopecia. (a) Before the treatment. (b) After the treatment. (c) Trichoscan evaluation. Patient with a very good result.**

Table 17.5 Alopecia Areata

	SVF	ADSCs
# Patients, 6 men, 9 women–Chronic AA, multiple patches	15	15
Score efficacy (average)	Very good: 2 patients Good: 2 patients Poor : 1 patient No result: 10 patients	Very good: 2 patients Good: 3 patients Poor : 4 patients No result: 5 patients
Side effects	No side effects	No side effects

We need further controlled studies to verify the proper efficacy of this technique in AGA.

In alopecia areata, using VSF we had four patients with very good/good results (resolution of hair disease, 26,6%) and no side effects in all the patients (Figure 17.21), The immunosuppressive effects of ADSCs and neoangiogenesis could be the therapeutic pathway of this treatment in this autoimmune disease.[47]

The ADSCs, in alopecia areata, gave a better but non-significant result in respect to VSF, with very good/good results in five patients (resolution of hair disease, 33.3%). In this group we had five poor results, more than in the

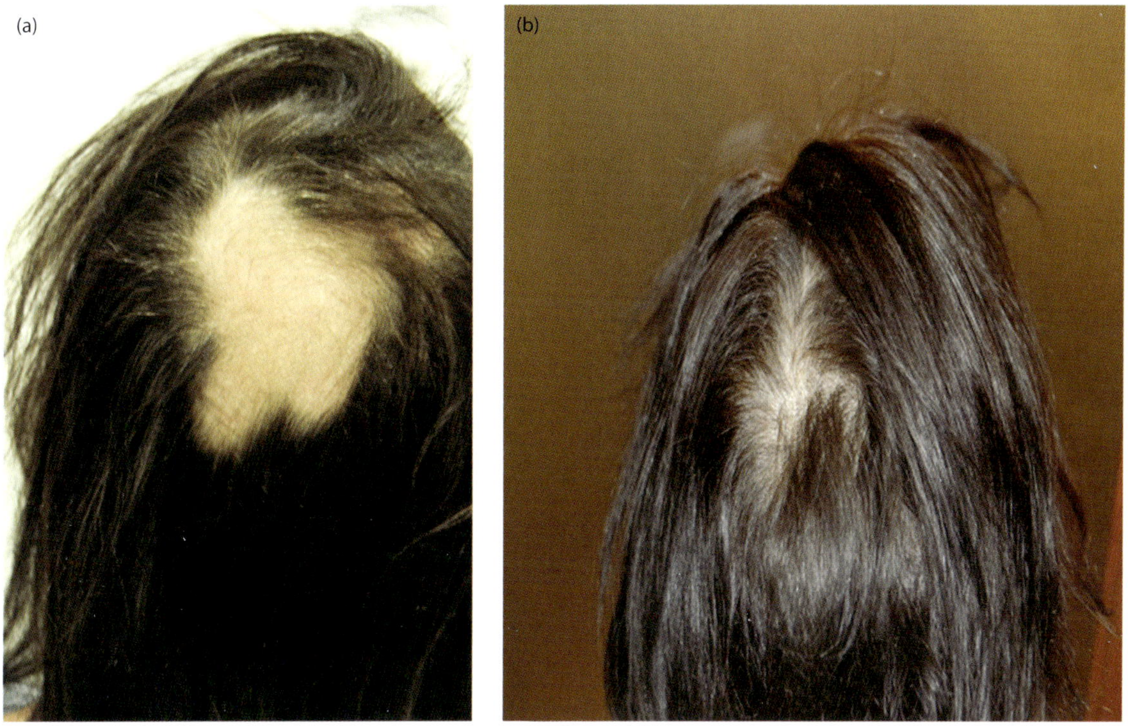

Figure 17.21 **Male androgenic alopecia. (a) Before and (b) result with stem cells treatment ADSC.**

SVF group. In no patients did we note any side effects (Figure 17.22).

We need further controlled studies to verify the proper efficacy of this technique in alopecia areata.

NEW HORIZON: DERMAL PAPILLA CLONING

Hair follicles also contain stem cells, and some researchers predict research on these follicle stem cells may lead to successes in treating baldness through the activation of already existing stem cells in the scalp.

So the second source of stem cells could be the hair follicle itself: we know that the cycling activities of the hair follicle are controlled by a group of specialized mesenchymal cells located in the dermal papilla

It was demonstrated many years ago that adult rodent dermal papilla could be removed from the hair follicle and transplanted into recipient skin, where they were able to induce de novo follicle development and hair growth. Further investigations in humans were unsuccessful because when dermal papilla cells are removed from their hair-follicle microenvironment and grown in culture, they lose key inductive properties. A recent study opens new perspectives demonstrating that in manipulating cell culture conditions in order to grow dermal papilla cells in a 3D spheroid environment, it becomes possible to induce a partial restoration of inductive capability, and that human dermal papilla cells, when grown as spheroids, are capable of inducing de novo hair follicles in human skin. It is the so called "community effect" phenomenon that occurs when groups of cells use close contact interactions to maintain their collective identity. The physical manipulation of dermal papilla is not enough to induce follicles, whose reactivation requires communications from the epidermis, surrounding adipocytes, and the whole follicle environment; each of these cues has the potential to translate to genetic changes in hair follicle and dermal papilla.[61]

SUMMARY

The most researched and publicized medical treatment available for male pattern baldness is 5% minoxidil lotion, and 2% minoxidil for female baldness. The first signs of improvement generally appear after 3 months of therapy. The side effects of minoxidil are minimal, but include itching, eczema, and hypertrichosis (the latter is more common in female patients). For male baldness, finasteride taken orally and daily (1 mg) works by inhibiting the 5α-reductase from forming DHT. The decreased DHT levels allow some intermediate follicles to enlarge and regrow normal terminal hairs. Side effects may include decreased libido. Cyproterone acetate (in Europe) can effectively block the increased levels of male hormones that cause hair loss in some women. Spironolactone (in

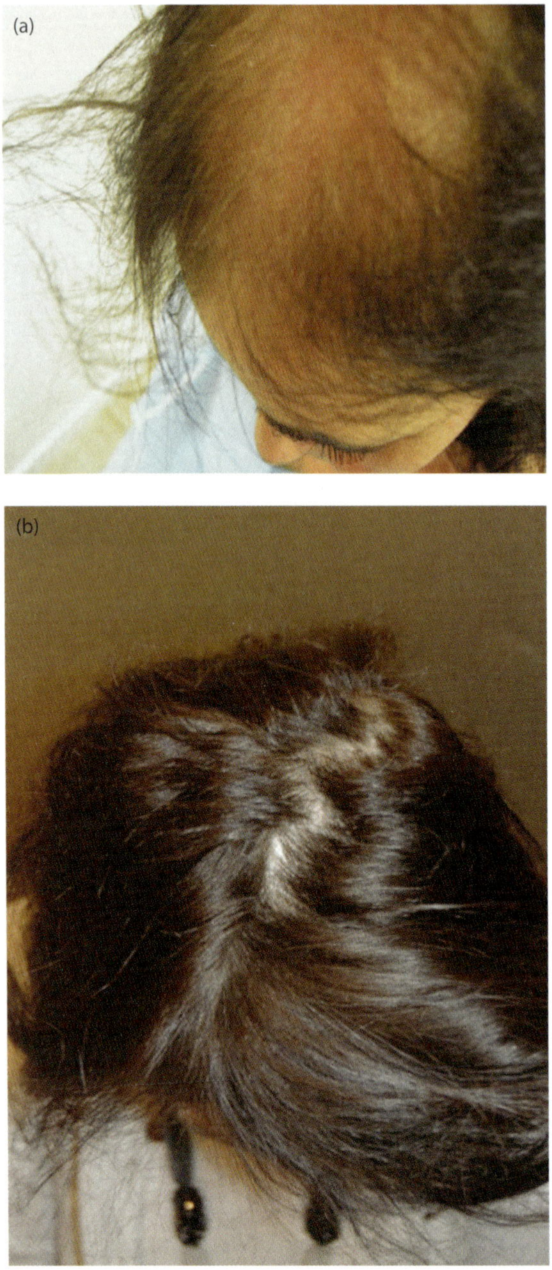

Figure 17.22 **Female androgenic alopecia. (a) Before and (b) result with stem cells treatment SVF.**

the United States) appears to be a competitive inhibitor of DHT-receptor binding.

The medical treatment has to be daily, and if the patient stops, the enhancement soon disappears. Also, many dermatologists do not agree to long-term prescriptions with hormonal therapy. New interest in preventing hair loss and baldness has been stimulated by cellular therapy, which normalizes hair loss and reverses hair miniaturization of male and female baldness. The actual protocol is two sessions with 3 months between them and then once every year.

We have to keep in mind that the PRP does not generate new follicles, it just helps to recover and stimulate follicles in apoptosis. It allows us to save a heritage that seemed lost and keep it. This is the reason why this treatment must be started early (at stage 3 for men and stage 2 for women).

The PRP is an interesting alternative for patients who cannot benefit from classical treatment (side effects) or do not want to take long-term hormonal therapy.

During the past 7 years, the authors have performed over 5000 surgical and nonsurgical treatments utilizing autologous PRP in hair loss treatments and have not incurred any adverse side effects. In the final analysis, the use of biologic cellular therapy may be the safest, most versatile, promising paradigm in hair restoration. While this may, or may not be true, only time and critical review will tell.

REFERENCES

1. Rosenthal AR, Harbury C, Egbert PR, Rubenstein E. Use of a platelet-fibrinogen-thrombin mixture as a corneal adhesive: Experiments with sutureless lamellar keratoplasty in the rabbit. *Invest Ophthalmol.* 1975;14(11):872–875.
2. Marx RE, Carlson ER, Eichstaedt RM, Schimmele SR, Strauss JE, Georgeff KR Platelet-rich plasma: Growth factor enhancement for bone grafts. *Oral Surg Oral Med Oral Pathol Oral Radiol Endod.* 1998;85:638–646.
3. Wieman TJ, Smiell JM, Su Y. Efficacy and safety of a topical gel formulation of recombinant human platelet-derived growth factor-BB (becaplermin) in patients with chronic neuropathic diabetic ulcers. A phase III randomized placebo-controlled double-blind study. *Diabetes Care.* 1998;21:822–827.
4. Raffoul W, Guerid S, Darwich S, Berger M, Hayoz D, Benathan M. Impact of platelets concentrate and keratinocyte suspension on wound healing—A prospective randomized trial. ResearchGate, 2008.
5. Bhanot S, Alex JC. Current applications of platelet gels in facial plastic surgery. *Facial Plastic* Surg. 2002;18:27–33.
6. Peerbooms JC, Sluimer J, Bruijn DJ, Gosens T. Positive effect of an autologous platelet concentrate in lateral epicondylitis in a double-blind randomized controlled trial: Platelet-rich plasma versus corticosteroid injection with a 1-year follow-up. *Am J Sports Med.* 2010;38(2):255–262.
7. Mishra A. Treatment of chronic elbow tendinosis with buffered platelet-rich plasma. *Am J Sports Med.* 2006;34(11):1774–1778.
8. Carter MJ, Fyling CP, Parnell LK. Use of platelet rich plasma gel on wound healing: A systematic review of meta-analysis. *J Plastic Surg.* 2011;11:e38.

9. Takakura N, Yoshida H, Kunisada T, Nishikawa S, Shin-Ich. Involvement of platelet derived growth factor receptor-a in hair canal formation. *J Invest Dermatol.* 1996;107:770–777.
10. Mazzucco BL. Tissue regeneration and in loco administration of platelet derivatives: Clinical outcome heterogeneous products and heterogeneity of the effectors mechanisms. *Transfusion.* 2005;45(11): 1759–1767.
11. Yano K, Brown L, Detmar M. Control of hair growth and follicle size by VEGF-mediated angiogenesis. *J Clin Invest.* 2001;107(4):409–417.
12. Mak, King-lun, Kingston, Chan SY. Epidermal growth factor as a biologic switch in hair growth cycle [published online April 24, 2003]. *J Biol Chem.* 2003;278:26120–26126.
13. Weger N, Schlake T. IGF-I signalling controls the hair growth cycle and the differentiation of hair shafts. *J Invest Dermatol.* 2005;125:873–882.
14. Mak, King-lun, Kingston. A transgenic mouse model to study the role of epidermal growth factor (EGF) in hair and skin development. University of Hong Kong (Pokfulam Road, Hong Kong), 2002.
15. Peters EMJ, Paus R, Klapp BF, Arck PC. Neuroimmunological hair growth control is stress-sensitive: An old paradigm revisited. *Experimental Dermatol.* 2006;15(1):1–13.
16. Li ZJ, Choi HI, Choi D-K et al. Autologous platelet-rich plasma: A potential therapeutic tool for promoting hair growth. *Dermatol Surg* 2012;38(7pt1):1040–1046.
17. Hoffmann R, Happle R. Current understanding of androgenetic alopecia. Part II: Clinical aspects and treatment. *Eur J Dermatol.* 2000;10(5):410–417, Articles FMC.
18. Sorbellini E, Trink A, Rinaldi F. Experimental clinical assessment of the use of platelet-rich plasma in dermatology and rationale for its use in the treatment of non-scarring alopecia. *La Medicina Estetica 35 Year* October 4, 2011.
19. Takikawa, M Md, Nakamura S, Nakamura S et al. Enhanced effect of platelet-rich plasma containing a new carrier on hair growth. *Dermatol Surg.* 2011;37(12):1721–1729.
20. Greco J, Brandt R. The effects of autologus platelet rich plasma and various growth factors on non-transplanted miniaturized hair. *Hair Transplant Forum Intl.* 2009;19:49–50.
21. Amgar G, Bouhanna P. Objective evaluation of autologous Platelet Rich Plasma injection in androgenic alopecia. *PRIME.* 2013;3(4):20–31.
22. Gilhar A, Etzioni A, Paus R. Alopecia areata. *N Engl J Med.* 2012;366:1515–1525.
23. Alkhalifah A, Alsantali A, Wang E et al. Alopecia areata update: Part I. Clinical picture, histopathology, and pathogenesis. *J Am Acad Dermatol.* 2010;62:177–188, quiz 89–90.
24. Alkhalifah A. Topical and intralesional therapies for alopecia areata. *Dermatol Ther.* 2011;24:355–363.
25. Rogers N. Commentary on autologous platelet-rich plasma: A potential therapeutic tool for promoting hair growth. *Dermatol Surg.* 2012;38:1047–1048.
26. Uebel CO, da Silva JB, Cantarelli D et al. The role of platelet plasma growth factors in male pattern baldness surgery. *Plast Reconstr Surg.* 2006;118:1458–1466, discussion 67.
27. Trink A, Sorbellini E, Bezzola P et al. A randomized, double-blind, placebo- and active-controlled, half-head study to evaluate the effects of platelet-rich plasma on alopecia areata. *Br J Dermatol.* 2013;169(3):690–694.
28. Alkhalifah A, Alsantali A, Wang E et al. Alopecia areata update: Part II. Treatment. *J Am Acad Dermatol.* 2010;62:191–202, quiz 3–4.
29. Lee JW, Kim BJ, Kim MN et al. The efficacy of autologous platelet rich plasma combined with ablative carbon dioxide fractional resurfacing for acne scars: A simultaneous split-face trial. *Dermatol Surg.* 2011;37:931–938.
30. Chen TM, Tsai JC, Burnouf T. A novel technique combining platelet gel, skin graft, and fibrin glue for healing recalcitrant lower extremity ulcers. *Dermatol Surg.* 2010;36:453–460.
31. El-Sharkawy H, Kantarci A, Deady J et al. Platelet-rich plasma: Growth factors and pro- and anti-inflammatory properties. *J Periodontol.* 2007;78:661–669.
32. Reese RJ. Autologous platelet rich plasma (PRP): What do we know? Important concepts relevant to hair restoration surgery. *Hair Transplant Forum Int.* 2010;14–17.
33. Uebel CO. Presented at the Annual Scientific Meeting of the American Society of Plastic Surgeons, Philadelphia, PA, October 9–13, 2004.
34. Perez-Meza D. Part II The use of autologous rich and poor plasma to enhance the wound healing and hair growth in hair restoration surgery. In: Programs and Abstracts. 13th ISHRS annual meeting; Sydney, Australia, 2005.
35. Greco J, Brandt R. Our preliminary experiences and extended applications for the use of autologus platelet rich plasma in hair transplant surgery. *Hair Transplant Forum Intl.* 2007;17:131–132.
36. Declair V. The importance of growth factors in wound healing. *Ostomy Wound Manage.* 1999;45:64–68.
37. Choi Y, Fuchs, E. TGF-beta and retinoic acid regulation of growth and modifiers of differentiation human epidermal cells. *Crell Regal.* January/February 2010.
38. Ross R. Platelet-derived growth factor. *Am Rev Med.* 1986;38:71–79.
39. Pierce GF, Mustoe TA, Lingelbach J, Masakowski VR, Gramates PP, Deuel TF. Transforming growth factor B reverses the glucocorticoid-induced wound-healing defect in rats: Possible regulation in microphages by platelet-derived growth factor. *Proc Natl Acad Sci.* 1989;86:2229–2233.

40. Yong M et al. Promotional effects of plate-rich-plasma on hair follicle reconstitution *in vivo*. *Dermatol Surg.* 2013;39(12):1868–1876.
41. Pittenger MF et al. Multilineage potential of adult human mesenchymal stem cells. *Science.* 1999;284(5411):143–147.
42. Garza LA, Cotsarelis G et al. Bald scalp in men with androgenic alopecia retains hair follicle stem cells but lacks CD 200- rich and CD34-positive hair follicle progenitor cells. *J Clin Invest.* 2011;121(2):613–622.
43. Greber B, Schöler H. A breakthrough in stem cell research? Reprogramming somatic cells into pluripotent stem cells. *Bundesgesundheitsblatt Gesundheitsforschung Gesundheitsschutz.* 2008;51(9):1005–1013.
44. Giakoumopoulos M, Golos TG. Embryonic stem cell-derived trophoblast differentiation: A comparative review of the biology, function, and signaling mechanism. *J Endocrinol.* 2013;216(3):R33–R45.
45. Jiang Y et al. Pluripotency of mesenchymal stem cells derived from adult marrow. *Nature.* 2002;418:41–49.
46. Roobrouck VD et al. Self-renewal and differentiation capacity of young and aged stem cells. *Exp Cell Res.* 2008;314(9):1937–1944.
47. Ringden O, Le Blanc K et al. Mesenchymal stem cells for treatment of therapy-resistent graft-versus-host disease. *Transplantation.* 2006;81(10):1390–1397.
48. Ratajczak MZ et al. A hypothesis for an embryonic origin of pluripotent Oct-4(+) stem cells in adult bone marrow and other tissues. *Leukemia.* 2007;21(5):860–867.
49. Castilla et al. Adipose-derived stromal cells: Their identity and uses in clinical trials, an update. *World J Stem Cells.* 2011;3(4):25–33.
50. Sheng L et al. Adipose tissue-derived stem cells (ADSCs) transplantation promotes regeneration of expanded skin using a tissue expansion model. *Wound Repair Regen.* 2013;21(5):746–754.
51. Lee EY et al. Hypoxia-enhanced wound healing function of adipose-derived stem cells: Increase in stem cell proliferation and up-regulation of VEGF and bFGF. *Wound Repair Regen.* 2009;17(4):540–547.
52. Cai L et al. IFATS collection: Human adipose tissue-derived stem cells induce angiogenesis and nerve sprouting following myocardial infarction, in conjunction with potent preservation of cardiac function. *Stem Cells.* 2009;27:230–237.
53. Lu F et al. Improved viability of random pattern skin flaps through the use of adipose-derived stem cells. *Plast Reconstr Surg.* 2008;121:50–58.
54. Nakagami H et al. Novel autologous cell therapy in ischemic limb disease through growth factor secretion by cultured adipose tissue-derived stem cells. *Arterioscler Thromb Vasc Biol.* 2005;25(12):2542–2547.
55. Ferrara N, Alitalo K. Clinical applications of angiogenic growth factors and their inhibitors. *Nat Med.* 1999;5:1359–1364.
56. Hebda PA, Klingbeil CK, Abraham JA, Fidders JC. Basic fibroblast growth factor stimulation of epidermal wound healing in pigs. *J Invest Dermatol.* 1990;95:626–631.
57. Park BS et al. Hair growth stimulate by conditioned medium of adipose-derived stem cells is enhanced by hypoxia: Evidence of increased growth factor secretion. *Biomed Res.* 2010;31(1):27–34.
58. Gentile et al. Concise review: Adipose derived stromal vascular fraction cells and platelet rich plasma: Basic and clinical implications for tissue engineering therapies in regenerative surgery. *Stem Cells Transl Med.* 2012;1(3):230–236.
59. Kurita M et al. Influences of centrifugation on cells and tissues in liposuction aspirates: Optimized centrifugation for lipotransfer and cell isolation. *Plast Reconstr Surg.* 2008;121(3):1033–1041.
60. Sterodimas A, de Faria J, Nicaretta B, Pitanguy I. Tissue engineering with adipose-derived stem cells (ADSCs): Current and future applications. *J Plast Reconstr Aesthet Surg.* 2010;63(11):1886–1892.
61. Higgins C, Christiano AM et al. Microenvironmental programming by three-dimensional culture enables dermal papilla cells to induce *de novo* human hair-follicle growth [published online October 21, 2013]. *Proc Natl Acad Sci USA.* 2013;110(49):19679–19688.

18 Adjuvant therapy for alopecia: Synthetic hair implant, dermopigmentation, hair prosthesis, and hair camouflage

Pierre Bouhanna and Sophie Casadio

In modern times, wigs, hairpieces, extensions, and scalp-covering cosmetics are used either to change the appearance of a hairstyle or to camouflage hair loss. Scalp prostheses enable patients to maintain the normal appearance of hair. Alternatively some patients choose to wear a wig or hairpiece in lieu of medical or surgical treatment. Wigs or hairpieces can be very useful in helping patients cope with various forms of alopecia, such as chemotherapy for cancer. Hair prostheses can be introduced while outlining medical and surgical options for therapy. Synthetic hair implants actually have few to no indications due to complications. Perhaps in the future synthetic implants will be better tolerated. Hair cosmetics may be an option to camouflage the areas of thinning. The dermopigmentation, and more precisely micropigmentation, is a good option for definitive and stabilized hair and body hair alopecia.

HAIR PROSTHESIS

Hair types

The type of hair used in wigs and hair extensions is of two categories: human and synthetic.

Human hair

Human hair is most expensive, but also the most durable and versatile material for good construction. Human hair comes from all over the world: China, India, Indonesia, and European countries.

Synthetic hair

Synthetic hair fibers offer the advantage of limitless supply, low cost, and great texture and color diversity. The newest man-made fibers are lightweight, durable, color and fade resistant, and have excellent curl retention properties.

Wigs

Full human-hair wigs are the most like natural scalp hair, and with proper care can last for years. However, realism and durability come at significant expense. For people with permanent scalp hair loss, a full custom designed scalp prosthesis may be required. For people with thinning hair due to androgenetic alopecia or stable patches of hair loss due to scarring alopecia, a hairpiece or a partial wig may be appropriate.

Hand-tied wigs are labor intensive and pricey but offer the most natural appearance because the hair can be parted or blown in different directions. Wefts are multiple hairs that are machine-sewed together at one end to make a long curtain of hair.

Machine-sewed wigs and hairpieces are less expensive than hand-tied versions but have a less natural appearance (Figure 18.1a and b).

Caps are the base to which strands or wefts of hair are attached to make a wig. A properly sized wig should fit securely on the head and be able to withstand normal head movement and a reasonable amounts of wind. The choice of wig attachment depends on comfort, style, and the amount of hair underneath.

Removable wigs may be attached with clips and combs to underlying natural scalp hair. Other attachment options include adhesives, double-sided tape, silicone strips, snaps, and Velcro (Figure 18.2a and b).

For patients with total scalp-hair loss, a vacuum-attached wig may be a consideration. This type of wig can only be attached to the scalp if it is completely bare, as in alopecia totalis or universalis. Patients that suffer from medical hair-loss conditions may qualify for public and private health insurances for the purchase of a hair prosthesis.

Hairpieces

Hairpieces are not designed to cover the entire scalp. They may be made out of human or synthetic hair.

The base is then clipped, pinned, taped, or glued to the scalp, and the natural scalp hair is styled under or around the piece.

The result gives the appearance of a thicker, fuller head of hair. A small hairpiece that covers a specific area of thinning due to cicatricial alopecia can be color-matched and integrated with the natural growth hair.

Modern hairpieces and toupees offer a natural-appearing option for men who want to camouflage hair loss. Toupees are constructed in the same way as hairpieces, and the natural occipital hair is left free. Toupees can be attached to the scalp with clips, combs, bonding agents, or double-sided tape. The wearer can shampoo and style the hairpiece as he or she would his or her own hair. Bonding agents may cause irritation, pruritus, or a contact allergy.[1]

HAIR EXTENSIONS

Hair extensions add length and volume to an existing style. Hair extensions are attached to natural scalp locks. There must be a sufficient and stable amount of natural growth hair to attach the extensions. Hair extensions can be either human or synthetic. Depending on the method

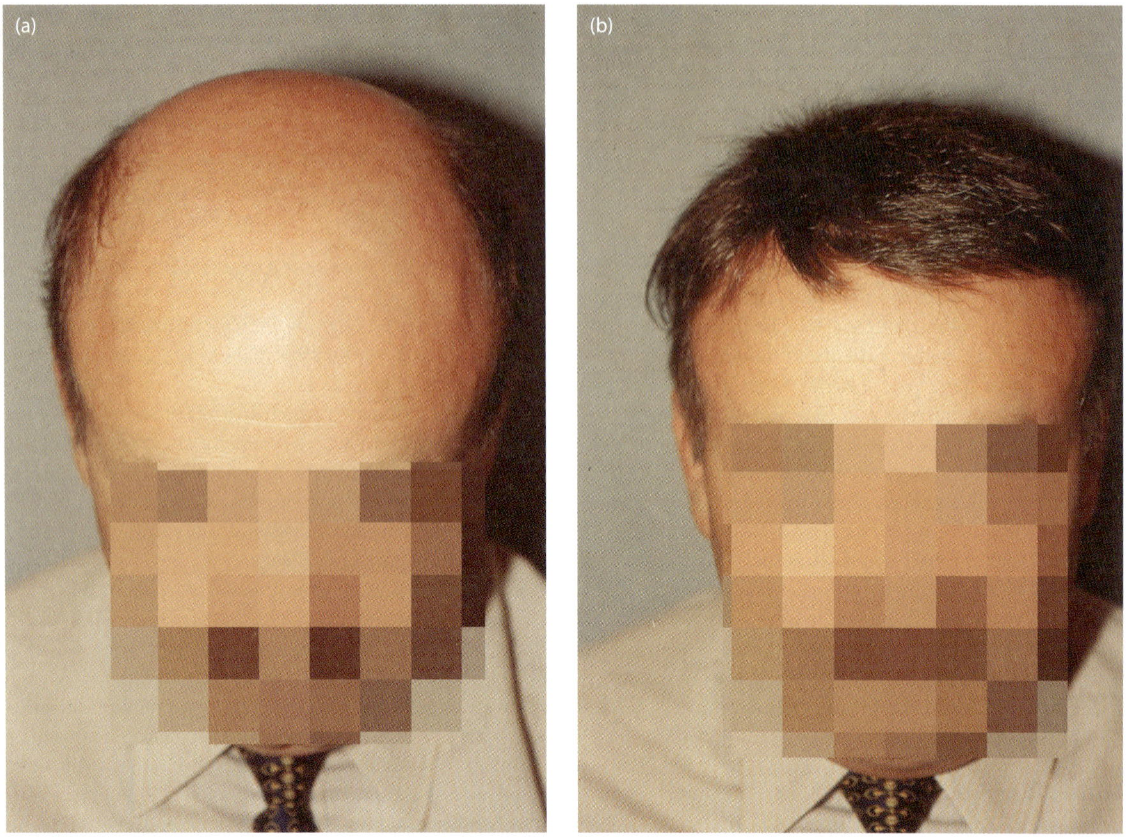

Figure 18.1 **Male androgenetic alopecia (a) before and (b) after wearing a wig.**

of attachment, human-hair extensions can be washed and styled along with the natural scalp hair.

The simplest hair extensions have plastic or metal clips. When the natural scalp hair grows past a few millimeters, the weaved-in hair tracks need to be tightened or replaced. Hair can be glued in close approximation to the corn-rowed scalp hair. A newer method of attaching hair extensions involves strand-to-strand hair bonding. A heated instrument, similar to a glue gun, melts and fuses the extension strands onto the scalp hair.

Braids

Braided hair extensions ensure that all braids are of a uniform width and length. A variety of braided styles are available, and different materials are used to achieve specific looks.

Problems associated with hair extensions

Traction alopecia has been associated with extensions attached to relaxed hair. Braiding can cause breakage, irreversible traction alopecia (Figure 18.3), and traction folliculitis.[2,3]

SYNTHETIC HAIR IMPLANT (HIS)

Different types of synthetic implant hair have been proposed for many years by American, Japanese, and Italian laboratories. Nearly all have been abandoned by most experts because of the extent of side effects.

The material most often used is polyester fiber of 80–100 mm in diameter. The root or knot of the synthetic hair may be of very varied appearance. The scalp area destroyed around each implant varies from 0.05 to 0.9 mm^2 depending on the procedure used.

Bouhanna[4,5] carried out a follow-up on 16 selected patients implanted as a test of 60 Japanese Nido synthetic hairs with clinical and macrophotographic assessment for 6 months.

The fiber was made of polyethylene terephthalate, 0.09 mm in diameter, with an alpha-type loop at its end (Figure 18.4). This fiber was implanted on the galea after traversing the epidermis, dermis, and hypodermis with a special 0.23 mm needle (Figure 18.5).

The synthetic hairs were implanted on four areas of 0.25 cm^2 localized by tattooing in each of the 16 patients (Figure 18.6a and b). They were counted in three successive macrophotographs on days 90 and 180. Tolerance

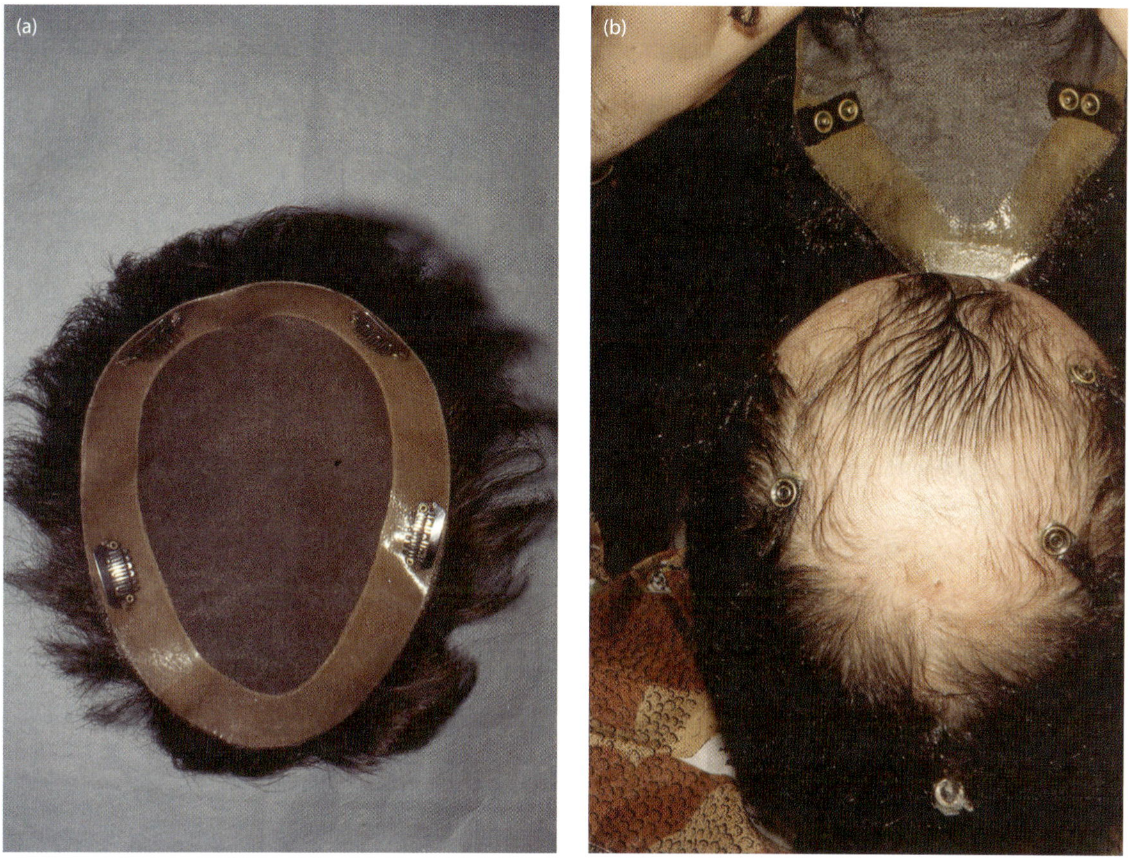

Figure 18.2 (a) Wig. (b) Wig attached with clips.

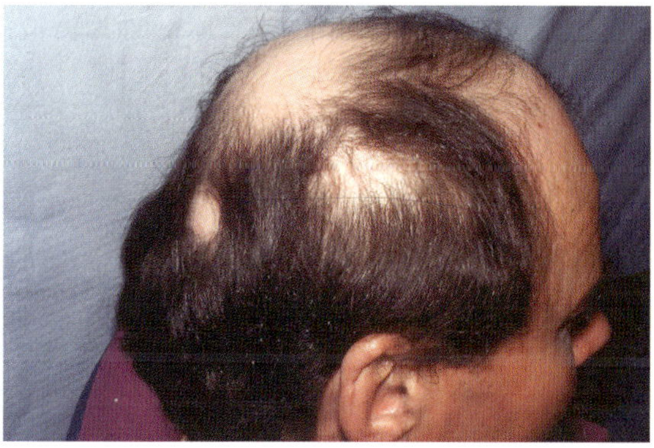

Figure 18.3 Traction alopecia due to the clips of the wig.

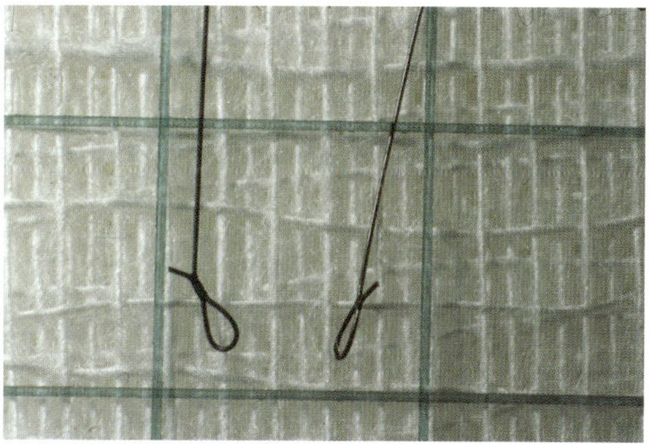

Figure 18.4 Synthetic fiber with an alpha loop at the end to allow retention.

was assessed as poor, moderate, good, or excellent. Complications such as folliculitis, seborrhoic dermatitis, follicular seborrhoic deposits (Figure 18.7), and scar pits (Figure 18.8) were assessed.

Results

- A mean density per square centimeter of implanted hairs varying from 137.48 at day 0 to 116.64 at day 90 and 90.5 at day 180.

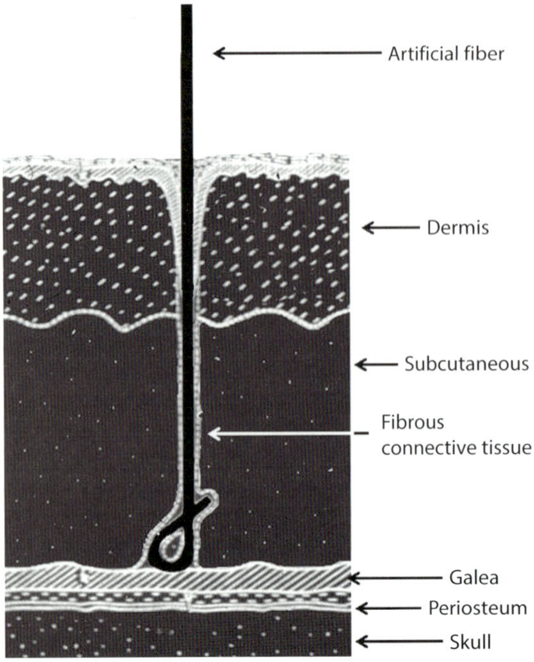

Figure 18.5 **Implantation of a synthetic fiber deep to the galea.**

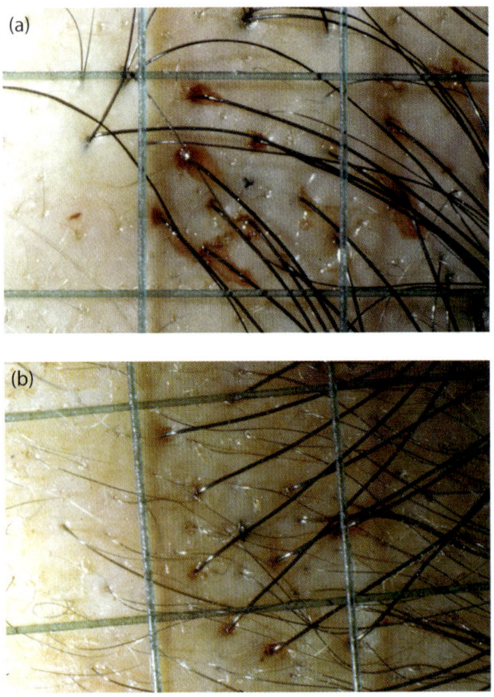

Figure 18.6 **(a) Synthetic hair fibers immediately after the implantation on a 0.25 cm² area. (b) Same implanted area 3 months later.**

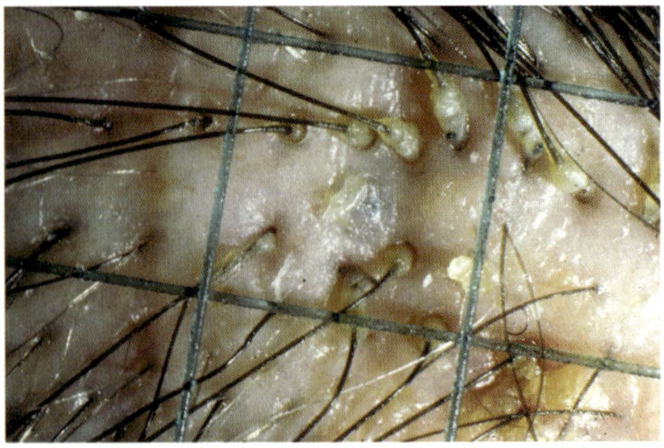

Figure 18.7 **Seborrheic deposits at the emergence of the fiber.**

- A mean percentage of fixation of 84.84% at 2 months and 65.82% at 6 months.
- A mean incidence of complications of 31.25% for folliculitis, 6.25% for seborrhoic dermatitis, 6.25% for scar piting and 43.7% for follicular seborrhoic deposits, due essentially to inadequately repeated local care using shampoo.

The mean percentage of tolerance was excellent in 31.25% of cases, good in 25% and moderate in 43.75%; there were no bad results. During the 6 month of follow-up of this study, no foreign body granuloma reaction was found (Figures 18.9 and 18.10a and b). The study was too short to provide a complete assessment of this procedure, as we have reported various complications such as foreign body granuloma outside this series.

According to Di Gregorio,[6] Hanke,[7] Lepaw,[8] and Schwartz,[9] different synthetic hairs gave different degrees of complications after implantation: foreign body granulomas, secondary infective pustules, residual scars, etc.

Apart from the local and general contraindications to this treatment, we advise a preliminary test with few

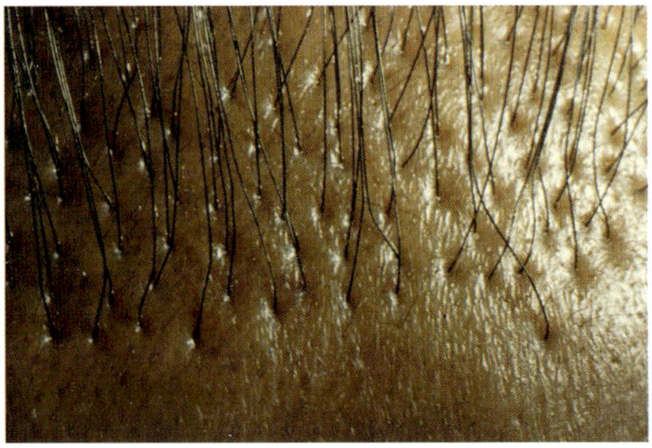

Figure 18.8 **Scar pits at the emergence of the fiber.**

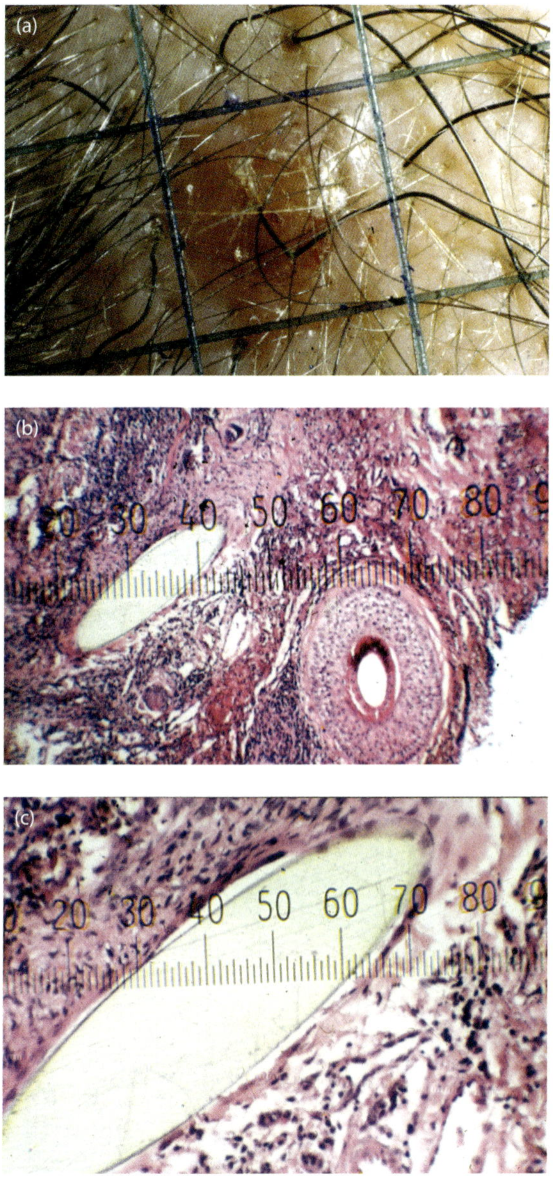

Figure 18.9 **(a) Foreign body granuloma around a synthetic hair fiber. (b,c) Histological aspect of the foreign body granuloma around the synthetic hair fiber and a normal hair on the right.**

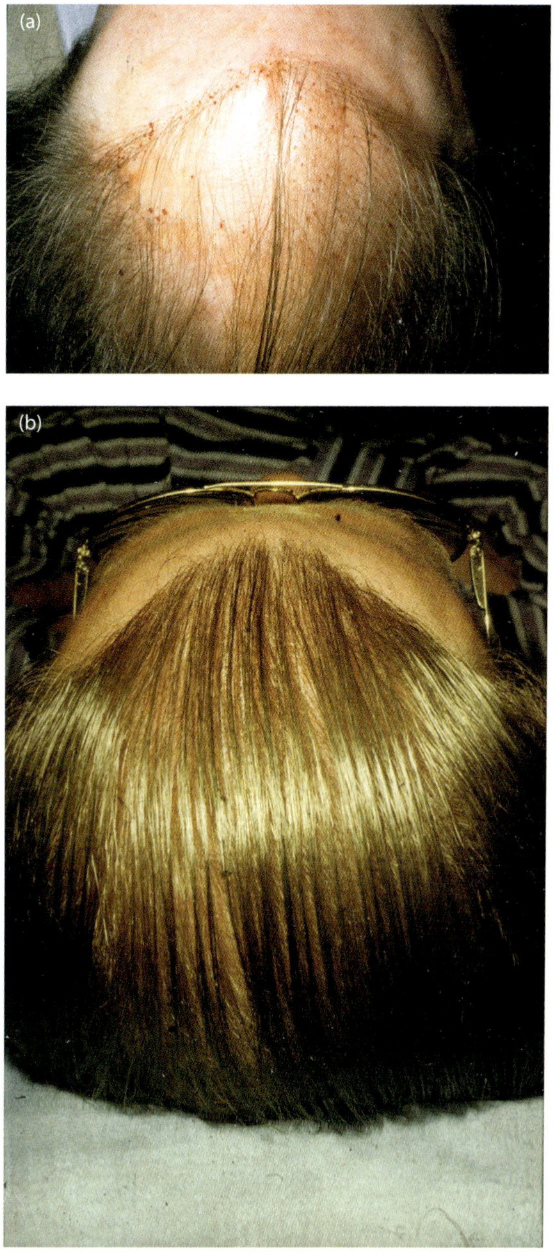

Figure 18.10 **(a) Immediate aspect after implantation of 500 synthetic hairs on a male with androgenetic alopecia. (b) Immediate aspect after implantation of 2000 synthetic hairs on the same patient.**

synthetic hairs (10–20) over a monitoring period of 6 months.

Conclusion

Synthetic hairs are of variable reliability, durability, and tolerance depending on the procedure selected. The indications for this treatment seem to be contraindications to surgical techniques using the patient's own hair, which alone guarantees a definitive and unconstrained result. The patient applying for this treatment must be told of the different complications and of the inevitable rejection of the implanted synthetic hairs in the near or long term. In the near future we are looking for a new synthetic hair implant with perhaps a better tolerance and less rejection.

HAIR CAMOUFLAGE

For many patients with thinning hair due to androgenetic alopecia, the most noticeable areas are the frontal and vertex scalp. As the hair density decreases, spaces between individual hairs increase and the scalp becomes more apparent. Hair cosmetics may be an option to camouflage the areas of thinning so that the area appears less noticeable (Figure 18.11a and b). Several products are available, including powder (Dermatch, synthetic fibers, cotton fibers, etc.) Toppik Hair Building Fibers that sprinkle out of a can and cover the thin areas and Good Looking Hair (GLH) Thickener Spray (Ronco, Inc.). Some clinicians recommended using camouflage makeup, such as Dermablend (L'Oreal). Hair cosmetics are relatively easy to apply. Most products are safe to use and rarely cause irritation. They can be used in post-op after hair transplantation during the delay of regrowth.

SCALP DERMOPIGMENTATION: DR. SOPHIE CASADIO

For the last 20 years, we have been using dermography to rebuild areas of damaged skin caused by accidents or pathologies.[10]

Now, the technique can be removed from reconstructive surgery (in particular in breast cancer and scars caused by burns) and moved to hair and body hair.

The dermopigmentation is a medicosurgical act of an implant into the mid-dermis.[11] The micropigmentation is a specialized treatment especially suited to hairy areas. It reproduces the appearance of body/head hair and requires a precise pigment implant specification as well as use of microneedles, which also have to comply with a precise and particular specification.

Tools and materials

Pigment implants

They are nontoxic, nonallergenic, biocompatible, made in a special "white room," sterilized following a very strict validated industrial method used only for this particular purpose, and certified by the CEIIb's standards and medical directives (Figure 18.12).[12,13]

They are minerals or organics but in any case they are made up of a chromophore (colorant), a dispersant, and an additive (Figure 18.13).

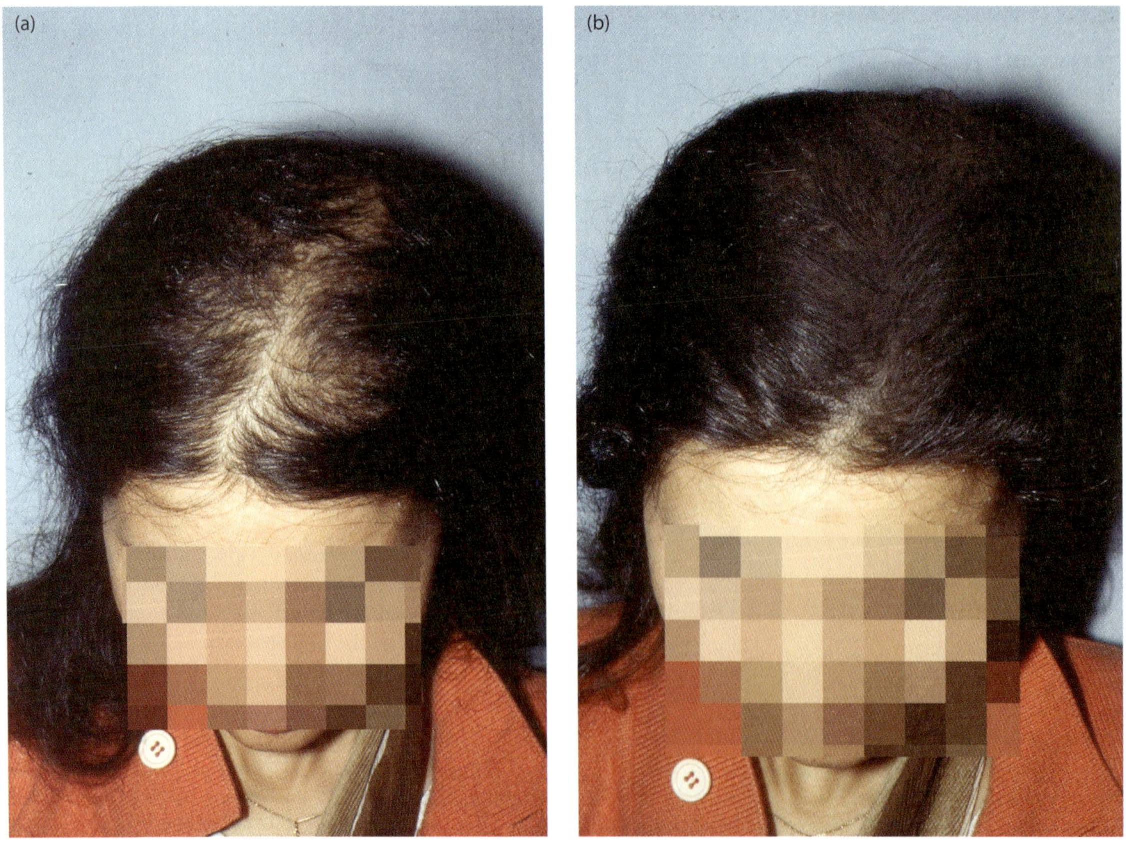

Figure 18.11 (a,b) Female androgenetic alopecia immediately after a hair powder camouflage.

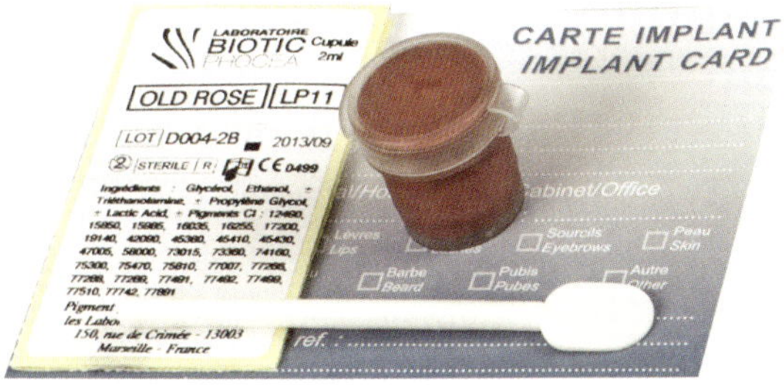

Figure 18.12 **Dermopigmentation implant card.**

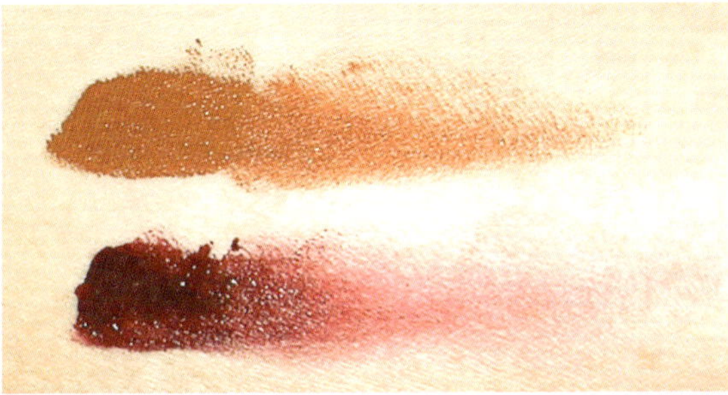

Figure 18.13 **Mineral or organic pigments for dermopigmentation.**

Their progressive fading out allows us to foresee the bleaching of the hair or the change in hair color in women in particular (Figure 18.14).

The dermograph

It is made of two pieces: one hand tool and a regulator (Figure 18.15).

1. The one hand tool is a very practical "pen" which leans against the anatomical snuffbox. It is composed of a sealed sterilized sleeve with a cog ring which allows the control and the setting of the needles' depth.
2. The regulator (Figure 18.16) is made of electronic components with a dual display offering security, quality, and ease of use.

The speed can be easily regulated: it can go from 50 to 180 shots per second.

Needles

Specific needles are used for specified tasks. Only used once, they are put together in a "disposable cartridge," and their number and layout depend on the work to be achieved: dots, lineage, and topping (coloring).

Technique and particularity of the skin

While the pigmentation is in the hairy area and if we want to reproduce the dotting effect of a hair, we need to obey specific technical rules. The penetration of the dermis must be perpendicular to the surface of the skin. It will therefore give a dotted aspect; however, if the angle of penetration is less than 90°, the needle will go through all dermo-epidermal layers and print on its way a line rather than a dot (Figure 18.17).

Another technique can be applied in order to give a high or low light effect by reproducing a multiple hair aspect: one can use different colored pigments in order to give a "scratch" look.

The lineage can be used for a line; one can use its density to realize the required gradient.

One can use (Figure 18.18):

- Dots.
- Lineage or hint used for eyeliners and masking scars.
- The "scratch impression" will give a gradual spread of color aspect if only used superficially: a high or low light effect is often used for eyebrows.
- Coloring or "topping" is used for the mammary areola.

The present contributors are dermatological criteria as discussed below.

MINERALS	ORGANIC
Opaque, high covering power	Transparent, with natural aspect
Dull and broken (off) colours	Bright colours
Unstable colours	Stable colours
Persistant	Fade away

Figure 18.14 **Pigments characters.**

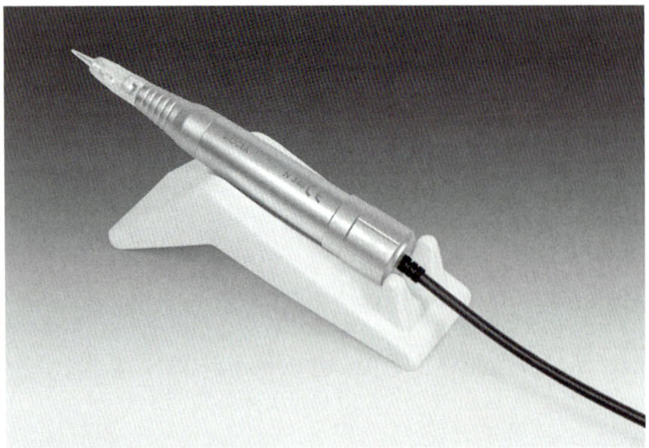

Figure 18.15 **Hand tool.**

Skin colors and depth

The different skin colors or phototypes do not all react the same way following their skin's chromatic composition: a Caucasian phototype might not react identically to an Asian or African type.

The color of the skin is the result of quantitative and qualitative elements. Melanin, eumelanin, and beta-carotene in various proportions make the skin aspect.

This is why one will need to juxtapose red, yellow, and blue pigments in variable but reliable and reproducible proportions.

The practitioner's experience will help in choosing the proper pigmented color from the chromatic circle reference: the color wheel (Figure 18.19).

One needs to know that some people have a natural tendency to influence the implanted color: warm or cold. This will result in a chromatic instability.

The depth of the work will be determined by the area of implantation: the quantity of epidermal cells and the thickness of the dermis vary. For example, we have to implant differently in the sole of the foot compared to the eyelid.

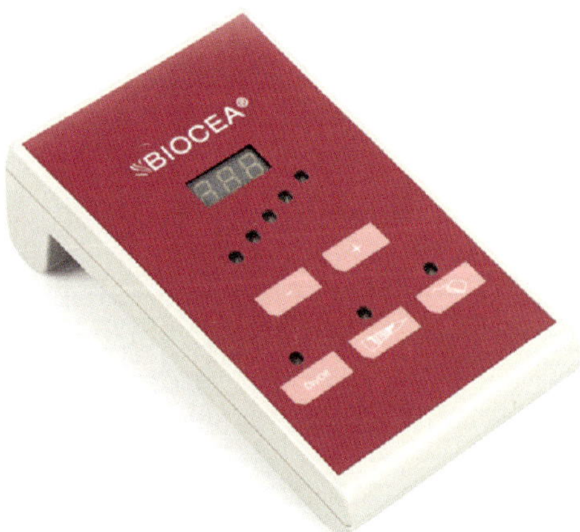

Figure 18.16 **Regulator.**

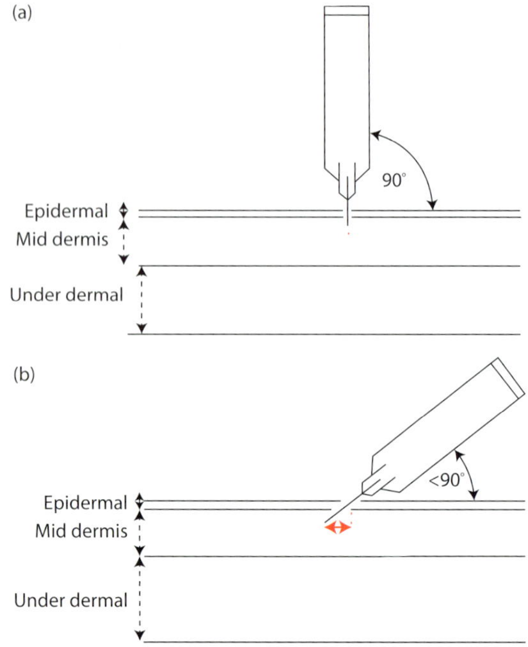

Figure 18.17 **Technical rules. (a) Pigmented aspect is a dot. (b) Pigmented aspect is a line.**

Histology

The pigment must be introduced in the mid-dermis.

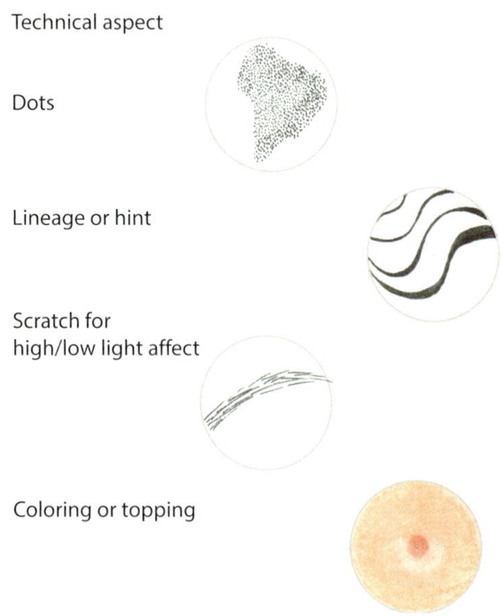

Figure 18.18 **Technical aspect.**

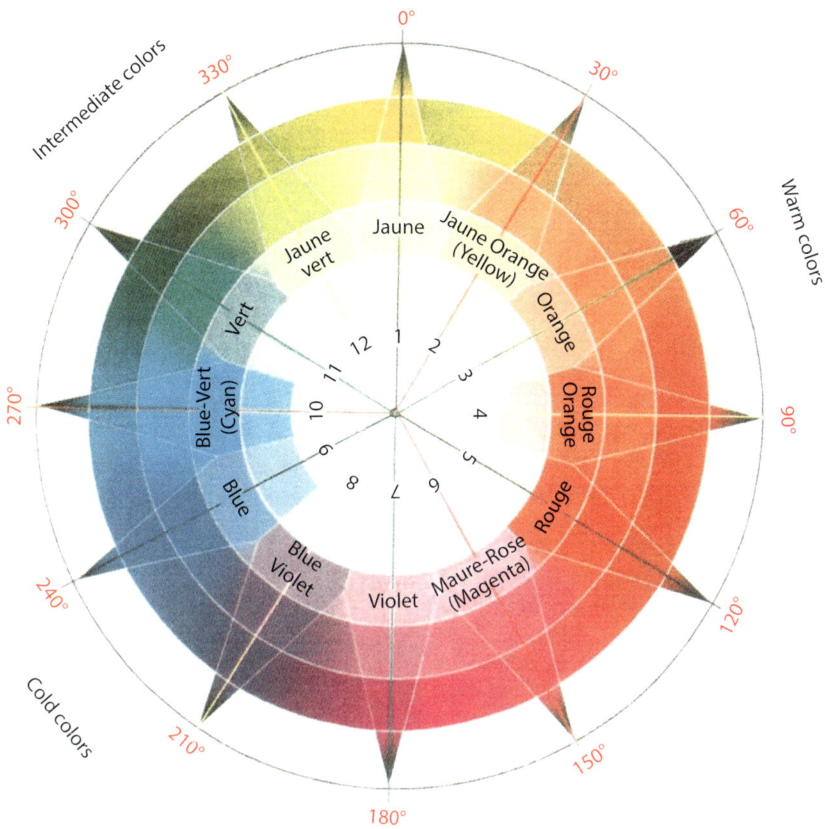

Figure 18.19 **Color wheel is an illustration of the relation between colors.**

A superficial implantation (as done in aesthetic makeup in beauty institutes) is painless but could rapidly fade away and disappear when the epidermis cells change at the next cell renewal.

To start with, when an implant is introduced into the dermis, some will naturally be eliminated in the healing process, and some others will be considered by the body cells as an intrusion. The immune system can then eliminate up to 30% of it. It often occurs between the day 7 and day 21.

Once it has healed, the epidermis is reconstituted "ad integrum" so it appears through transparency under the dermis: it is stored in the papillary dermis near blood vessels (Figure 18.20).

Definition, contraindications, and complications

Dermopigmentation of head hair or micropigmentation of hairy areas, also named trichopigmentation, follows an international process of scalp micropigmentation which is used for:

- Head scars caused by accidents or from transplant donor areas.
- Scars through beards or moustaches.
- Head hair rarefactions, temporary or definitive, dermal pathologies or lichen.
- Alopecia androgenetic capillary rarefactions.

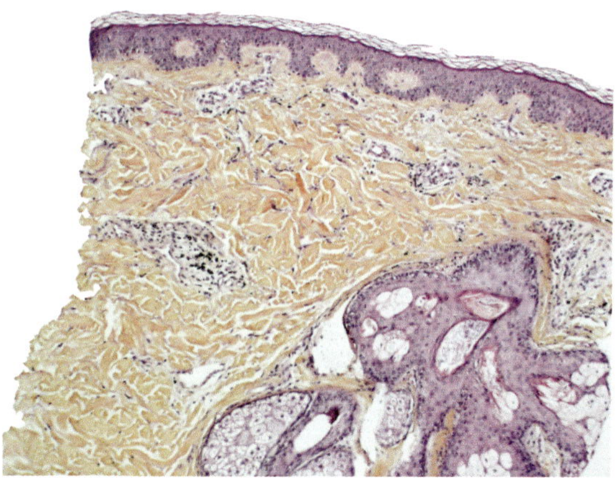

Figure 18.20 **Vertical histological section of the superficial and the mid-dermis showing the pigment implant.**

- Eyebrows.
- Eyelids or lashlids (ciliary border).

Contraindications: If one proceeds following the previous description, contraindications are only relative: kidney failure and hepatic (encephalopathy) and autoimmune disorders.

Pigmentations can only be attained on healthy skin, without progressive diseases and with special precautions for diabetic or arteritic patients or ones with heart valve diseases.

The use of nonallergenic pigments removes the risk of allergies in atopic patients. A test can, however, be performed (in 20 years of practice the author has never come across an allergy following the above procedures).

Complications: When the skin has been broken, one can expect some side effects: inflammation, redness, and bruising.

Rules are the same for dermography, but they will resolve themselves within a few days.

It is possible for the color to change because of a chemical reaction called *oxidoreduction*.

The patient, even aware, might have been exposed to ultraviolet (UV) light. One can try to "mask" or neutralize this change, which demands an excellent command of the color wheel mentioned above.

Another side effect could be a spread of color called the *blotting paper appearance*, with its pigment diffusion in deep dermis or under dermal due to bad operating technique (Figure 18.21).

Extremely rarely a granuloma could appear which will spontaneously disappear within a few weeks.

European Forensic Aspects: A decree dated January 6, 1962, was modified by a decree dated February 19, 2008, which determined the level of skills in the trade according to interventions on the skin. From the article L.312 Code of Public Health: all medical acts that require breaking the skin can only be performed by people from the medical profession or paramedics under a doctor's responsibility.

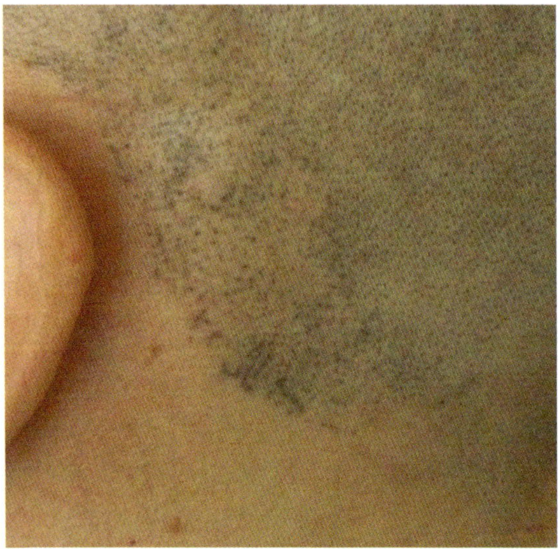

Figure 18.21 **Blotting paper affect.**

Technical achievements

Head hair scars

Just like donor transplant areas, it is a sunless area that causes the skin to be extremely fair[14,15] (Figure 18.22a and b).

The technique must reproduce, as finely as is necessary, the density and the implantation of the hair in order to fit into the healthy hair thickness (Figure 18.22b).

Beard and moustache scars

The particularity of this area is its permanent exposure to the sun which gives the scar a whiter aspect (Figure 18.23a and b). The treatment therefore has to be done in two steps:

- The first one concentrates on matching the scar's color with the surrounding skin color as it is usually slightly darker. A "topping" of the same skin color is necessary; the operation might have to be repeated to obtain the same color all around.
- The second step is purely a micropigmentation work: once one has reached the skin color required, the hair can then be micropigmented following the previous technique (Figure 18.24a and b).

Head hair rarefactions, alopecia, and lichen

Micropigmentation can trick the eye by giving a hairy effect enabling us to hide some hairless areas (Figure 18.25a and b).[16,17]

This requires a precise move and fine precision on the depth of the implant.

Two side effects can easily occur:

- The pigment can be diffused in the deep dermis (as mentioned above, the blotting paper effect) following its thinning engendered by a local cortisone treatment, for example, in lichen of the scalp.
- The color can turn due to a chemical reaction (oxidoreduction) from mineral components of the pigment implant.

A thorough study of the phototype is necessary to choose the right color in order to correct or neutralize the area if that risk is likely to happen.

This technique is used for patients who suffer from male pattern baldness or for those who are awaiting a transplant or who are in the process of hair micrografts. It is used on the area pending a transplant or the area that needs redensifying, or simply if it is desired to give the

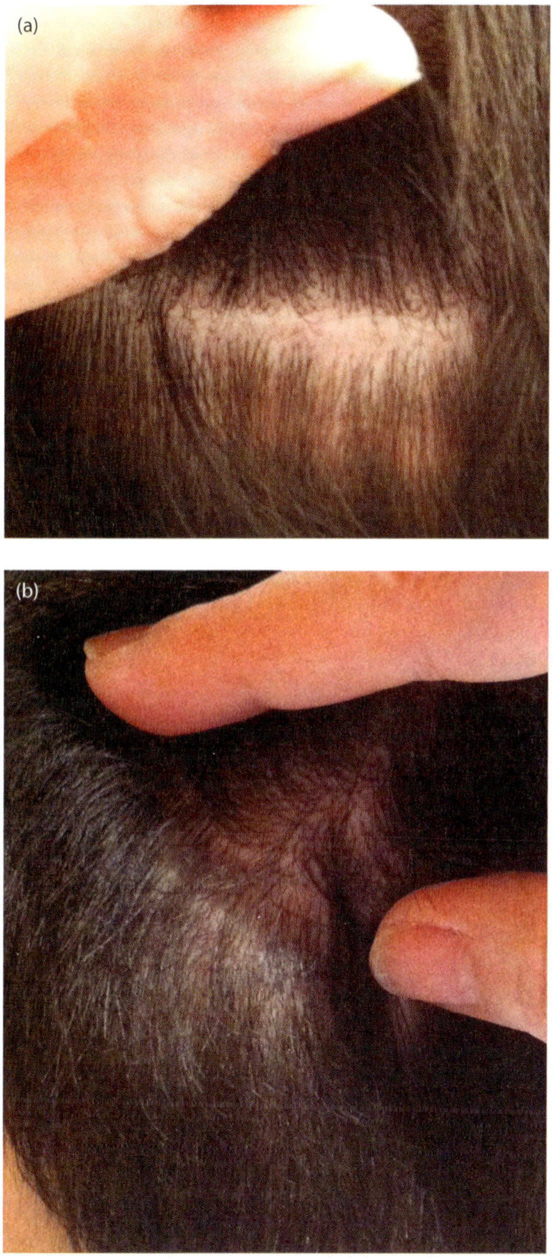

Figure 18.22 **Donor transplant scar (a) before and (b) after pigmentation.**

impression of a shortly shaved head, depending on the actual fashion.

Eyebrows

They frame the face and are essential to facial expression: happiness, sorrow, concentration, relaxation, etc.[18,19]

This explains why its neutral layout is so important so as to keep a natural expression when there is one.

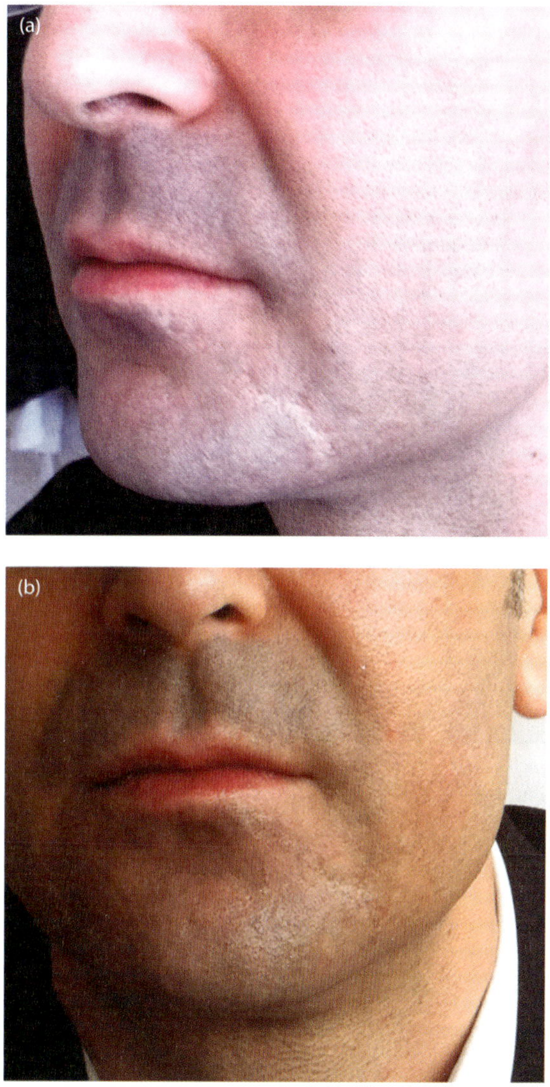

Figure 18.23 **Beard scar (a) before and (b) after pigmentation.**

1. *Dermography can offer:* Reconstruction of the eyebrows can be accomplished. They are organs that also age with the rest of the face. They can get whiter and the layout thinner. Dermography can redesign an eyebrow's layout and proceed to a slight high or low light affect giving its original hairy impression.
2. *Hiding a scar:* Like any other hairy areas, eyebrows can get scarred from burns or accidents. Dermography can therefore hide a scar by using the same technique as used in sunless areas.
3. *Eyebrows reconstruction:* This can be accomplished after a repeated epilation or after medical treatments (chemotherapy, hormonal therapy) (Figure 18.26a and b).

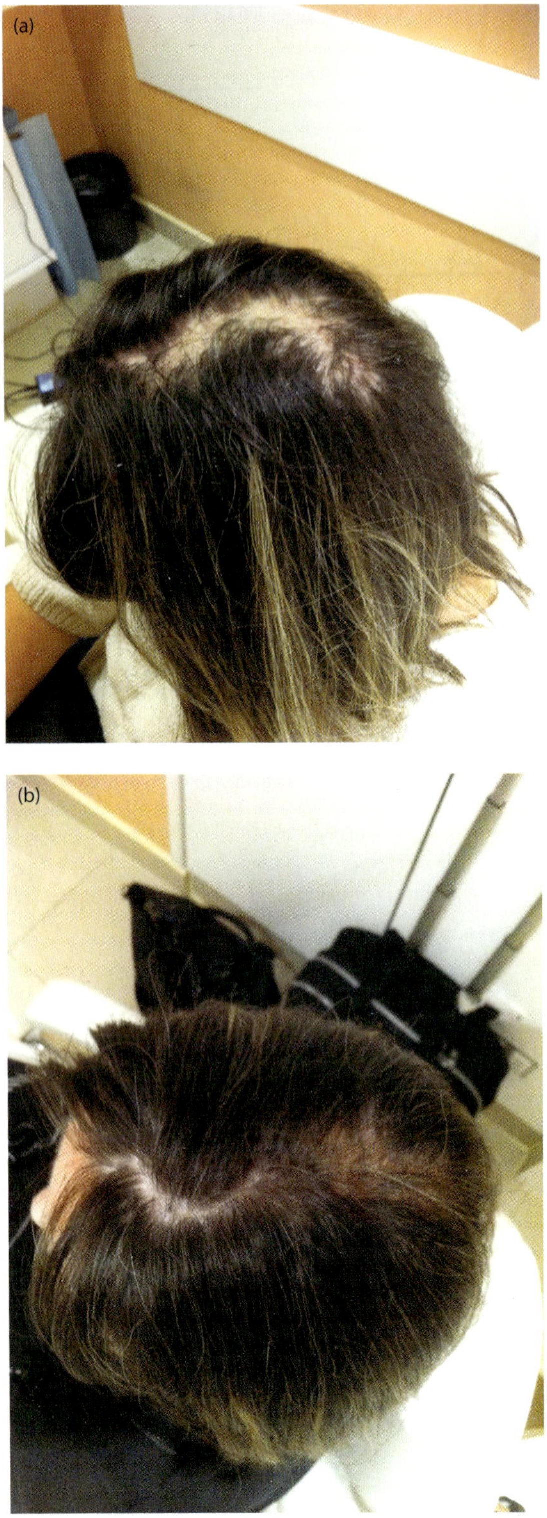

Figure 18.24 **Cicatricial alopecia due to a lichen (a) before and (b) after densification.**

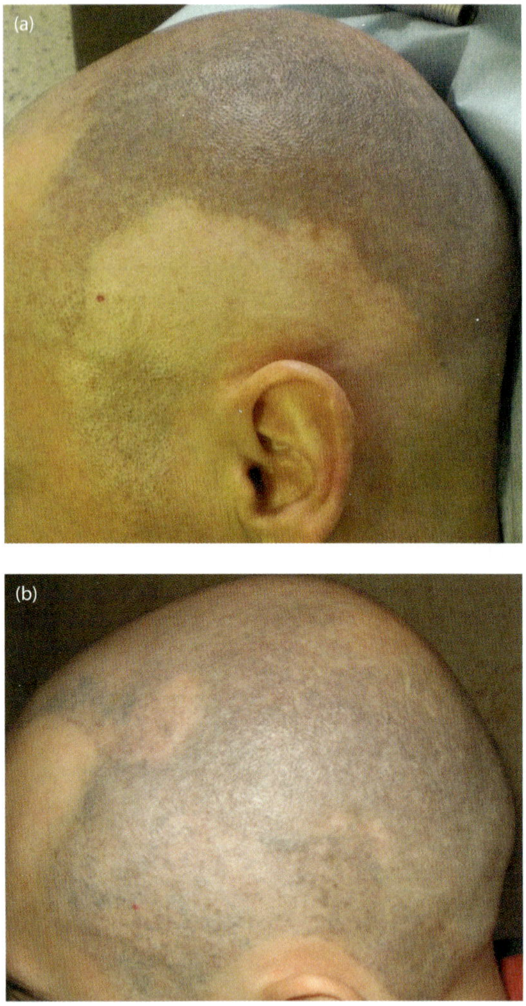

Figure 18.25 **Temporal alopecia areata (a) before and (b) after micropigmentation.**

Eyelashes

The edge of the eyelashes can rarefy due to different factors: one would be chemotherapy. The ciliary area can then be redensified: "type lash liner." The dermopigmentation method uses "close points" (which can vary depending on the density requested).

One can also accomplish a complete makeup-type eyeliner; the method then used is a lineage type.

The rebuild of a ciliary line can also be obtained on a grafted eyelid (Figure 18.27a and b).

Anesthesia

Anesthesia has a fundamental role in dermography. Indeed, the pain will produce an oxidative stress that might cause an oxidoreduction of the pigment and

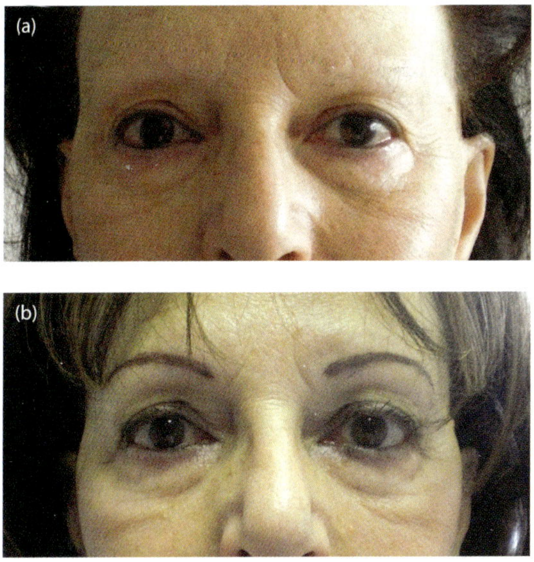

Figure 18.26 **Eyebrow alopecia (a) before and (b) after pigmentation.**

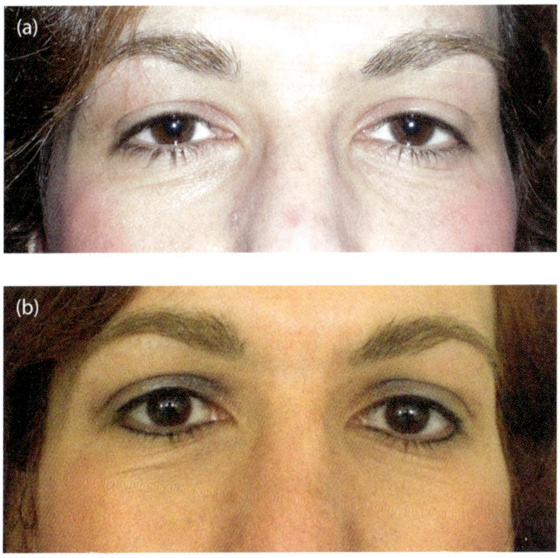

Figure 18.27 **Eyelids (a) before and (b) after pigmentation.**

therefore engender the oxidation of the mineral pigments and produce a color change.

This explains why we use "lidocaine" for skin pigmentation and "xylocaine" by intradermal injections for eyelids and eyebrows.

Conclusion

Dermopigmentation, or dermography or trichopigmentation or micropigmentation, are adapted processes of yesteryear's primitive tattoos.

For the last 20 years, its use in medicine and surgery as well as its research to date, allow its use in dermatological pathological treatments. Before, this was not possible, and its use enables us to improve the appearance and therefore the quality of our patients' lives, which are often extremely affected by their look.

After thousands of areola nipple reconstructions, eyebrows, eyelashes, outlines, and recoloring of the lips after accidents or pathologies, thanks to the technical progress, we now have power tools, needles, and biochemistry pigments which have enabled us to successfully achieve great results in hairy areas. We anticipate more to come in the future.

CONCLUSION

Wigs, hairpieces, and scalp-covering cosmetics are important and often underutilized tools in helping patients with hair loss or alopecia. Dermopigmentation, if well handled, used alone or in combination with hair surgery, becomes a good indication for definitive alopecia or body hair alopecia. Synthetic hair implants should become a useful tool for the treatment of some definitive alopecia if we observe a decrease of the rejection and the complications and an increase of the tolerance.

REFERENCES

1. Wakelin S. Contact anaphylaxis from natural rubber latex used as an adhesive for hair extensions. *Br J Dermatol.* 2002;146(2):340–341.
2. Khumalo NP, Jessop S, Gumedze F et al. Hairdressing is associated with scalp disease in African schoolchildren. *Br J Dermatol.* 2007;157(1):106–110.
3. Grimes PE. Skin and hair cosmetic issues in women of color. *Dermatol Clin.* 2000;18(4):659–665.
4. Bouhanna P. Clinical and macrophotographical study of the percutaneous implantation of synthetic hair. In: Van Neste D, La Chapelle JM, Antoine JL, eds. *Trends in Human Hair Growth and Alopecia Research.* Boston, MA: Kluwer Academic Publishers; 1989:257–265.
5. Bouhanna P. Accessory techniques. In: Bouhanna P, Dardour JC, eds. *Hair Replacement Surgery. Textbook and Atlas.* Berlin, Germany: Springer-Verlag; 1996: 174–187.
6. Di Gregorio VR, Rauscher G. Experience with the complications of synthetic hair transplantations. *Plast Reconstr Surg.* 1981;68(4):498–504.
7. Hanke CW, Bergfeld WF. Fiber implantation for pattern baldness. *J Am Acad Dermatol.* 1981;4:278–283.
8. Lepaw MI. Hair implant complications. *Cutis.* 1972; 9:304.
9. Schwartz RS, Downham TF. Dangers of synthetic fiber implantation for male pattern baldness. *Cutis.* 1980;25:491–492.

Dermopigmentation References

10. Casadio S. Le tatouage médical: pour oublier la maladie. *Quotidien du Médecin*. 2004;7496:14.
11. Casadio S. La dermopigmentation, reconnue d'intérêt thérapeutique et de pratique médicale obligatoire. *Quotidien du Médecin*. 2006;7864:10.
12. Grognard C. *Tatouage et maquillage réparateurs*. Collection dermatologie esthétique, Paris, France: Arnette Blackwell; 2008.
13. Tiziano JP, Semeria E, Levy JL. *la dermographie, technique du tatouage*. Marseille, France: Solal; 1990.
14. Casadio S. Dermographie des zones pileuses. *Revue dermatologique du cheveu*. 2007;15:6–12.
15. Bernstein R. Scalp Micropigmentation (Scalp Tattooing) at the 2012 ISHRS (International Society of Hair Restoration surgery) Scientific Meeting, Bahamas.
16. Pak JP, Kim J, Rassman WR. Scalp Micropigmentation (SMP*). A valuable technique for use in hair loss. In: *Hair Transplant 360*. Vol. 3. New Delhi, India: Jaypee Brothers Medical Publishers; 2013:349–357.
17. Rassman WR. Scalp Micropigmentation: Facial plastic surgery. In: *Hair Loss and Replacement for Dummies*. Clinics of North America, Pending publication; 2012.
18. Casadio S, Béchaux S. Micropigmentation du cuir chevelu et des zones pileuses, une solution pour les dermatologues. *Nouv Dermatol*. 2003;32:418–422.
19. Casadio S. Dermopigmentation for head hair and vellus areas. *1st I.C.H.S; 1st AMEC (Anti Aging Medicine European Congress)*, Paris, France; October 12, 2013.

19 Hair cosmetology

Claude Bouillon and Michèle Verschoore

CLEANSING HAIR AND SCALP

Shampooing is a basic hygiene measure worldwide, yet performed in various ways from one individual to another or from one place to another. Hair cleaning is more frequent where water is abundant or where it is considered as a symbol of purification, like in Japan and Korea.

The word *shampoo* comes from the Hindi "Champo," meaning to massage, to knead. It still fits such a traditional way as practiced by hairdressers in China, involving a prolonged massaging with pure shampoo prior to adding water, a procedure called "dry wash" by the Chinese people.

The frequency of shampooing largely increased in parallel to improved housing and living standards. In Europe, it reaches three times weekly on average, and about one out of four among the population, especially younger men (<30 years), shampoo their hair daily. Eighty percent of people in the United States and 90% of those in Japan declare washing their hair twice daily on average. With regard to gender, the shampooing procedure is less frequent among women who view time-consuming hair-drying and management of long hair,

The primary function of shampoo is to cleanse both hair and scalp, which requires this product to be versatile enough to fulfill a variety of demands:

- To remove rapidly and efficiently the soil from hair without damaging the latter when rubbing onto hair and with no irritant effect upon eyes, scalp, and hands.
- To correctly clean with a widely variable amount depending on the user (from few grams to dozens), irrespective of the nature and the amount of soil, the condition and characteristics of hair (sparse or dense, dry or not, short or long, straight or frizzy, etc), different scalp conditions (seborrhea, dandruff), and using tap waters of varying hardness.
- To develop enough foam, since perceived as evidence of cleaning efficiency, a key aspect.

But the expectations of a consumer, more acute for women with regard to longer hair, lie far beyond efficient cleaning and pleasant in-use qualities, aesthetic appearance, liquid, gel, or cream, smooth and abundant foam, and easy rinsing. The shampoo must transform the head of hair, yielding lively and bright hair.

Changing and beautifying hair condition may encompass a variety of aspects according to the user:

- To provide ease of entangling of wet hair
- To enhance wet hair feel
- To ease combing of hair when dried
- To impart volume, body, spring, manageability, and suppleness
- To reduce flyaways
- To bring a silky feel
- Not to reveal drawbacks when frequently used
- To meet specific needs, such as clearing a scalp condition or maintaining a hairstyle

In brief, these items compose a huge diversity of requirements and/or expectations, often conflicting and not easy to reconcile, that make the development of a quality shampoo an intricate achievement. This also explains the wide range of shampoos designed to most appropriately solve the various and varying compromises like a magic wand.

From a consumer viewpoint, in addition to its foaming properties (rapidity to develop, density), the fragrance (fruity, floral, or woody) introduced within a shampoo plays a crucial role in its marketing/consumer acceptance. Both hedonic properties during shampooing and residual fragrance(s) left on a dried head of hair are such key factors that despite its best cleansing and conditioning properties, an inappropriately fragranced shampoo is promised very low commercial attainment.

CLEANSING FUNCTION OF SHAMPOO

Hair soil consists of lipids of the daily gram range, mostly originating from sebum released through follicular outlets[1] and trapped mineral and organic air pollutants, scalp keratin debris, hair dressing deposits, and a significant number of resident and transient members of scalp flora (bacteria and yeasts). Table 19.1 gathers the overall ranges of quantitative key factors involved in or eliminated during the act of shampooing, according to individual daily life routines and specificities (hair length, hair shapes, dandruff, etc.).

The role of a cleansing or detergent agent is to weaken the adhesive forces that stick the soil to hair and scalp, then transfer it into water medium and disperse it within while avoiding any redeposit onto the hair.[2] This process is performed by surfactants, dual-faceted agents

Table 19.1 Major Elements of Skin and Hair Involved and Eliminated during the Act of Shampooing

Scalp surface (adult)	600–700 cm^2
Hair surface (according to hair length)	0.5–6 m^2
Sebum on scalp and hair (daily amount)	0.5–2 grams
Keratin debris and scales	5–50 milligrams (including squames/dandruff)
Volume of water used, rinsing included	20–50 L
Amount of shampoo used (one to two successive times)	2–30 grams
Total time of shampooing	1–5 minutes
Time to dry (hair dryer)	5–30 minutes, according to length

(i.e., endowed with dual affinity). These are composed of a long hydrocarbon chain (10–14 carbon atoms), so-called fatty chain with hydrophobic/lipophilic properties, and a polar hydrophilic head group. The lipophilic part of the surfactant shows high affinity toward lipids and links to the soil, whereas the polar head is water soluble and transfers the soil into water when rinsing.

Soap (Figure 19.1), a salt of fatty acid mixture produced by saponification of plant oils and fats by strong alkaline agents (sodium or potassium hydroxide), was the first detergent used for hair cleansing.[3] To make it soluble in water and avoid acid release, however, soap requires an increase in pH toward an alkaline level, hence possibly altering the hair surface. Moreover, in the presence of hard water, insoluble calcium salts are formed leaving deposits on hair and causing hair to look dull.

R–COOH **Fatty acid** $R = CH_3–(CH_2)_n$ $n > 10$

$R–COOH^- Na^+$ **Soap** e.g., Sodium (Na) salt of fatty acid

Example of soap from natural plant oil/butter:

Cocoa butter: Triglyceride of palmitic acid (26%), stearic acid (34.5%) and oleic acid (34.5%)

$CH_2–O–CO–(CH_2)_{14}–CH_3$ Palmitate
|
$CH–O–CO–(CH_2)_{16}–CH_3$ Stearate
|
$CH_2–O–CO–(CH_2)_7–CH{=}CH–(CH_2)_7–CH_3$ Oleate

Cocoa soap: Mix of sodium palmitate (26%), stearate (34.5%) and oleate (34.5%)

Palmitic and stearic acids are saturated fatty acids while oleic acid has one C=C double bond and therefore falls into unsaturated acid class.

Figure 19.1 Soaps.

$R–O–SO_3^- Na^+$ Fatty alcohol sulfate $R = C_{12–14}$ linear chain (or R = 12–14 carbon chain)

$R–O–(CH_2–CH_2–O)_n – SO_3^-Na^+$ Ethersulfate of ethoxylated fatty alcohol

$R–O–CH_2–CH_2–O–CH_2–CH_2–O\,H$ Ethoxylated fatty alcohol with 2 ethoxy (OE) groups (n = 2)

Figure 19.2 **Fatty alcohol sulfates and ethersulfates.**

These drawbacks have been erased in replacing soaps by other anionic surfactants, the linear fatty alcohol sulfates, or the ethersulfates of ethoxylated fatty alcohols (Figure 19.2) which both offer good foaming, emulsifying, and cleansing powers, and biodegradability as well. The rather poor cosmetic properties of these highly suitable hair cleansing agents have led to them being combined with amphoteric surfactant (such as betaines, for example), the fatty chain of which ends with both anionic and cationic sites (Figure 19.3). Amphoteric surfactants form complexes with anionic surfactants, improve foam tightness and softness, and reduce the tendency of anionics to adsorb onto proteins.

Progress in research and formulation has allowed shampoos that are very mild on the skin and eye to be developed, involving anionic surfactants such as sulfosuccinates, sarcosinates, taurates, glutamates, polyethoxylated fatty acids, or *N*-acylpeptide salts.[4]

FORMULATING SHAMPOO

The development of a cleansing base is the prime goal that needs to be optimized according to the versatile or specific features of the shampoo that are desired. It must be suitable for hair and scalp condition, frequency of use, and hair care or styling routine. The goal is to efficiently and rapidly clean without drying, keeping unaltered normal scalp homeostasis, given that the scalp is more sensitive than the hair to degreasing action. Requirements also entail lubricating hair while removing soil (i.e., replacing soil by conditioning material that enhances hair condition), another challenge.

In-use properties are brought by a variety of additives affording pleasant texture and feel when carrying out the

$$CH_3–(CH_2)_{11}–CO–NH–(CH_2)_3–{}^{+}N(CH_3)_2–CH_2–COO^-$$

Figure 19.3 **Amphoteric surfactant (cocoamidopropylbetaine). At neutral pH it behaves like an internal salt (ammonium carboxylate).**

cleansing operation. To the detergent/cleansing ingredients which account for 10%–20% of the shampoo product, thickening agents are added to providing controlled flow, easy measuring out in the hollow of the hand, easy spreading, and easy distribution into the hair without altering foam. Some of these enhance foam smoothness and stability, whereas others show critical thresholds to prevent fall in foam and product consistency, notably with hard water. Pearlescents such as ethyleneglycol distearate provide micrometric crystal particles whose size, density, and arrangement lend an opaque, shiny, or creamy appearance.

Choosing the conditioning ingredients and defining their right proportions, however, has become the most tricky step when designing and developing a shampoo. The purpose is to bring to hair ease of untangling, soft touch, gloss, and reduced flyaway. Conditioning agents should help to gain a smoother, even hair shaft with tighter adhesiveness of cuticle scales to minimize friction. A large variety of ingredients, mentioned below in the section dedicated to hair care products, may be introduced into the formula of a shampoo as far as they are compatible with the cleansing base. The contribution of such ingredients in a shampoo product of course does not compare with that in a product fully designed for hair care only or a specific after-shampoo rinse, due to different, hardly reconcilable, if not antonymic, functions to be achieved at the same time within a single operating procedure instead of two, separately performed. This way, however, the selected conditioning ingredients can play a significant role in the aesthetic appearance, condition, and manageability of hair after shampooing.

The initial breakthrough in conditioning shampoos came with the availability of cationic polymers (PC) with high affinity for damaged hair that, unlike dedicated cationic surfactants, are compatible with anionic surfactants used in shampoos. The mechanisms of PC interaction with, and effect upon, the hair shaft are described in the section dealing with hair care. These PCs form soluble complexes with anionic surfactants by adjusting either or both concentrations and possibly adding amphoteric or nonionic surfactant. When diluted with water, the structure of these complexes changes, leading to phase separation and polymer deposit onto hair, a sequence of intricate micelle formation, air/liquid, and liquid/hair substrate interaction processes.[5] Most used cationic polymers are cellulose and guar gum derivatives. These improve hair untangling and combing considerably, while affording a clearly soft feel. They also impart dense, smooth foam. Most dramatic effects of these PCs are obtained upon dry and sun or oxidation damaged hairs. Less efficient on unaltered or slightly damaged hair due to reduced affinity (low ionic character/charges), they may have some build-up effect, and are not easy to rinse off with frequent shampooing.

A second breakthrough arose from the introduction of silicones of polydimethylsiloxane type (Figure 19.4) which impart a silky feel to hair and protect the hair surface with a hydrophobic film. However, silicone polymers are insoluble in the aqueous vehicle of shampoos, an aspect that raised a major issue and subsequently delayed their use in such an application. The formulation process had to be devised for homogeneous and stable dispersions in surfactant solutions to be achieved without altering their detergent and foaming properties. Such dispersions could be further stabilized through adding pearlescent agents to thickened solutions of cleansing bases. They gave rise to so-called "2 in 1" shampoos.

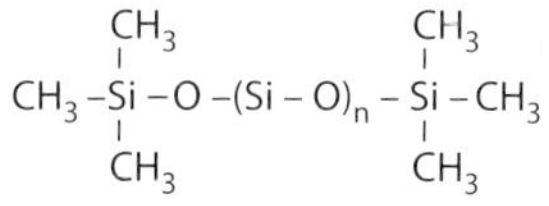

Figure 19.4 **Polydimethylsiloxanes (dimethicones). The viscosity of dimethicones used in conditioning shampoos is 50,000–1,000,000 mm^2/s.**

A further step forward consisted in combining polydimethylsiloxanes (PDMS) and selected cationic polymers, thereby optimizing beneficial effects. For example, PDMS adsorption onto hair can be strengthened by PC, whereas PC inhibits potential build-up of PDMS with repeated shampooing. On the other hand, PDMS favors an even deposit of PC along the hair shaft. The strong interdependence between PC and PMDS has been particularly accounted for in most performing conditioning shampoos, as well as the use of PDMS derivatives having cationic groups such as amodimethicones (Figure 19.5).[6]

Developing such shampoos requires PDMS technology and industrial processing to be perfectly mastered in addition to a tremendous contribution from research investigations.

TYPES OF SHAMPOO

A variety of shampoos ranging from general use to hair- or scalp-specific conditions are available on the market. They are most often presented in opaque liquid form of varying viscosities, or in cream form for dry, damaged hair. Other forms are gels or clear liquids, with minimal ingredient content for hair care with the exception of some cationic polymer for easier combing of wet hair. The main types are as follows.

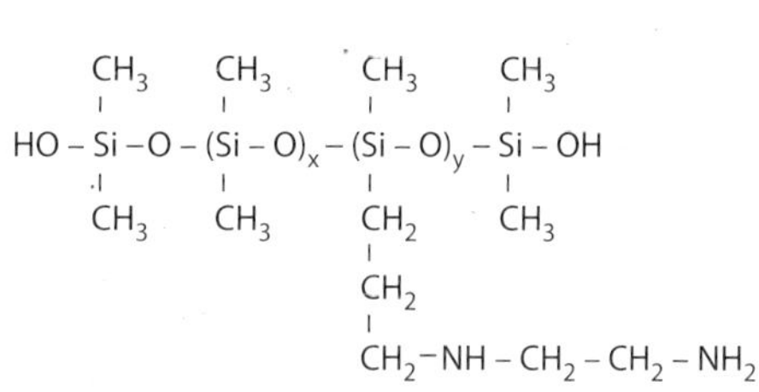

Figure 19.5 **Amodimethicones.**

Shampoos for general use

Family shampoos are required to foam and cleanse the hair well, without excessive detergency, and to provide easy untangling and hair shine while being cost-effective, with an image of softness.

Mild shampoos for frequent use

The development of personal hygiene, practicing sport or exercise, living in a highly polluted city, or humid ambient air result in increasingly frequent shampooing. Regardless of the issue, be it excessive sweating, greasy hair, density of airborne pollutant particles, or coating related to leave-on hair care or dressing products, the need for detergency is not as high when shampooing every second day or less, but high enough for cleansing hair likely more exposed or prone to collect more soil. This type of shampoo is based upon the combination of anionic and amphoteric surfactants selected for suitable mildness and tolerance. Another requirement is fine tuning its conditioning potency (i.e., favoring ease of combing and yielding a beautiful head of hair but without causing any buildup of polymer film deposit and its resulting effect of weighing hair down).

Conditioning shampoos

These shampoos are tailor-made for achieving the dual function of a shampoo and a conditioner. Targeting increasingly high expectations in terms of beautifully changing hair appearance, condition, and touch, they must yield closer to the performance of two separately applied products with distinct functions and abundant water rinsing in between a single operation using a multifunctional product. In addition to cleansing and foaming properties, conditioning shampoos (Figure 19.6) must hold the capacity of correcting fairly efficiently the flaws inherent to some types of hair. The formula of such products is highly sophisticated, requiring subtle adjustment of detergent and conditioning actions to ensure during shampooing both clear soil extraction/dispersion and sequential microdeposit of cationic/silicone polymer softening film along each hair.

Conditioning shampoos for fine hair are designed to provide body, spring, and bounce, whereas dry hairs need easy disentangling, reduced friction, lubrication, and shine. Cationic polymers or PDMS may have a negative impact on the rate of regreasing of greasy hairs post shampooing. Therefore, dedicated shampoos must impart volume and lightness, and delay weighing down by sebum uptake. When targeting dyed or lightened hairs, conditioning shampoos should bring suppleness, control, and easy combing and brushing, and also enhance vividness of the coloring.

Styling shampoos

These aim at helping to impart and sustain a hairstyle post shampooing. Anionic, amphoteric, and nonionic polymers are combined with conditioning high-molecular-weight cationic polymers according to a carefully adjusted measuring out depending on type of hair. PCs with weak ionic charge are favored to avoid excessive bonding to hair and risk of hair being weighed down.

Specific shampoos for scalp condition

Intended for dandruff or greasy scalp, such shampoos aim at clearing scalp conditions and mitigating associated unaesthetical aspects. When developing a shampoo

Ingredient	Amount w/w %
Sodium lauryl ether sulfate	15
Cocoamidopropyl betaine	3
Fatty acid ethanolamide	2
Ethyleneglycol distearate	2
Cationic polymer	0.2
Polydimethylsiloxane	1
Fragrance	0.5
Preservative qsp	
Water	qsp 100
pH adjusted at 7	

Figure 19.6 **Basic formula of a conditioning shampoo. Cleansing base includes anionic and amphoteric surfactants. A thickener and a pearlescent agent are added for foaming consistency, appearance, and quality in use. (Adapted from Tan Tai Ho L; Ho Tan Tai ed.** ***Formulating Detergents and Personal Care Products: A [Complete] Guide to Product Development.*** **Urbana, IL: AOCS Press; 2000.)**

for greasy scalp and hair, the prime focus is on defining the most suitable blend of surfactants (i.e., the cleansing base).

Dandruff is a most common scalp disorder, shared by about 45% of the human population, irrespective of gender and ethnicity,[8] mainly in large urban cities, where psychological stress is prevalent. The central inducer of this scaly disorder is the resident yeast *Malassezia* sp., the proliferation of which accounts for 75% of scalp microflora in dandruff conditions, initiating a micro-inflammatory process. The latter causes persistent itching, increased epidermal turnover, and impaired keratinocyte maturation, as reflected by scale production (33.2 mg/2 days vs. 8.1 on nondandruff scalp) and an elevated parakeratotic index (18.4 vs. 3.9)—that is, the percentage of corneocytes which retain a nucleus.[9] The inducing yeast colonizes the stratum disjunctum releasing lipase and lipoxygenase that degrade sebum components, used as nutrients.

Efficient and safe antifungal agents are available, mainly zinc pyrithione (ZPT), piroctone olamine, selenium sulfide, climbazole, and ketoconazole, used at 0.5–1.5 g% in anti-dandruff shampoos. Regular application (i.e., twice a week) of such active ingredients within a mild cleansing base significantly eliminates the symptoms and improves scalp condition.

Improved hair density or thickness was reported following daily use of antidandruff shampoo in men with alopecia.[10]

Shampoos for babies and children

The purpose here is to ensure an optimal mildness and comfort to skin and eyes. The composition is therefore based upon nonionic surfactants (about 10%) such as fatty acid esters of highly ethoxylated glycerol or sorbitan (e.g., copra monoglycerides with 30 ethoxy groups, palm glycerides with 200 ethoxy groups, sorbitan [20 ethoxy groups] monolaurate) (Figure 19.7). These surfactants favor the formation of large micelles that hardly adsorb onto proteins, and in particular onto the surface of mucous lachrymal membrane, thus avoiding any eye tingling, watering, or dislike.

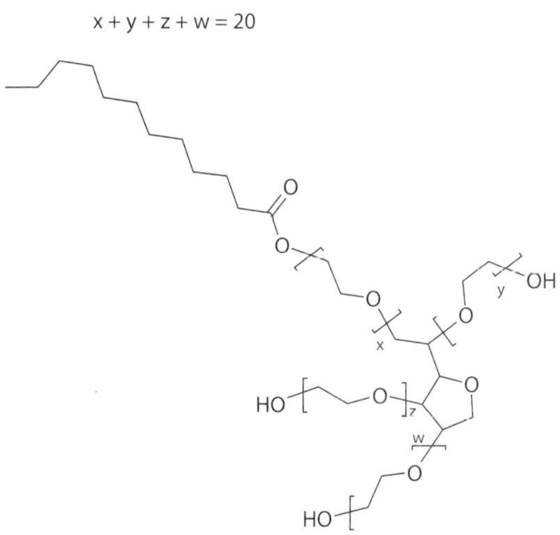

Figure 19.7 **Sorbitan monolaurate (20 OE).**

HAIR CONDITIONERS

The prime target of hair care products is correcting deterioration of the hair surface and protecting it from weathering or any further external assault.

The hair surface is the outer part of the cuticle, a thick sheath that tightly wraps the core of the hair, or cortex which is the key mechanical structure and strength of the fiber. The hair cuticle is made up of superimposed layers (7–10 at the proximal end, decreasing toward the distal end and in short cycling hairs) of flat inert cells/scales covering each other like roof tiles. Hair structure is composed of keratin proteins characterized by a high overall sulfur content. Among the 18 amino acids included in the keratin polypeptide sequence, one of them, cystine, has a disulfide linkage and amounts to 20%–30% of the proteinaceous material in the outermost layer of the cuticle.[11] Natural hair is covered by a long lipid chain, mainly 18-methyl eicosanoic acid (MEA) covalently bound by a thioester linkage.[12]

The hair surface undergoes multiple physical and chemical stresses depending upon hair routines and exposures. Frequent and daily mechanical handling such as brushing and combing erodes and uplifts cuticle scales and breaks cell edges producing a jagged surface. Frequent, hot blow drying combined with brushing makes hair dry and brittle. Environmental factors, primarily sun exposure, change the chemical balance of the hair surface through cleaving intra- and interkeratin chain disulfide linkages and thus giving rise to numerous strong sulfonic acid groups by the photo-oxidation process (Figure 19.8). The highly cystine-rich surface of hair takes on a strong anionic character, dramatically changing interactions, hair/hair included. Lipid MEA coating also vanishes, leaving hair rough and poorly lubricated.

Upon contact with such damaged hair, cationics become strongly attracted. An electrochemical bond is created between the positive (cationic) group and a negative (anionic) site/group of the hair surface. In the presence of a cationic surfactant (Figure 19.9a), which is composed of a cationic hydrophilic group at the end of a lipophilic (hydrocarbon) chain, the electrostatic bonding of the cationic group to the hair surface anionic site/group leads to the deposit of a monomolecular layer of surfactant fatty chain onto hair (Figure 19.9b). As a consequence, hair touch and surface properties are drastically altered. The extremely thin lipid chain coating lubricates the damaged area. The friction coefficient is considerably decreased. Following application of cationic surfactant, hair roughness vanishes, as does

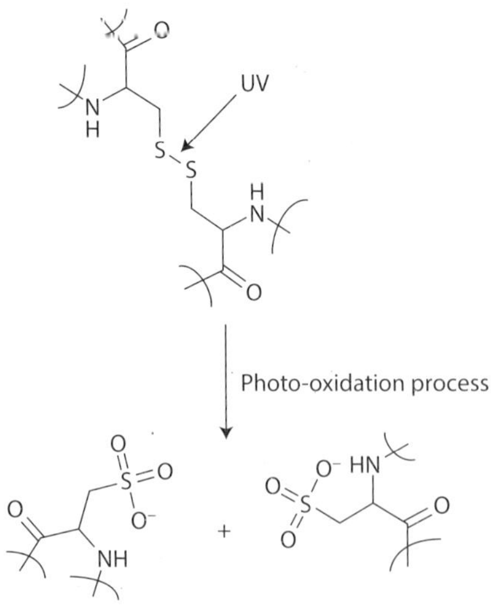

Figure 19.8 **Cystine linkage between two keratin polypeptide chains. UV-induced radical cleavage of disulfide bond and photo-oxidative conversion into sulfionic groups.**

flyaway behavior, as a result of charge neutralization. Hairs, then, gain a soft feel.

Fixing the cationic surfactant takes place where an anionic (sulfonic) group is present. The more altered the hair surface, the more numerous are the anionic groups and the more cationic surfactant molecules are bound to the hair surface. As a result, an even hair surface is regained, every damaged site being neutralized and smoothed over. Rinsing with water removes unneeded cationic surfactant, leaving hair with appropriate care where needed. It is worth emphasizing that cationic surfactants used for hair care and beauty are devoid of detergent properties. They compose hydrocarbon (fatty) chains clearly longer than those of anionic, amphoteric, and nonionic surfactants used for hair cleansing (i.e., 17–20 carbon atoms instead of 12–14). They are consequently endowed with radically different properties.

Being most suitable for hairs with surfaces that exhibit behavior and interactions altered by acquired anionic character, conditioning cationic surfactants allow damaged areas to be protected (negatively charged) site by site, leveling out the surface. Rid of rough patches, the latter becomes amazingly easy to comb through. These cationic surfactants that show potent conditioners, however, cannot improve hair consistency, and most are incompatible with anionic surfactants used in shampoos and various hair products. When mixed, they form complexes that abolish their respective properties, and hence, the tremendous step forward brought by another category of ingredients mentioned in the previous sections (i.e., cationic polymers).

In the structure of a cationic polymer, the functional groups prone to bind to the hair surface are not at the end of a lipophilic chain but instead are grafted to or located along a macromolecular chain (Figure 19.10). As a result, while being attracted by anionic groups and readily taken up by an anionic hair surface, they stretch over the hair a continuous film with multiple binding sites, whereby surface properties are transformed. In addition to covering and smoothing hair, cationic polymer imparts texture and body without weighing hair down. The hair surface becomes even, soft, protected all along from external assaults, while hair is easy to disentangle and dress.

Most frailty hairs are fine, or very curly hairs at twisting points where the cortex, which endows hair with outstanding mechanical properties and resilience, is highly reduced. The finer the hair, the lower is the mass that most composes the cuticle. Surface alterations consequently affect the whole hair. Flyaways and lack of control are major issues for fine hair, lacking body and firmness. More porous, such hair easily breaks, and the friction coefficient is high. Cationic polymers substantially benefit this type of hair.

Cationic polymers for hair conditioning are polysaccharides derived from cellulose, guar, starch, chitosan, or a variety of vinyl, allyl, acrylate, and methacrylate copolymers.

Another major hair condition contributor, as highlighted in the paragraph dedicated to shampoos, is the

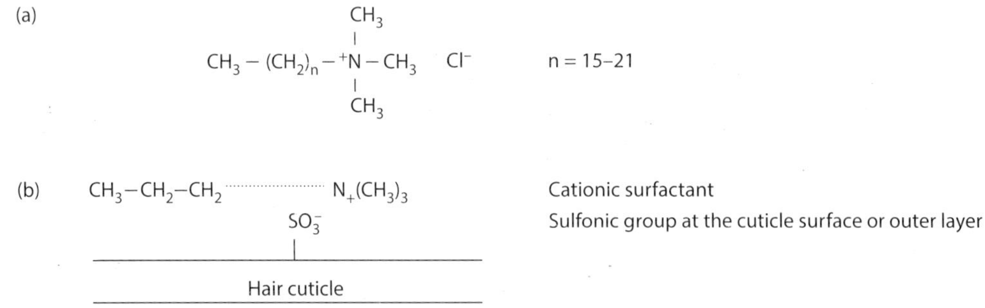

Figure 19.9 (a) **Cationic surfactant (e.g., cetyltrimethylammonium chloride, *n* = 15). (b) Electrostatic bonds between cationic surfactant and anionic group at the hair surface.**

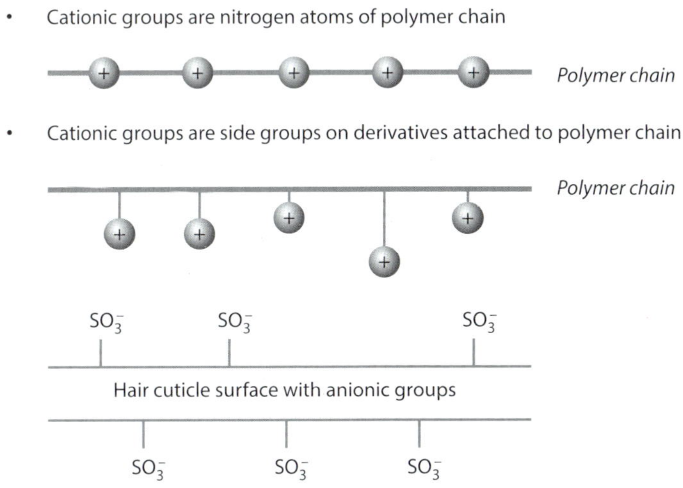

Figure 19.10 **Cationic polymers.**

field of silicone polymers. First used for their nongreasiness and light feel, these have met with outstanding diversity of applications and cosmetic development on account of low surface tension, despite viscosity that may be high, hydrophobic behavior, weak cohesive forces, and being chemically inert. Whereas PCs are most suitable for hairs prone to interact following oxidative damage to epicuticle layers, PDMS provide optimal benefits to natural, undamaged, or physically impaired hairs, yielding a smooth feel from root to tip and lightweight, nimbled hairs. These silicone polymers spread a thin, uniform, hydrophobic deposit on the hair, smoothing out the whole hair shaft, split end included (Figure 19.11a), enhancing sheen and gloss, and steadily protecting it when combing.

To prevent buildup and undesired hair-appearance possibly resulting from repeated applications, hair conditioners require a meticulous, thorough development taking into account type of hair, targeted effects and benefits, frequency of use, and hair routines (waving, coloring, lightening, straightening, relaxing). Hair conditioning agents must be blended with the most adequate vehicles able to boost, extend, and magnify their effects and favor pleasantness in use, comprehensive distribution within

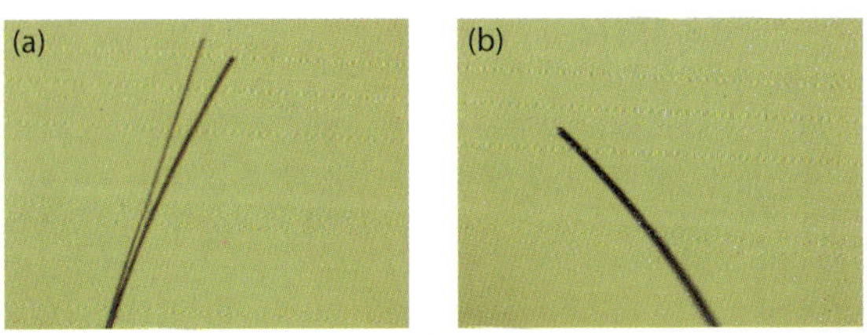

Figure 19.11 **Hair split end (a) before (b) after applying a conditioning serum based upon silicone derivatives.**

the head of hair, and the whole range of care and beauty contributions with added benefits. Hence, among the palette of ingredients that are used to improve hair condition, the following can be mentioned:

- Fatty materials such as fatty alcohols, natural oils (e.g., olive, almond, avocado, karite, monoi, corn), or waxes (e.g., jojoba, beeswax) that have been traditionally used in all civilizations for lubricating, nourishing hair, and providing sheen; fatty acids (e.g., oleic, linoleic, linolenic, behenic); ethoxylated derivatives; ceramides such as *N*-oleoyl sphinganine, shown to restore damaged hair cuticles through strengthening interscale junction and protecting the hair shaft from brushing and sun-induced damage.[13]
- Protein hydrolysates (e.g., silk, wool, collagen, soybean, oat, wheat).

Hair conditioners include a large variety of products to suitably meet the changing and diverse needs or demands according to the type, abundance, and condition of hair, preferred texture, intended frequency of application, and level of expected performance.

Most are rinsed off after being left on the hair for some time, generally a few minutes, or longer in the case of deep conditioners. Practically, they are presented as:

- *Conditioning creams or emulsions*: Of common use, applied after shampooing, these are of varying viscosity (i.e., fluid lotions, gel emulsions, or creams such as untangling balms). They usually contain cationic surfactant and fatty alcohols, readily spread onto the head of hair where they are left 1 or 2 minutes, then rinsed off. They are intended for normal, dry, or very dry hair to which they provide manageability, suppleness, ease of combing, and shine.

- *Deep conditioners*: These are thick creams for intensive care of damaged or very dry hair with high friction coefficient. For less frequent use (e.g., once a week), they contain more conditioning agents and are left on the hair for a prolonged time (10–15 minutes). Silicone polymers and cationic surfactants are often combined to obtain synergetic repairing effects, help to recover tightly adhesive scales, smooth over the hair shaft, and impart lightness.
- *Lotions or fluid gels*: Of light texture, clear or opaque, without fatty ingredients, they are aqueous solutions of cationic surfactant and/or PC intended for normal or fine hair or hair with a greasy tendency. The target is to afford lightness, volume, control, and sheen with no perception of deposit that could detract from the look of the hair.
- *Oils*: Plant oils have long been used as nutrients to protect, beautify, lubricate, and give shine to hair. Clear, translucent emulsions are now available where oils are combined with cationics and silicones, can impregnate the outer layers of cuticle and resist removal by shampoos.[14]

Leave-on conditioners

Other hair care and beauty products are designed to be kept in the hair after application. They aim at facilitating combing (combing aids) and affording sheen and smoothness to hair. They contain cationic surfactants or polymers in a lower amount than products to be rinsed post application. Various silicones are also widely used, such as cationic amodimethicones or ethoxylated silicones. They are presented as aerosol foams or creams and gel emulsions of various viscosities.

Oils and serums

Originally and essentially water-free products containing oils and/or silicone derivatives, they are used for nourishing and protecting very dry hair exposed to sun, air conditioning, salt water, drying wind, or climate. Silicone derivatives, less oily and of widely varying texture, are used in a variety of serums for smoothing hairs or repairing damaged areas such as split ends (Figure 19.11b). Aqueous serums containing cationic and/or silicone derivatives are also proposed.

Hairstyling products

The basic ingredient in hairstyling and hair-dressing products is anionic film-forming polymer that gives hold to hair shape through sheathing the hair shaft.[15] A thin, fluid coating maintains the hairstyle in an inconspicuous way, looking natural. It also helps the hairstyle keep its shape in a humid atmosphere. The deposited film must be hard and resistant enough when passing the brush through, for example. Depending on the expected effect, a given polymer or a combination of polymers is chosen, together with additives to increase film hardness or give some flexibility or favor hair sticking together to yield stranded effects. Water-soluble polymers are preferred for easy removal by shampooing. Anionic polymer can be combined with cationic polymer, taking advantage of the affinity of the latter toward hair and conditioning properties, providing a soft feel and possibly synergetic hold. Silicone derivatives are often added to improve hair shaft condition, reduce friction, make brushing easier, and contribute to smoother hair. Lubricants such as ceramide may also be introduced, and polyols (e.g., glycerol) as well to reduce dry feel.[16]

Spreadability is a critical point. The texture of the product is a decisive factor. Most commonly, aqueous or aqueous alcoholic lotions are applied to the hair using a spray, or are thickened with gelling agents such as guar gum derivatives.

EVALUATION OF HAIR SURFACE CONDITION AND CARE-INDUCED CHANGES

A variety of techniques have been studied and developed for assessing the condition of the hair surface and most closely reflecting the sensory and visual appreciation of the consumers following hair-conditioning product applications.[17] Confocal laser scanning microscopy was used to generate high-resolution three-dimensional (3D) images of polymer deposits on hair before and after shampooing.[18,19] The availability of atomic force microscopes was a further significant advance in providing hair surface images of very high spatial resolution, down to the nanometer, and allowing friction or viscoelastic properties to be measured.[20,21] The effects produced by hair-conditioning or styling products or shampoos can be thoroughly explored, as well as the interactions and friction forces at the nano level.[22–24]

Other devices measure the wet and dry combing forces[25,26] or hair brittleness[27] on hair swatches or hair in vivo in real-life conditions before and after hair product applications. Electrostatic charges (flyaway) developed during combing, and the antistatic effect of hair conditioners, can be recorded by automated or manual tensile combs.[28,29] Other techniques for characterizing the hair surface properties include potent analytical methods, such as secondary ion mass spectroscopy (SIMS),[13,30,31] x-ray photoelectron microscopy,[32,33] and dynamic electronic and permeability analysis.[34,35]

A video method addressing the difficult issue of dynamic properties of hairs in relation to visual perception of the head of hair moving in real-life conditions was recently published.[36]

Appraising shine or luster, a key attribute of hair visual appearance and beauty perception, has been another major challenge. Many authors have used a goniophotometer, recording the multiangular distribution of reflected light when hair is illuminated with white light or a laser beam at a 30° angle. Reflected light includes specular, internal, and diffuse reflections. Various formulas have been proposed for calculating shine from data obtained from a single hair or tresses of aligned hairs.[37–40] A new approach involves taking images of hair using a fast video camera with high polarization contrast, called SAMBA, and analyzing these with a specific algorithm to calculate luster.[41,42] Results were shown to be in agreement with the subjective evaluation of consumers.[41,43]

REFERENCES

1. Piérard-Franchimont C, Piérard G. Seborrhea. In: Bouillon C, Wilkinson J, eds. *The Science of Hair Care*. 2nd edn. Boca Raton, FL: Taylor & Francis; 2005:587–590.
2. Beauquey B. Scalp and hair hygiene: Shampoos. In: Bouillon C, Wilkinson J, eds. *The Science of Hair Care*. 2nd edn. Boca Raton, FL: Taylor & Francis; 2005:94–105.
3. Wolf R, Wolf D, Tüzün B, Tüzün Y. Soaps, shampoos and detergents. *Clin Dermatol*. 2001;19:393–397.
4. Beauquey B. Scalp and hair hygiene: Shampoos. In: Bouillon C, Wilkinson J, eds. *The Science of Hair Care*. 2nd edn. Boca Raton, FL: Taylor & Francis; 2005:84–93.
5. Goddard ED. Polymers/surfactant interaction in applied systems, principles of polymer science and technology. In: Goddard ED, Grubber JV, eds. *Cosmetics and Personal Care*. New York, NY: Marcel Dekker; 1999.
6. Dubief C, Mellul M, Loussouarn G, Saint-Léger D. Hair care products. In: Bouillon C, Wilkinson J, eds. *The Science of Hair Care*. 2nd edn. Boca Raton, FL: Taylor & Francis; 2005:146–150.
7. Tan Tai Ho L; Ho Tan Tai ed. *Formulating Detergents and Personal Care Products: A [Complete] Guide to Product Development*. Urbana, IL: AOCS Press; 2000.
8. Saint-Léger D, Clavaud C, Breton L, Talwar S. The human scalp and related cosmetic care products. In: Chakaravarthi S, Verschoore M, eds. *Basic Science for Modern Cosmetology*. New Delhi, India: Jaypee Brothers Medical; 2014:167–178.
9. Saint-Léger D. Dandruff (pytyriasis capitis simplex): Of yeasts and men. In: Bouillon C, Wilkinson J, eds. *The Science of Hair Care*. 2nd edn. Boca Raton, FL: Taylor & Francis; 2005:618–619.
10. Berger RS, Fu JL, Smiles KA et al. The effects of minoxidil, 1% pyrithione zinc and a combination of both on hair density in a randomized control trial. *Brit J Dermatol*. 2003;149(2):354–362.
11. Swift JA. Minimum depth electron probe X-ray microanalysis as a means for determining the sulfur content of the human hair surface. *Scanning*. 1979;2:83–88.
12. Swift JA. Human hair cuticle: Biology conspired to the owner's advantage. *J Cosmet Sci*. 1999;50:23–47.
13. Braida D, Dubief C, Lang G et al. Ceramide: A new approach to hair protection and conditioning. *Cosmet Toiletries*. 1994;109:49–57.
14. Dubief C, Mellul M, Loussouarn G, Saint-Léger D. Hair care products. In: Bouillon C, Wilkinson J, eds. *The Science of Hair Care*. 2nd edn. Boca Raton, FL: Taylor & Francis; 2005:159–162.
15. Beitone R, Sturla JM, Paty H et al. Temporary restyling of the hair. In: Bouillon C, Wilkinson J, eds. *The Science of Hair Care*. 2nd edn. Boca Raton, FL: Taylor & Francis; 2005:188–191.
16. Beitone R, Sturla JM, Paty H et al. Temporary restyling of the hair. In: Bouillon C, Wilkinson J, eds. *The Science of Hair Care*. 2nd edn. Boca Raton, FL: Taylor & Francis; 2005:173–180.
17. Franbourg A, Leroy F, Braida D. Evaluation of hair product efficacy. In: Bouillon C, Wilkinson J, eds. *The Science of Hair Care*. 2nd edn. Boca Raton, FL: Taylor & Francis; 2005:388–454.
18. Corcuff P, Gremillet P, Jourlin M et al. 3D reconstruction of human hair by confocal microscopy. *J Soc Cosmet Chem*. 1993;44:1–12.
19. Hadjur C, Madry G Daty G, et al. Cosmetic assessment of the human hair by confocal microscopy. *Scanning*. 2002;24:59–64.
20. Luengo G, Leroy F. The science of beauty on a small scale. Nano-technologies applied to cosmetic science. In: Bhushan B, Fuchs H, Hosaka S, eds. *Applied Scanning Probe Methods*. Amsterdam, The Netherlands: Elsevier; 2004:363–386.
21. Smith JR. Use of atomic force microscopy for high-resolution non-invasive structural studies of human hair. *J Soc Cosmet Chem*. 1997;48:199–208.
22. Yahagi K. Silicones as conditioning agents in shampoos. *J Soc Cosmet Chem*. 1992;43:275–284.
23. McMullen RL, Jachowicz J, Kelty SP. Correlation of AFM/LFM with combing forces of human hair. *J Cosmet Sci*. 2000;51:334–335.
24. Hossel P, Dieing R Norenberg R et al. Conditioning polymers in today's shampoo formulations—Efficacy, mechanism, and test methods. *Int J Cosmet Sci*. 2000;22:1–10.
25. Kamath YK, Weigmann HD. Measurement of combing forces. *J Soc Cosmet Chem*. 1986;37:111–124.
26. Bauer D, Beck JP, Monnais C et al. Contribution to the quantification of the conditioning effects of hair dyes. *Int J Cosmet Sci*. 1983;5:113–129.
27. Haake HM, Marten S, Seipel W et al. Hair breakage and how to counteract. *J Cosmet Sci*. 2009;60:143–151.
28. Lunn AC, Evans RE. The electrostatic properties of human hair. *J Soc Cosmet Chem*. 1977;28:549–569.
29. Wis-Surel G, Jachowicz J, Garcia M. Triboelectric charge distributions generated during combing of hair tresses. *J Soc Cosmet Chem*. 1987;38:341–350.
30. Dalton JS, Allen GC, Heard PJ et al. Advancements in spectroscopic and microscopic techniques for

investigating the adsorption of conditioning polymers onto human hair. *J Cosmet Sci.* 2000;51:275–287.
31. Bernard BA, Franbourg A, François AM et al. Ceramide binding to African-American hair fibre correlates with resistance to hair breakage. *Int J Cosmet Sci.* 2002;24:1–12.
32. Goddard ED, Harris WC. An ESCA study on the substantivity of conditioning polymers on hair substrates. *J Soc Cosmet Chem.* 1987;38:233–246.
33. Beard BC, Hare J. Surface interactions of quaternary amines with hair. *J Surfact Detergents.* 2002; 5:145–151.
34. Jachowitz J, Williams C. Fingerprinting of cosmetic formulations by dynamic electrokinetic and permeability analysis. I. Shampoos. *J Soc Cosmet Chem.* 1994;45:309–336.
35. Jachowitz J, Fingerprinting of cosmetic formulations by dynamic electrokinetic and permeability analysis. II. Hair conditioners. *J Soc Cosmet Chem.* 1995;46:110–116.
36. Galliano A, Lheur M, Santoprete R. Analyzing the movement of a hair swatch using video and image analysis: A promising technique for exploring the dynamic properties of hair. *Int J Cosmet Sci.* 2015;37(1):56–62.
37. Guiolet A, Garson LC, Lévêque JL. Study of the optical properties of human hair. *Int J Cosmet Sci.* 1987;9(3):111–124.
38. Reich C, Robbins CR. Light scattering and shine measurements of human hair: A sensitive probe of the hair surface. *J Soc Cosmet Chem.* 1993;44:221–234.
39. Czepluch W, Hohm G, Tolkiehn K. Gloss of surfaces: Problems of visual evaluation and possibilities for goniophotometric measurements of treated strands. *J Soc Cosmet Chem.* 1993;44:299–318.
40. Nagase S, Satoh N, Nakamura K. Influence of internal structure of hair fiber on hair appearance. II. Consideration of the visual perception mechanism of hair appearance. *J Cosmet Sci.* 2002;53(6):387–402.
41. Lefaudeux N, Lechocinski N, Clemenceau P et al. New luster formula for the characterization of hair tresses using polarization imaging. *J Cosmet Sci.* 2009;60(2):153–169.
42. Gao T, Pareira A, Zhu S. Study of hair shine and hair surface smoothness. *J Cosmet Sci.* 2009;60(2): 187–197.
43. Lim JM, Chang MY, Park ME, et al. A study correlating between instrumental and consumers' subjective luster values in oriental hair tresses. *J Cosmet Sci.* 2006;57(6):485–495.

Index